Atlas of Neuroanatomy for Communic Science and Disorders

Second Edition

Edited by
Leonard L. LaPointe

Based on the work of
Michael Schuenke
Erik Schulte
Udo Schumacher

Illustrations by
Markus Voll
Karl Wesker

458 illustrations

Thieme
New York • Stuttgart • Delhi • Rio de Janeiro

Based on the work of Michael Schuenke, MD, PhD, Erik Schulte, MD, and Udo Schumacher, MD

Leonard L. LaPointe
Francis Eppes Distinguished Professor
School of Communication Science and Disorders
Florida State University
Tallahassee, Florida
32306-1200

Michael Schuenke, MD, PhD
Institute of Anatomy
Christian Albrecht University Kiel
Otto-Hahn-Platz 8
D-24118 Kiel

Erik Schulte, MD
Department of Functional and Clinical Anatomy
Johannes Gutenberg University
Saarstrasse 19-21
D-55099 Mainz

Udo Schumacher, MD, FRCPath, CBiol, FIBiol, DSc
Institute of Anatomy II: Experimental Morphology
Center for Experimental Medicine
University Medical Center Hamburg-Eppendorf
Martinistrasse 52
D-20246 Hamburg

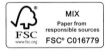

MIX
Paper from responsible sources
FSC® C016779
www.fsc.org

© 2019 Thieme Medical Publishers, Inc.

Thieme Publishers New York
333 Seventh Avenue, New York, NY 10001 USA
+1 800 782 3488, customerservice@thieme.com

Thieme Publishers Stuttgart
Rüdigerstrasse 14, 70469 Stuttgart, Germany
+49 [0]711 8931 421, customerservice@thieme.de

Thieme Publishers Delhi
A-12, Second Floor, Sector-2, Noida-201301
Uttar Pradesh, India
+91 120 45 566 00, customerservice@thieme.in

Thieme Publishers Rio de Janeiro,
Thieme Publicações Ltda.
Edifício Rodolpho de Paoli, 25° andar
Av. Nilo Peçanha, 50 – Sala 2508
Rio de Janeiro 20020-906, Brasil
+55 21 3172 2297

Illustrators: Markus Voll and Karl Wesker
Cover design: Thieme Publishing Group
Typesetting by DiTech Process Solutions, India

Printed in India by Replika Press Pvt. Ltd.

ISBN 978-1-62623-875-6

Also available as an e-book:
eISBN 978-1-62623-876-3

Acquisitions Editor: Delia K. DeTurris
Managing Editor: Prakash Naorem
Director, Editorial Services: Mary Jo Casey
Production Editor: Shivika
International Production Director: Andreas Schabert
Editorial Director: Sue Hodgson
International Marketing Director: Fiona Henderson
International Sales Director: Louisa Turrell
Senior Vice President and Chief Operating
   Officer: Sarah Vanderbilt
President: Brian D. Scanlan

Library of Congress Cataloging-in-Publication Data

Names: LaPointe, Leonard L., editor. | Based on (work): Schuenke, Michael. Thieme atlas of anatomy.
Title: Atlas of neuroanatomy for communication science and disorders / edited by Leonard L. LaPointe ; based on the work of Michael Schuenke, Erik Schulte, Udo Schumacher ; illustrations by Markus Voll, Karl Wesker.
Description: Second edition. | New York : Thieme, [2018] | Includes bibliographical references and index. |
Identifiers: LCCN 2018012517 (print) | LCCN 2018012738 (ebook) | ISBN 9781626238763 | ISBN 9781626238756 (softcover) | ISBN 9781626238763 (eISBN)
Subjects: | MESH: Communication Disorders—physiopathology | Central Nervous System—anatomy & histology | Nervous System Physiological Phenomena | Atlases
Classification: LCC RC423 (ebook) | LCC RC423 (print) | NLM WL 17 | DDC 612.8/2078—dc23
LC record available at https://lccn.loc.gov/2018012517

Important note: Medicine is an ever-changing science undergoing continual development. Research and clinical experience are continually expanding our knowledge, in particular our knowledge of proper treatment and drug therapy. Insofar as this book mentions any dosage or application, readers may rest assured that the authors, editors, and publishers have made every effort to ensure that such references are in accordance with **the state of knowledge at the time of production of the book**.

Nevertheless, this does not involve, imply, or express any guarantee or responsibility on the part of the publishers in respect to any dosage instructions and forms of applications stated in the book. **Every user is requested to examine carefully** the manufacturers' leaflets accompanying each drug and to check, if necessary in consultation with a physician or specialist, whether the dosage schedules mentioned therein or the contraindications stated by the manufacturers differ from the statements made in the present book. Such examination is particularly important with drugs that are either rarely used or have been newly released on the market. Every dosage schedule or every form of application used is entirely at the user's own risk and responsibility. The authors and publishers request every user to report to the publishers any discrepancies or inaccuracies noticed. If errors in this work are found after publication, errata will be posted at www.thieme.com on the product description page.

Some of the product names, patents, and registered designs referred to in this book are in fact registered trademarks or proprietary names even though specific reference to this fact is not always made in the text. Therefore, the appearance of a name without designation as proprietary is not to be construed as a representation by the publisher that it is in the public domain.

5 4 3 2 1

To my children, of whom I am most proud. To Christopher, who has dedicated his life to helping to save this fractured planet, and to Adrienne and her husband Captain Thomas King, who have shown extraordinary persistence and courage and are role models for all who must face medical and health crises. These children share my values and my sense of humor, which is a blessing and a curse.

Contents

Contents

Foreword

Atlas, the Greek titan, supported the heavens. This edition of the *Atlas of Neuroanatomy for Communication Science and Disorders* supports a foundation for understanding the neurology of human communication, and for understanding why, when things go wrong with the machinery of the brain, our ability to communicate can go awry.

For students with a primary interest in communication and its disorders, the first encounter with neuroanatomy is rarely enjoyable, and its relevance may not be readily apparent. For communication scientists, speech–language pathologists, and those in related research and clinical disciplines, knowing neuroanatomy can be fundamental and essential for day-to-day work. These realities make having a focused, user-friendly tool for learning an important commodity. This second edition—which incorporates updates in text and illustrations that reflect advances in neuroscience—more than meets that standard.

The illustrations by Markus Voll and Karl Wesker, acquired from the pages of the Thieme Atlas of Anatomy volumes, are exquisitely rendered from multiple visual perspectives and with a level of detail that is well-tuned to the intended audience. The supporting text, originally written by Michael Schuenke, Erik Schulte, and Udo Schumacher, provides an excellent guide to the topography and its functions, and nicely balances the need for a broad overview with a special focus on the functional neuroanatomy of speech and language. The framework provided by Dr. LaPointe in the introductory text in Chapter 1 and the concluding text in Chapter 7 provide an eloquent and substantive rationale for attending to the contents of this unique resource.

The many enduring contributions of Dr. LaPointe, a valued colleague and friend, align perfectly with the high quality of this book. I suspect this atlas will sustain its value well into the careers of those who study the neurologic underpinnings of communication or who care for people for whom those underpinnings have come undone.

Joseph R. Duffy, Ph.D.
Emeritus Consultant and Professor
Division of Speech Pathology
Department of Neurology
Mayo Clinic and Mayo Clinic College of Medicine and Science
Rochester, Minnesota

1 Introduction and Brain Basics*

The brain is a modest yet spectacular thing. In this three and a half pounds of gelatinous squish tissue rests everything that we are or have ever been. The brain is the seat and soul of our fears, joys, achievements, relationships, creativity, happiness, sadness, identity, memory, and history. The brain allows us to acquire language, interact with one another, cajole and console, cheer, thank, joke, sing off key, talk to the animals, and aspire. The miracle of language makes us human, more so than the opposable thumb and the ability to conceptualize death and subsequently fear it. Pessimists among us would cite that the brain is inextricably linked to abilities to lie, steal, cheat, go to war, and ruin our nest. However, for all human foibles, there is ample evidence that language and intraspecies communication is responsible for the sum of human achievements, altruism, and decency. Debates on what makes us human have boiled for generations, but always atop the list of human attributes is language and sophisticated communication.[1] The brain has been rhapsodized in poem and song, and been called everything from an "enchanted loom that weaves a never-ending stream of dissolving patterns" to "a computer on steroids".[2,3]

Diane Ackerman described the brain as follows[4]:

Shaped a little like a loaf of French country bread, our brain is a crowded chemistry lab, bustling with nonstop neural conversations. Imagine the brain, that shiny mound of being, that mouse-gray parliament of cells, that dream factory, that petit tyrant inside a ball of bone, that huddle of neurons calling all the plays, that little everywhere, that fickle pleasure dome, that wrinkled wardrobe of selves stuffed into the skull like too many clothes into a gym bag.

What a poetic and rapturous characterization of what used to be regarded as something that showed no more capacity for thought than a cake of suet or a bowl of curds. How times have changed. The brain in all its wonder forms the infrastructure for all that will be discussed in this book. Herewith we present an abbreviated introduction and summary of some brain basics.

The brain and the human nervous system are vital to the perception and production of processes that take place inside (enteroception) or outside (exteroception) the body. Not the least of these processes is internal and external communication. The brain keeps us in touch with our environment. It allows all of our sensory perceptions (e.g., taste a hot fudge sundae, hear the chirping of a Carolina Wren, view the sunset at Cape San Bias, touch Annie the Golden Retriever's soft head) and everything we do to move or communicate within the environment (e.g., swim to the raft at Sawyer Lake, hit a drop shot in tennis, do a full twisting dismount from the pommel horse, operate the lever of the recliner chair, fuss with the remote control, or pick up the baby

and realize that she needs a change). More to our specialty areas of human exchanges of information and feelings, the brain is responsible for the vast spectrum of human communication such as writing a poem; apologizing; texting the important message that you are in the produce section of the market, near the broccoli, and will be right home; or telling your daughter that you love her.

Given the diversity of these perceptual and production tasks, the human body has evolved an intricately complex nervous system that can be subdivided and discussed in various ways.[5] The principles of classification vary. A common one is to divide the nervous system morphologically into a peripheral nervous system (PNS) and a central nervous system (CNS). The brain and spinal cord comprise the CNS; they are seamlessly interconnected in a functional unit. The PNS is formed by the nerves that emerge from the brain and spinal cord (cranial and spinal nerves) and are distributed into the periphery of our vast collection of muscles, tissues, and organs. The brain and spinal cord consist of neurons, or brain cells, that have been characterized as gray matter or white matter.[5] The conducting part of a neuron, known as the axon, is covered by a fatty-like myelin sheath that looks white upon gross examination of a specimen and, hence, white matter. The cell bodies of neurons, on the other hand, are not covered with myelin and appear gray to the naked eye. To help protect the brain from external injury—which, of course, is not entirely possible in instances of slamming into a bridge abutment or drunkenly diving into the shallow end of the swimming pool from a balcony—the CNS is encased in bony structures (vertebrae and cranial bones). Between the bones and the CNS are coverings (meninges) of the brain and spinal cord. The meninges consist of three layers: pia mater ("pious mother"), arachnoid ("spider-like"), and dura mater ("tough mother").

The CNS can be further studied and divided into the telencephalon (new brain), diencephalon (between brain), and the brain stem. The telencephalon, which is composed of the cerebrum including the later evolved cerebral cortex, is of vital interest to us. The lobes of the mirror-like left and right hemispheres of the cerebral cortex are traditionally divided morphologically and functionally into the frontal lobes, temporal lobes, parietal lobes, occipital lobes, and the hidden insular lobes. Although the external surfaces of the left and right cortical hemispheres look alike, like sisters, they can be very different. We will discover this as the images and legends in this atlas unfold. Further, as a method of labeling morphological and functional areas of the cerebral cortex, a traditional numeric labeling system developed by Korbinian Brodmann is used in many anatomical and physiological depictions.

To appreciate human functional neuroanatomy and place it fully in the context of the human body, it is necessary to consider some general anatomical concepts and the neighborhoods

*Adapted from LaPointe LL. Brain basics. In: LaPointe LL, ed. Aphasia and Related Neurogenic Language Disorders. 4th ed. New York, NY: Thieme Medical Publishers; 2011.

wherein the nervous system resides; therefore, this atlas is divided into the following chapters:

- Chapter 1. Introduction and Brain Basics
- Chapter 2. General Anatomical Concepts (surface anatomy of the body, landmarks, and reference lines)
- Chapter 3. Head, Skull, Neck Anatomy
- Chapter 4. Anatomy of the Brain and Nervous Systems (central, peripheral, and autonomic)
- Chapter 5. Cranial Nerves
- Chapter 6. Blood Vessels, Vascular System
- Chapter 7. Functional and Dysfunctional Systems

As the story and images of the wonder of the human brain unfold, these image legends and notes on the structures will be biased toward how these structures are integrated into the function and dysfunction of human communication and its disorders. Basic anatomy and physiology of human communication and swallowing are related to the images in this atlas, as well as the neural mechanisms controlling speech, language, cognitive, and swallowing functions. In addition to the traditional acquired speech/language disorders of the nervous system (i.e., aphasia, neuromotor speech disorders), content also will include communication impairments caused by traumatic brain injury, multisystem blast injuries, and degenerative disorders of the nervous system.

Purpose and Intended Audience

The purpose of this work is to provide an atlas and reference work for undergraduate and graduate students as they learn to study and appreciate functional neuroanatomy, and to provide a reliable reference source for instructors and practitioners. The atlas is geared to the disciplines of communication science and disorders (speech–language pathology) and to students in neuroscience and neuropsychology, cognitive psychology, and rehabilitation science. It serves as a useful reference for medical and nursing students, and rehabilitation scientists and practitioners (physical therapy, occupational therapy, biomedical engineering, orthotics and prosthetics, kinesiology, and exercise science). Further, it functions as a beneficial reference for nursing and the medical specialties of neurology, neurosurgery, physical medicine and rehabilitation, and otolaryngology—particularly as they relate to the communication and cognitive disorders seen in their patients. This work avails itself to the vast and exquisite library of images in the Thieme Medical Publishers archive. These images have been used with permission, adapted in some cases, and embellished with legends and information relevant to the science of human communication and its disorders.

2 General Anatomical Concepts

2.1 The Human Body (Proportions, Surface Areas, and Body Weights)

2.1.1 Change in Body Proportions during Growth

While the head height in embryos at 2 months' gestation is equal to approximately half the total body length, it measures approximately one-fourth of the body length in newborns, one-sixth in a 6-year-old child, and one-eighth in an adult (**Fig. 2.1**).

2.1.2 Normal Body Proportions

In an adult, the midpoint of the total body height lies approximately at the level of the pubic symphysis, that is, there is a 1:1 ratio of upper to lower body height at that level (**Fig. 2.2**). The pelvis accounts for one-fifth of the upper body height, the thorax for two-fifths, and the head and neck for two-fifths. The lower body height is distributed equally between the thigh and leg (plus heel) at the joint space of the knee.

2.1.3 Span of the Outstretched Arms

The arm span from fingertip to fingertip (= 1 fathom) is slightly *greater* than the body height (~ 103% in women and 106% in men) (**Fig. 2.3**).

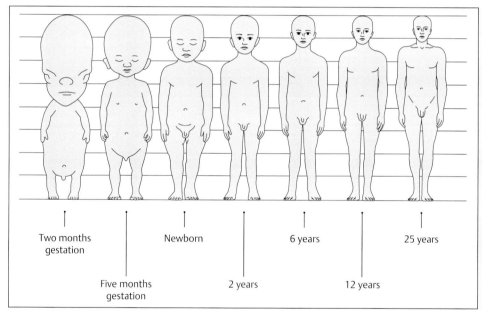

Two months gestation

Five months gestation

Newborn

2 years

6 years

12 years

25 years

Fig. 2.1 Change in body proportions during growth.

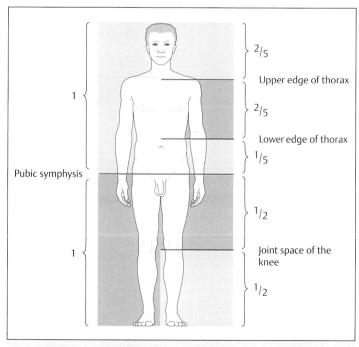

Pubic symphysis

1

1

$2/5$

Upper edge of thorax

$2/5$

Lower edge of thorax

$1/5$

$1/2$

Joint space of the knee

$1/2$

Fig. 2.2 Normal body proportions.

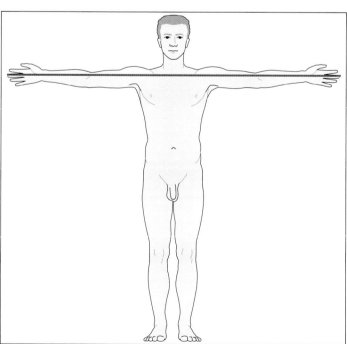

Fig. 2.3 Span of the outstretched arms.

2.1.4 Selected Body Measurements in the Standing and Sitting Human Being (Unclothed, 16–60 Years of Age)

The percentile values indicate what percentage in a population group are below the value stated for a particular body measurement. For example, the 95th percentile for body height in males 16 to 60 years of age is 184.1 cm, meaning that 95% of this population group are shorter than 184.1 cm, and 5% are taller (**Fig. 2.4, Table 2.1**).

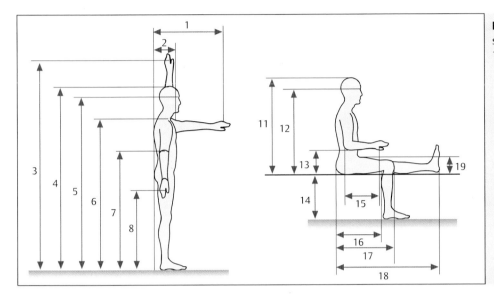

Fig. 2.4 Selected body measurements in the standing and sitting human being (unclothed, 16–60 years of age).

Table 2.1 Normative human measurements

| Measurements (in cm) | Percentiles | | | | | |
| | Male | | | Female | | |
	5th	50th	95th	5th	50th	95th
1 Forward reach	66.2	72.2	78.7	61.6	69.0	76.2
2 AP body thickness	23.2	27.6	31.8	23.8	28.5	35.7
3 Overhead reach (with both arms)	191.0	205.1	221.0	174.8	187.0	200.0
4 Body height	162.9	173.3	184.1	151.0	161.9	172.5
5 Ocular height	150.9	161.3	172.1	140.2	150.2	159.6
6 Shoulder height	134.9	144.5	154.2	123.4	133.9	143.6
7 Elbow-to-floor distance	102.1	109.6	117.9	95.7	103.0	110.0
8 Hand-to-floor distance	72.8	76.7	82.8	66.4	73.8	80.3
9 Shoulder width	31.0	34.4	36.8	31.4	35.8	40.5
10 Hip width, standing	36.7	39.8	42.8	32.3	35.5	38.8
11 Sitting body height (trunk height)	84.9	90.7	96.2	80.5	85.7	91.4
12 Ocular height while sitting	73.9	79.0	84.4	68.0	73.5	78.5
13 Elbow to sitting surface	19.3	23.0	28.0	19.1	23.3	27.8
14 Height of leg and foot (height of sitting surface)	39.9	44.2	48.0	35.1	39.5	43.4
15 Elbow to gripping axis	32.7	36.2	38.9	29.2	32.2	36.4
16 Sitting depth	45.2	50.0	55.2	42.6	48.4	53.2
17 Buttock-knee length	55.4	59.9	64.5	53.0	58.7	63.1
18 Buttock-leg length	96.4	103.5	112.5	95.5	104.4	112.6
19 Thigh height	11.7	13.6	15.7	11.8	14.4	17.3
20 Width above the elbow	39.9	45.1	51.2	37.0	45.6	54.4
21 Hip width, sitting	32.5	36.2	39.1	34.0	38.7	45.1

2.1.5 Distribution of Body Surface Area in Adults, Children, and Infants

According to the "rule of nines" described by Wallace (1950), the body surface area of adults over about 15 years of age (a) can be divided into units that are a *multiple* of 9%: the head and each arm account for 9% each, the front and back of the trunk and each leg account for 18% (2 × 9) each, and the external genitalia comprise 1%. In children (b) and infants (c), the rule of nines must be adjusted for age. *Note:* The rule of nines can be used in burn victims to provide a quick approximation of the area of skin that has been burned (**Fig. 2.5**).

2.1.6 Hand Area Rule

The percentage of the body surface affected by burns can be accurately estimated with the hand area rule, which states that the area of the patient's hand is approximately 1% of the patient's own total body surface area. The hand rule also applies to children, whose hands and total surface area are both proportionately smaller than in adults (**Fig. 2.6**).

2.1.7 Dependence of Relative Body Surface Area (Skin Surface Area) on Age, and Consequences

For progressively larger solid bodies, the surface area increases as the square of the radius, but the volume increases as the cube of the body's radius. Because of this basic geometrical relationship, smaller animals generally have a larger relative surface area than larger animals. A higher ratio of surface area to volume causes smaller animals to radiate relatively more body heat. As a result, small animals like mice and children tend to have a higher metabolic rate than larger animals like elephants and human adults (**Table 2.2**).

Table 2.2 Relative body weight and surface

Age	Body weight	Body surface area	Body surface area over body weight
	(kg)	(cm²)	(cm²/kg)
Newborn	3.4	2,100	617.6
6 months	7.5	3,500	466.7
1 year	9.3	4,100	440.9
4 years	15.5	6,500	419.4
10 years	30.5	10,500	344.3
Adult	70.0	18,100	258.6

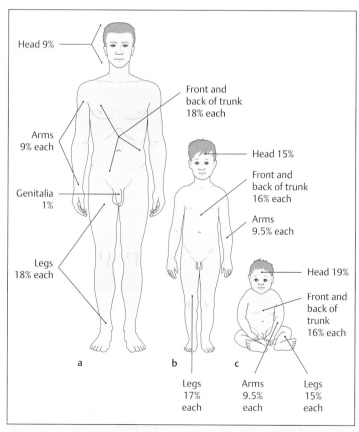

Fig. 2.5 Distribution of body surface area. **(a)** Adults. **(b)** Children. **(c)** Infants.

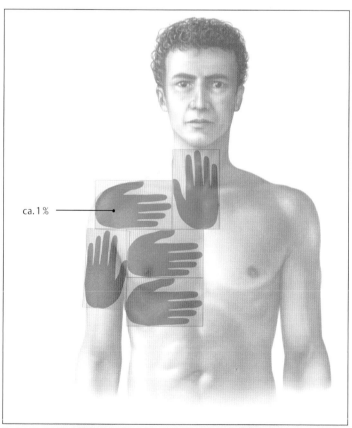

Fig. 2.6 Hand area rule.

2.1.8 Body Mass Index

In anthropometry, the body mass index (BMI) has become the international standard for evaluating body weight because it correlates relatively well with total body fat. BMI is defined as the body weight in kilograms divided by the square of the height in meters:

$$BMI = \frac{kg}{m^2}$$

Body mass and body weight are important to practitioners of speech–language pathology when significant weight loss caused by swallowing disorders is related to malnutrition. Under these circumstances, decisions on assessment and treatment of swallowing disorders must be undertaken (**Fig. 2.7**).

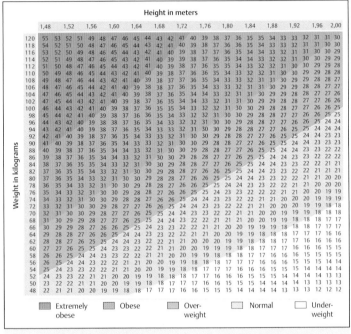

Fig. 2.7 Body mass index.

2.2 The Structural Design of the Human Body

2.2.1 Location of the Internal Organs

Lateral view (**Fig. 2.8**).

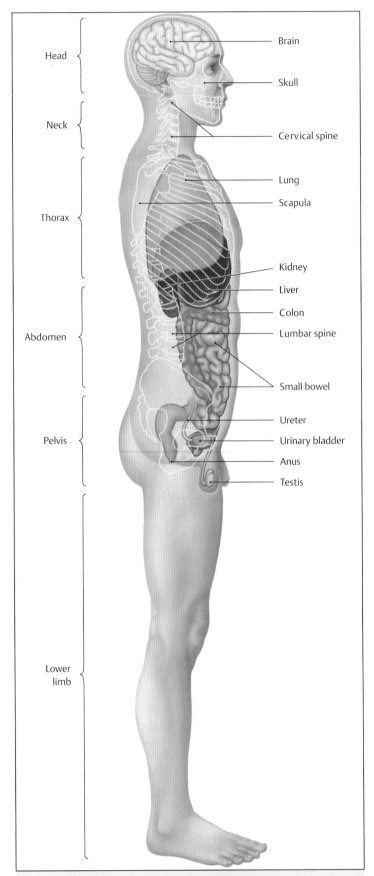

Fig. 2.8 Location of the internal organs.

2.2.2 Regional Subdivisions of the Body

Head

Neck

Trunk

- Thorax (chest)
- Abdomen
- Pelvis

Upper limb

- Shoulder girdle
- Free upper limb

Lower limb

- Pelvic girdle
- Free lower limb

2.2.3 Functional Subdivision by Organ Systems

Locomotor system (musculoskeletal system)

- Skeleton and skeletal connections (passive part)
- Striated skeletal musculature (active part)

Viscera

- Cardiovascular system
- Hemolymphatic system
- Endocrine system
- Respiratory system
- Digestive system
- Urinary system
- Male and female reproductive system

Nervous system

- Central and peripheral nervous system
- Sensory organs

Of all the functional systems of the human body, the sensory organs and central and peripheral nervous systems are mostly associated with human speech and language.

The skin and its appendages.

2.2.4 Serous Cavities and Connective Tissue Spaces

Organs and organ systems are embedded either in serous cavities or in connective tissue spaces of varying size. A serous cavity is a fully enclosed potential space that is lined by a shiny membrane (serosa) and contains a small amount of fluid. The serosa consists of two layers that are *usually* apposed (both layers are not *necessarily* in direct contact, as in the abdominal cavity): a visceral layer that directly invests the organ, and a parietal layer that lines the wall of the serous cavity.

Serous cavities

- Thoracic cavity (chest cavity) with the following:
  - The pleural cavity
  - The pericardial cavity
- Abdominopelvic cavity with the following:
  - The peritoneal cavity
  - The pelvic cavity

Connective tissue spaces

- Space between the middle and deep layers of cervical fascia
- Mediastinum
- Extraperitoneal space with the following:
  - The retroperitoneal space (retroperitoneum)
  - The subperitoneal space
- Bursa and synovial cavities

2.2.5 Selected Planes of Section Through the Human Body Superior View

See **Fig. 2.9** (see also Chapter 2.4).

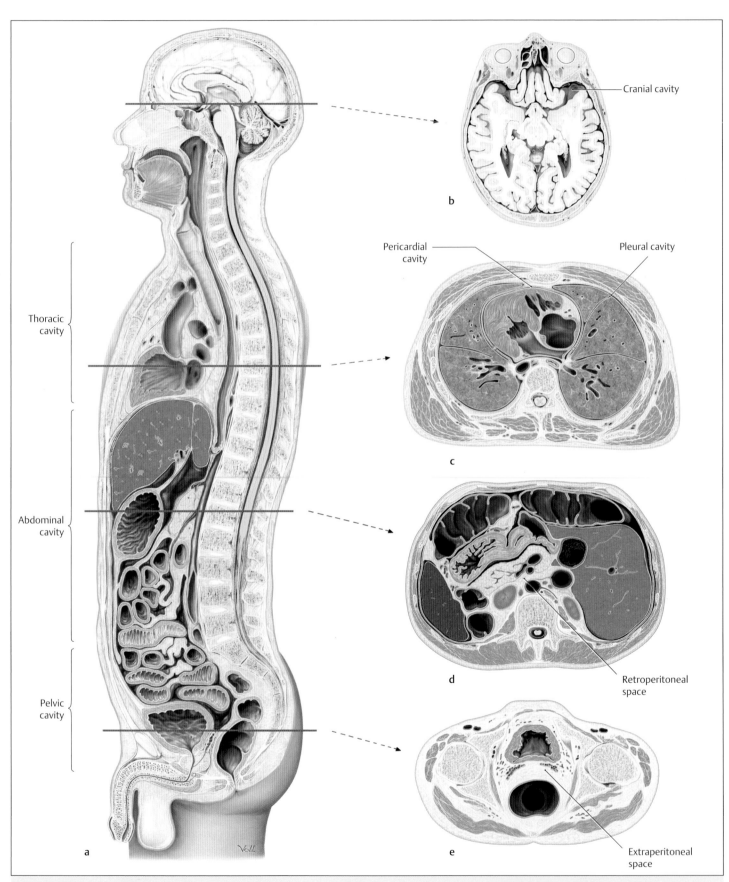

Fig. 2.9 Selected planes of section through the human body superior view. **(a)** Midsagittal section. **(b)** Cross-section at the level of the head. **(c)** Cross-section through the thorax. **(d)** Cross-section through the abdomen. **(e)** Cross-section through the lesser pelvis.

2.3 Body Surface Anatomy

2.3.1 Body Surface Anatomy of the Female (Anterior View)

Body surface anatomy deals with the surface anatomy of the living subject (**Fig. 2.10**). It plays an important role in classic methods of examination (inspection, palpation, percussion, auscultation, function testing), and so it has particular significance in clinical examination courses.

2.3.2 Body Surface Anatomy of the Female (Posterior View)

See **Fig. 2.11**.

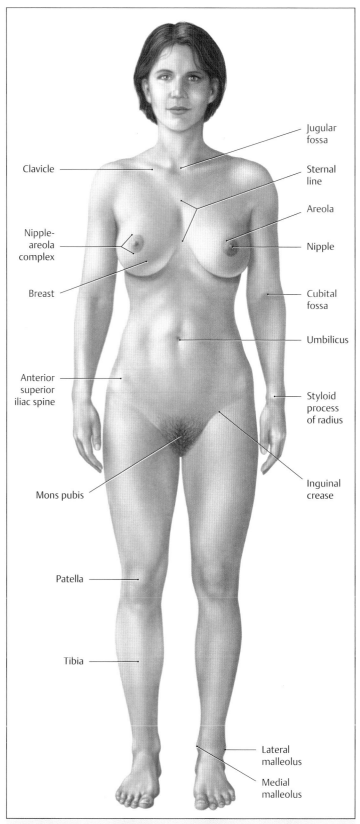

Fig. 2.10 Body surface anatomy of the female (anterior view).

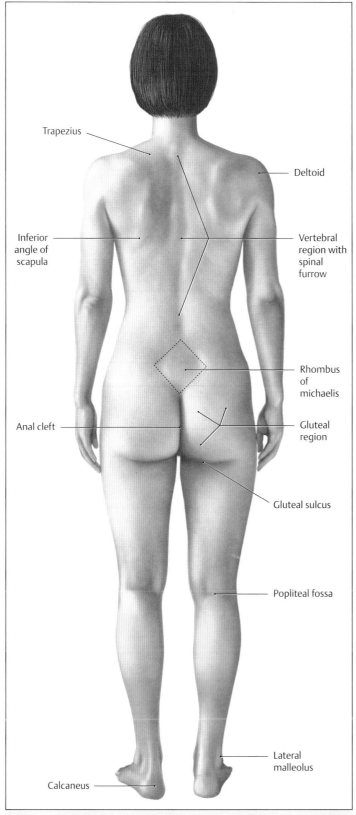

Fig. 2.11 Body surface anatomy of the female (posterior view).

2.3.3 Body Surface Anatomy of the Male (Anterior View)

See **Fig. 2.12**.

2.3.4 Body Surface Anatomy of the Male (Posterior View)

See **Fig. 2.13**.

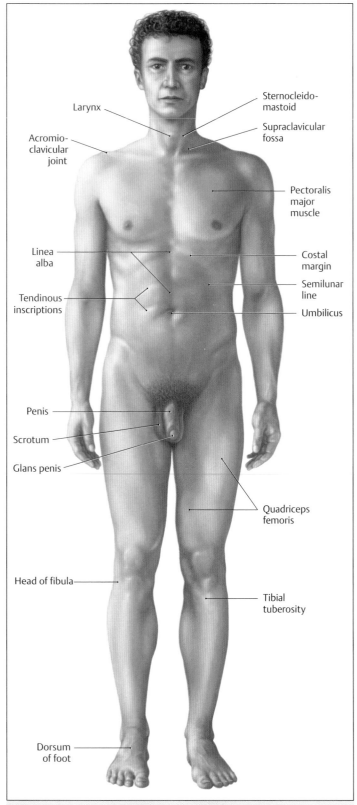

Fig. 2.12 Body surface anatomy of the male (anterior view).

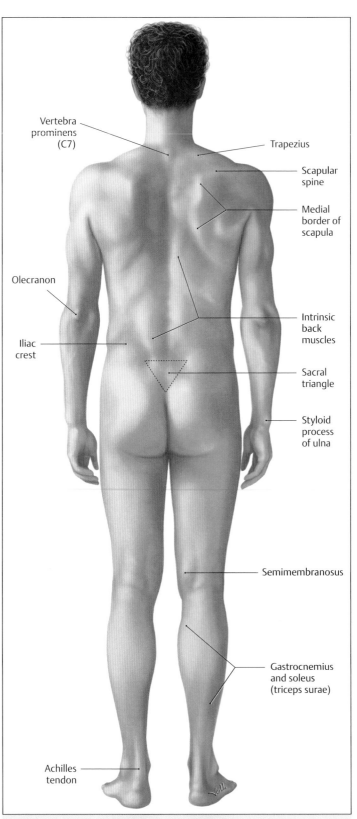

Fig. 2.13 Body surface anatomy of the male (posterior view).

2.4 Terms of Location and Direction, Cardinal Planes and Axes

2.4.1 General Terms of Location and Direction

See **Table 2.3**.

2.4.2 The Anatomical Body Position

The gaze is directed forward, the hands are supinated. The *right* half of the body is shown in light shading to demonstrate the skeleton.

Note that the designations "left" and "right" always refer to the patient. Understanding anatomical planes will facilitate learning terms related to position of structures relative to each other and movement of various parts of the body (**Fig. 2.14**).

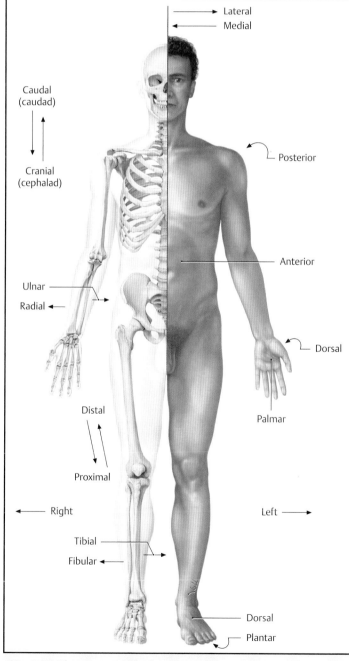

Fig. 2.14 The anatomical body position.

Table 2.3 Body planes, axes, and positional terms

Upper body (head, neck, and trunk)	
Cranial	Pertaining to, or located toward the head
Cephalad	Directed toward the head
Caudal	Pertaining to, or located toward the tail
Caudad	Directed toward the tail
Anterior	Pertaining to, or located toward, the front
	Synonym: Ventral (used for all animals)
Posterior	Pertaining to, or located toward, the back
	Synonym: Dorsal (used for all animals)
Superior	Upper or above
Inferior	Lower or below
Medius	Located in the middle
Flexor	Pertaining to a flexor muscle or surface
Extensor	Pertaining to an extensor muscle or surface
Axial	Pertaining to the axis of a structure
Transverse	Situated at right angles to the long axis of a structure
Longitudinal	Parallel to the long axis of a structure
Horizontal	Parallel to the plane of the horizon
Vertical	Perpendicular to the plane of the horizon
Medial	Toward the median plane
Lateral	Away from the medial plane (toward the side)
Median	Situated in the median plane or midline
Central	Situated at the center or interior of the body
Peripheral	Situated away from the center
Superficial	Situated near the surface
Deep	Situated deep beneath the surface
External	Outer or lateral
Internal	Inner or medial
Apical	Pertaining to the tip or apex
Basal	Pertaining to the bottom or base
Occipital	Pertaining to the back of the head
Temporal	Pertaining to the lateral region of the head (the temple)
Sagittal	Situated parallel to the sagittal suture
Coronal	Situated parallel to the coronal suture (pertaining to the crown of the head)
Rostral	Situated toward the nose or brow
Frontal	Pertaining to the forehead
Basilar	Pertaining to the skull base
Limbs	
Proximal	Close to or toward the trunk
Distal	Away from the trunk (toward the end of the limb)
Radial	Pertaining to the radius or the lateral side of the forearm
Ulnar	Pertaining to the ulna or the medial side of the forearm
Tibial	Pertaining to the tibia or the medial side of the leg
Fibular	Pertaining to the fibula or the lateral side of the leg
Palmar (volar)	Pertaining to the palm of the hand
Plantar	Pertaining to the sole of the foot
Dorsal	Pertaining to the back of the hand or top of the foot

2.4.3 Cardinal Planes and Axes in the Human Body (Neutral Position, Left Anterolateral View)

Although any number of planes and axes can be drawn through the human body, it is a standard practice to designate the *three cardinal planes* and *axes.* They are perpendicular to one another and are based on the three spatial coordinates (**Fig. 2.15**).

The Cardinal Body Planes

- **Sagittal plane:** Any *vertical* plane that is parallel to the sagittal suture of the skull, passing through the body from front to back. The *midsagittal plane* (= median plane) divides the body into equal left and right halves.
- **Coronal plane (frontal plane):** Any plane that is *parallel to the forehead* or to the coronal suture of the skull. In the standing position, it passes vertically through the body from side to side.
- **Transverse plane (axial plane):** Any *horizontal,* cross-sectional plane that divides the body into upper and lower portions. It is perpendicular to the longitudinal body axis.

The Cardinal Body Axes

- **Vertical or longitudinal axis:** In the standing position, this axis runs through the body *craniocaudally* and is perpendicular to the ground. It lies at the intersection of the coronal and sagittal planes.
- **Sagittal axis:** This axis runs *anteroposteriorly* from the front to back surface of the body (or from back to front) and lies at the intersection of the sagittal and transverse planes.
- **Transverse or horizontal axis:** This axis runs from side to side and lies at the intersection of the coronal and transverse planes.

2.4.4 Coronal and Sagittal Planes in the Skull

The coronal plane is named for the fact that it is parallel to the coronal suture, just as the sagittal plane is parallel to the sagittal suture. The cranial sutures serve as directional indicators, "sagittal" meaning in the direction of the sagittal suture, "coronal" in the direction of the coronal suture (**Fig. 2.16**).

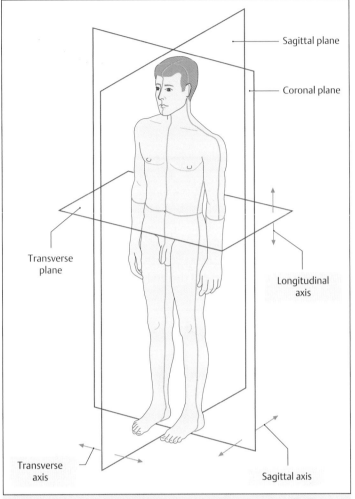

Fig. 2.15 Cardinal planes and axes in the human body (neutral position, left anterolateral view).

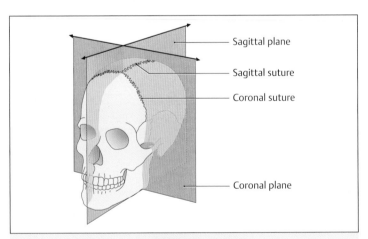

Fig. 2.16 Coronal and sagittal planes in the skull.

2.4.5 The Whole-Body Center of Gravity and the Line of Gravity

See **Fig. 2.17**.

- **Anterior view:** The line of gravity is directed vertically along the midsagittal plane, passing through the whole-body center of gravity below the sacral promontory at the level of the second sacral vertebra.

- **Lateral view:** The line of gravity passes through the external auditory canal, the dens of the axis (second cervical vertebra), the anatomical and functional junctions within the spinal column, the whole-body center of gravity, and through the hip, knee, and ankle joints (after Kummer).

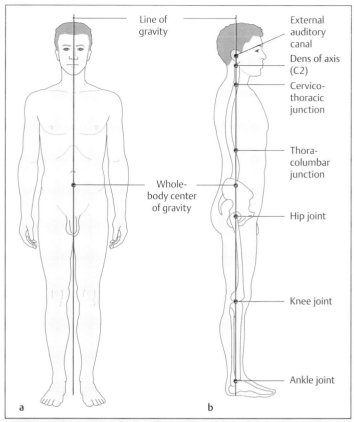

Fig. 2.17 The whole-body center of gravity and the line of gravity. **(a)** Anterior view. **(b)** Lateral view.

2.5 Body Surface Contours and Palpable Bony Prominences

Palpable bony prominences are important landmarks for anatomical orientation in the skeleton, as it is not always possible to palpate articulating skeletal structures (e.g., the hip joint). In these cases, the examiner must rely on palpable bony prominences as an indirect guide to the location of the inaccessible structure.

2.5.1 Surface Contours and Palpable Bony Prominences of the Face and Neck

Anterior view: These bony prominences are relative to traumatic injuries of the head and face and may impact speech function (**Fig. 2.18**).

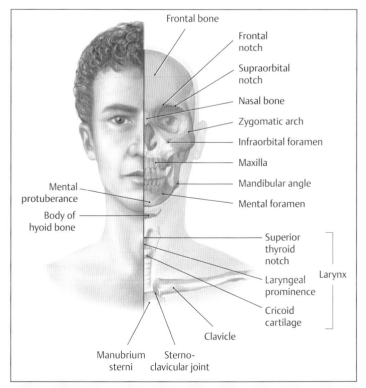

Fig. 2.18 Surface contours and palpable bony prominences (anterior view).

2.5.2 Surface Contours and Palpable Bony Prominences of the Trunk and Upper and Lower Limbs in the Female

Anterior view (**Fig. 2.19**).

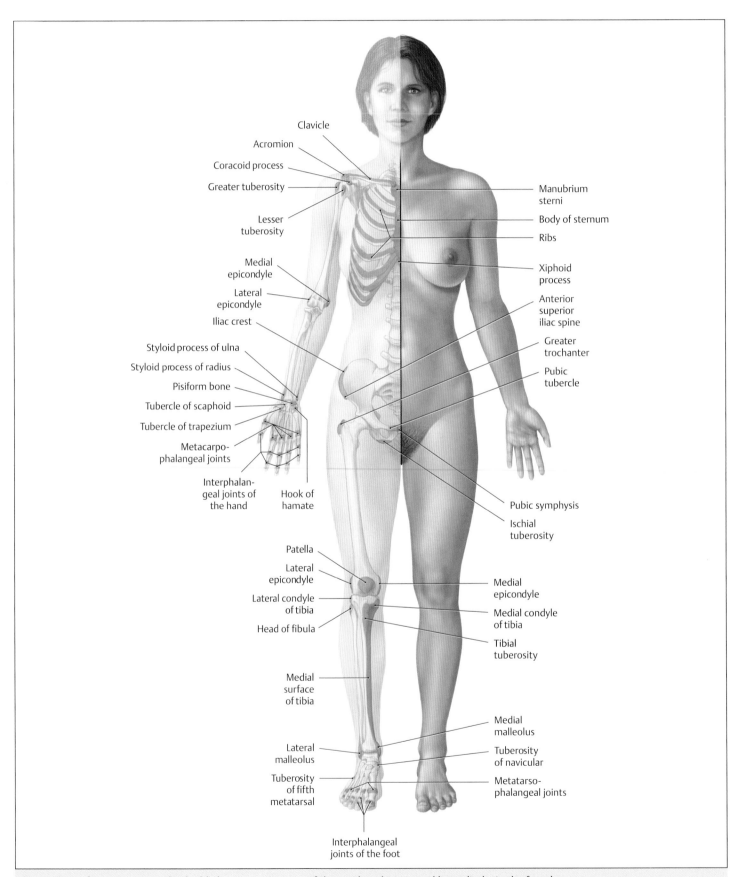

Clavicle

Acromion

Coracoid process

Greater tuberosity

Lesser tuberosity

Medial epicondyle

Lateral epicondyle

Iliac crest

Styloid process of ulna

Styloid process of radius

Pisiform bone

Tubercle of scaphoid

Tubercle of trapezium

Metacarpo-phalangeal joints

Interphalan-geal joints of the hand

Hook of hamate

Patella

Lateral epicondyle

Lateral condyle of tibia

Head of fibula

Medial surface of tibia

Lateral malleolus

Tuberosity of fifth metatarsal

Interphalangeal joints of the foot

Manubrium sterni

Body of sternum

Ribs

Xiphoid process

Anterior superior iliac spine

Greater trochanter

Pubic tubercle

Pubic symphysis

Ischial tuberosity

Medial epicondyle

Medial condyle of tibia

Tibial tuberosity

Medial malleolus

Tuberosity of navicular

Metatarso-phalangeal joints

Fig. 2.19 Surface contours and palpable bony prominences of the trunk and upper and lower limbs in the female.

2.5.3 Surface Contours and Palpable Bony Prominences of the Trunk and Upper and Lower Limbs in the Male

Posterior view (**Fig. 2.20**).

2.5.4 Surface Contours and Palpable Bony Prominences of the Face and Neck

Posterior view (**Fig. 2.21**).

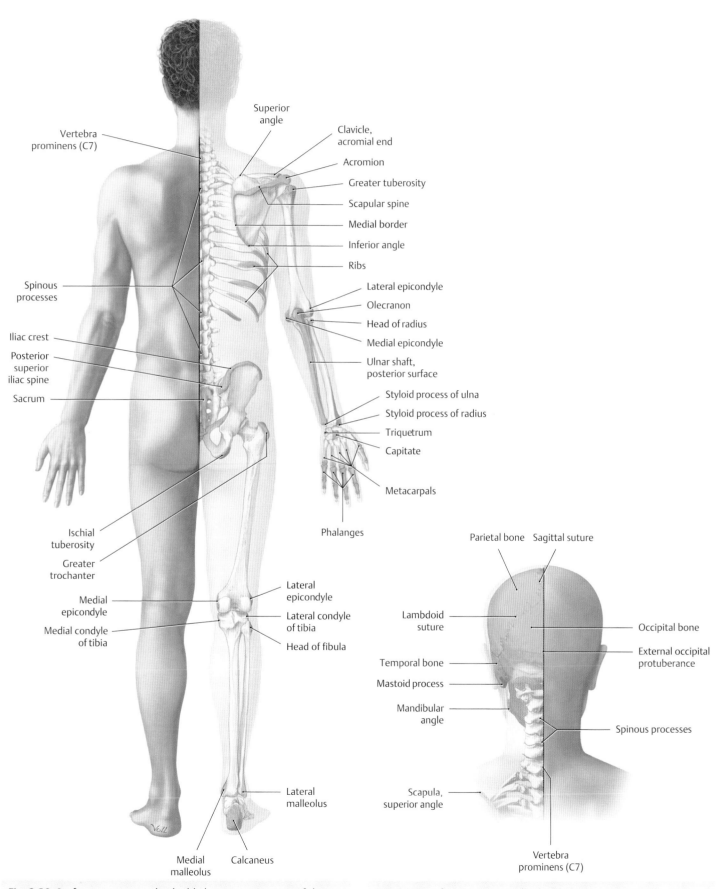

Fig. 2.20 Surface contours and palpable bony prominences of the trunk and upper and lower limbs in the male.

Fig. 2.21 Surface contours and palpable bony prominences (posterior view).

2.6 Topography and Structure of the Nervous System

2.6.1 Topography of the Nervous System

(a) Posterior view, (b) right lateral view.

The *central nervous system* (CNS), consisting of the brain (encephalon) and spinal cord, is shown in pink **Fig. 2.22**. The *peripheral nervous system* (PNS), consisting of nerves and ganglia, is shown in yellow. The nerves arising from the spinal cord leave their bony canal through the *intervertebral foramina* and are distributed to their target organs. The *spinal nerves* are formed in the foramina by the union of their dorsal (posterior) roots and ventral (anterior) roots. The small *spinal ganglion* in the intervertebral foramen appears as a slight swelling of the dorsal root (visible only in the posterior view).

In the limbs, the ventral rami of the spinal nerves come together to form plexuses. These plexuses then give rise to the peripheral nerves that supply the limbs.

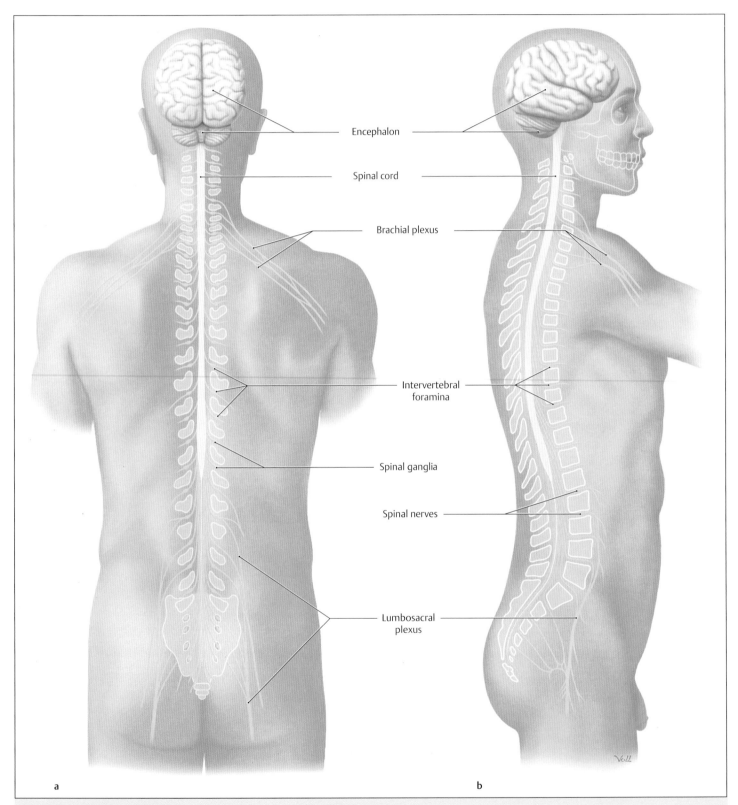

Encephalon

Spinal cord

Brachial plexus

Intervertebral foramina

Spinal ganglia

Spinal nerves

Lumbosacral plexus

a

b

Fig. 2.22 Topography of the nervous system. **(a)** Posterior view. **(b)** Right lateral view.

2.6.2 Spinal Nerves and Cranial Nerves

Anterior view: *Thirty-one pairs of spinal nerves* arise from the spinal cord in the *PNS*, compared with *12 pairs of cranial nerves* that arise from the brain. The cranial nerve pairs are traditionally designated by Roman numerals (**Fig. 2.23**).

2.6.3 Location and Designation of Spinal Cord Segments in Relation to the Spinal Canal

Right lateral view: The longitudinal growth of the spinal cord lags behind that of the spinal column, with the result that the cord extends only about to the level of the first lumbar vertebra (L1). *Note* that there are seven cervical vertebrae (C1–C7) but eight pairs of cervical nerves (C1–C8). The highest pair of cervical nerves exit the spinal canal superior to the first cervical vertebra. The remaining pairs of cervical nerves, like all the other spinal nerve pairs, exit inferior to the cervical vertebral body. The pair of coccygeal nerves (gray) has no clinical importance (**Fig. 2.24**).

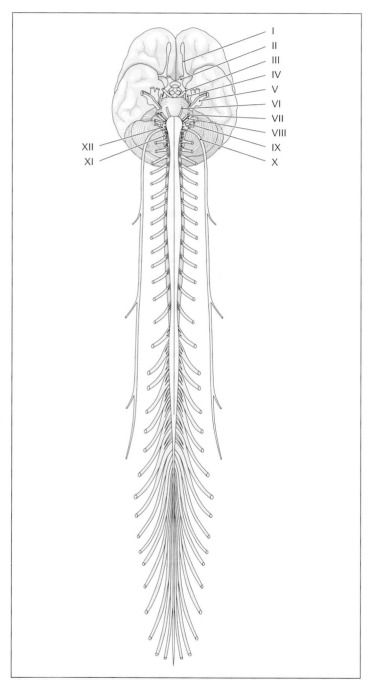

Fig. 2.23 Spinal nerves and cranial nerves.

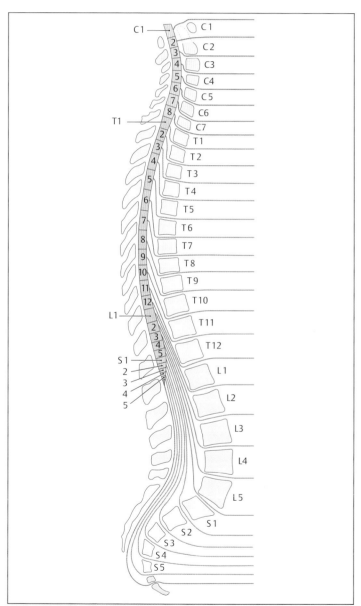

Fig. 2.24 Location and designation of spinal cord segments in relation to the spinal canal.

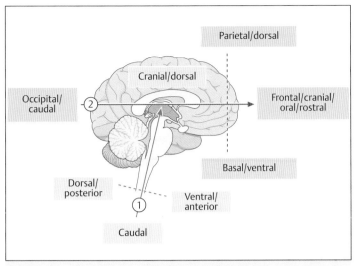

Fig. 2.25 Midsagittal section (right lateral view).

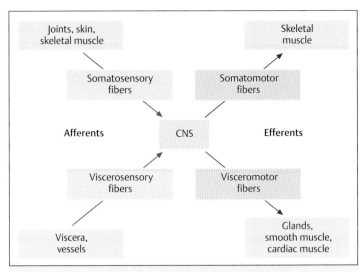

Fig. 2.26 Schematic representation of information flow in the nervous system.

2.6.4 Terms of Location and Direction in the CNS

Midsagittal section, right lateral view (**Fig. 2.25**).

Note two important axes:

① The almost vertical brainstem axis (corresponds approximately to the body axis).

② The horizontal axis through the diencephalon and telencephalon.

Keep these reference axes in mind when using directional terms in the CNS!

2.6.5 Schematic Representation of Information Flow in the Nervous System

The information encoded in nerve fibers is transmitted either *to the CNS* (brain and spinal cord) or *from the CNS* to the periphery (PNS, including the peripheral parts of the autonomic nervous system). Fibers that carry information to the CNS are called afferent fibers or *afferents* for short; fibers that carry signals away from the CNS are called efferent fibers or *efferents*. This afferent (input) and efferent (output) distinction is fundamental to understanding information flow to and from the brain. Afferent input is primarily sensory and efferent is motor, or related to movement (**Fig. 2.26**).

2.7 Cells of the Nervous System

2.7.1 The Nerve Cell (Neuron)

The neuron is the smallest functional unit of the nervous system. Neurons communicate with other nerve cells through synapses. The *synapses that end at nerve cells* usually do so at dendrites (as seen here). The transmitter substance that is released at the synapses to act on the dendrite membrane may have an *excitatory* or *inhibitory* action, meaning that the transmitter either increases or decreases the local action potential at the nerve cell membrane. All of the excitatory and inhibitory potentials of a nerve cell are integrated in the axon hillock. If the excitatory potentials predominate, the stimulus exceeds the excitation threshold of the neuron, causing the axon to fire (transmit an impulse) according to the all-or-nothing rule (**Fig. 2.27**).

2.7.2 Electron Microscopy of the Neuron

Electron microscopes are scientific instruments that use a beam of highly energetic electrons to examine objects on a very fine scale. The development of the electron microscope in the 1930s revolutionized biology, allowing organelles such as mitochondria and membranes to be seen in detail for the first time. With modern scanning electron microscopes, objects may be viewed from 25× to 250,000× their actual size. These advances have allowed

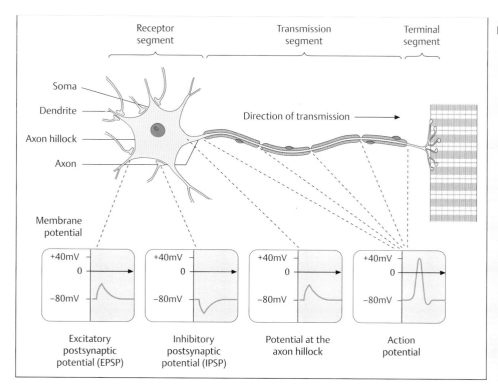

Fig. 2.27 The nerve cell (neuron).

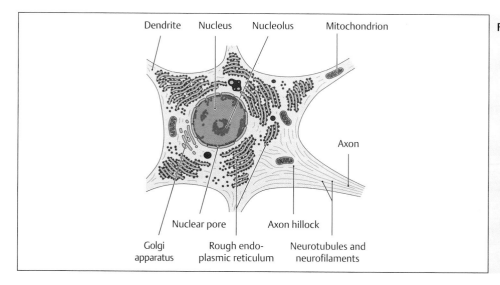

Fig. 2.28 Electron microscopy of the neuron.

details of neurons to be discovered. Neurons are rich in *rough endoplasmic reticulum* (protein synthesis, active metabolism). This endoplasmic reticulum (known also as *Nissl substance)* is easily demonstrated by light microscopy using cationic dyes, which bind to the phosphodiester backbone of the ribosomal RNAs. The distribution pattern of the Nissl substance is used in neuropathology to evaluate the functional integrity of neurons. Neurotubules and neurofilaments are collectively referred to as *neurofibrils* in light microscopy, as they are too fine to be identified as separate structures under a light microscope. Neurofibrils can be demonstrated in light microscopy by impregnating the nerve tissue with silver salts. This is of interest in neuropathology because the clumping of neurofibrils is an important histological feature of Alzheimer's disease. In fact, the presence of neurofibrillary tangles is one of several diagnostic signs of confirming Alzheimer's disease (**Fig. 2.28**).

2.7.3 Basic Forms of the Neuron and Its Functionally Adapted Variants

The horizontal line marks the region of the axon hillock, which represents the initial segment of the axon. (a) Multipolar neuron (multiple dendrites) with a *long* axon (= long transmission path). Examples are projection neurons such as alpha motor neurons in the spinal cord. (b) Multipolar neuron with a short axon (= short transmission path). Examples are interneurons like those in the gray matter of the brain and spinal cord. (c) Pyramidal cell: Dendrites are present only at the apex and base of the *tridentate* cell body, and the axon is long. Examples are efferent neurons of the cerebral motor system. (d) Purkinje's cell: An elaborately branched dendritic tree arises from a circumscribed site on the cell body. The Purkinje cell receives many synaptic contacts from afferents to the cerebellum and is also the efferent cell of the cerebellar cortex. (e) Bipolar neuron: The dendrite branches in the periphery. Examples are bipolar cells of the retina. (f) Pseudounipolar neuron: The dendrite and axon are not separated by a cell body. An example is the primary afferent (= first sensory) neuron in the spinal ganglion (**Fig. 2.29**).

2.7.4 Synaptic Patterns in a Small Group of Neurons

Axons can terminate at various sites on the target neuron and form synapses there. The synaptic patterns are described as axodendritic, axosomatic, or axoaxonal. Axodendritic synapses are the most common (see also Chapter 2.7.1) (**Fig. 2.30**).

2.7.5 Electron Microscopy of Synapses in the CNS

Synapses are the functional connection between two neurons. They consist of a presynaptic membrane, a synaptic cleft, and a postsynaptic membrane. In a *spine synapse* (1), the presynaptic knob (bouton) is in contact with a specialized protuberance (spine) of the target neuron. The side-by-side synapse of an axon with the flat surface of a target neuron is called a parallel contact or *bouton en passage* (2). The vesicles in the presynaptic expansion contain the neurotransmitters that are released into the synaptic cleft by exocytosis when the axon fires. From there the neurotransmitters diffuse to the postsynaptic membrane, where their receptors are located. A variety of drugs and toxins act upon synaptic transmission (antidepressants, muscle relaxants, toxic gases, botulinum toxin). The wondrous transmission of the action potential from one neuron to another has been referred to as the "synaptic kiss." It is faster than a speeding bullet (**Fig. 2.31**).

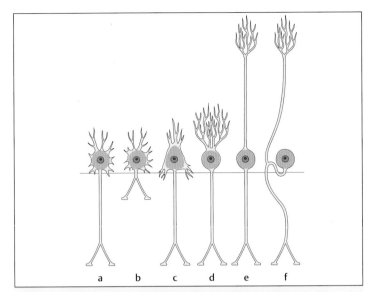

Fig. 2.29 Basic forms of the neuron and its functionally adapted variants. Multipolar neuron with (**a**) long axon, (**b**) short axon. (**c**) Pyramidal cell. (**d**) Purkinje's cell. (**e**) Bipolar neuron. (**f**) Pseudounipolar neuron.

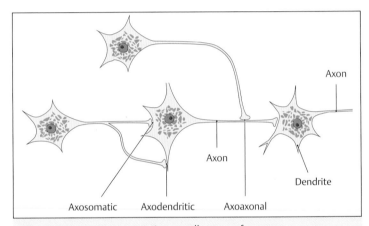

Fig. 2.30 Synaptic patterns in a small group of neurons.

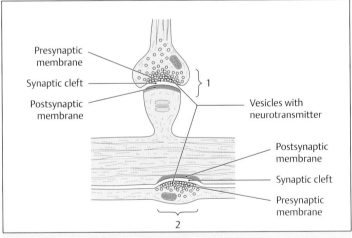

Fig. 2.31 Electron microscopy of synapses in the CNS.

2.7.6 Cells of the Neuroglia in the CNS

Neuroglial cells surround the neurons, providing them with structural and functional support (see **Table 2.4**). Various staining methods are available in light microscopy for selectively demonstrating different portions of the neuroglial cells: (a) Cell nuclei demonstrated with a basic stain. (b) Cell body demonstrated by silver impregnation (**Fig. 2.32**).

2.7.7 Summary: Cells of the CNS and PNS and Their Functional Importance

See **Table 2.4**.

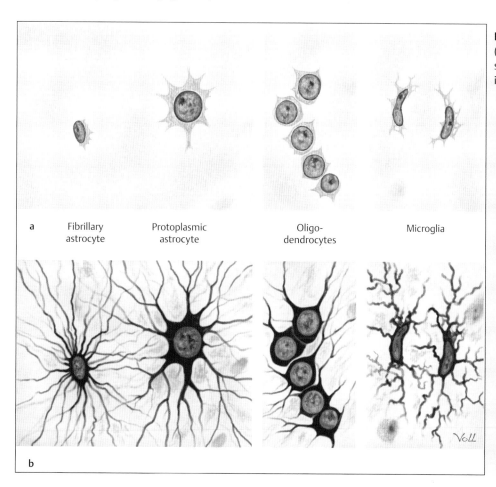

a   Fibrillary astrocyte   Protoplasmic astrocyte   Oligo-dendrocytes   Microglia

b

Fig. 2.32 Cells of the neuroglia in the CNS. (**a**) Cell nuclei demonstrated with a basic stain. (**b**) Cell body demonstrated by silver impregnation.

Table 2.4 Cells of the CNS and PNS and their functional importance

Type of cell	Function
Neurons (CNS and PNS)	1. Impulse formation
	2. Impulse conduction
	3. Information processing
Glial cells Astrocytes (CNS only)	1. Maintain a constant internal milieu in the CNS
	2. Contribute to the structure of the blood–brain barrier
	3. Phagocytize dead synapses
	4. Form scar tissue in the CNS
	5. (e.g., in multiple sclerosis or following a stroke)
Microglial cells (CNS only)	Phagocytosis ("macrophages of the brain")
Oligodendrocytes (CNS only)	Myelin sheath formation in the CNS
Schwann cells (PNS only)	Myelin sheath formation in the PNS
Satellite cells (PNS only)	Modified Schwann cells; surround the cell body of neurons in PNS ganglia

Abbreviations: CNS, central nervous system; PNS, peripheral nervous system.

2.8 Differences between the Central and Peripheral Nervous Systems

2.8.1 Myelination Differences in the PNS and CNS

The purpose of myelination is to provide the axons with electrical insulation, which significantly increases the nerve conduction velocity. The very lipid-rich membranes of myelinating cells are wrapped around the axons to produce this insulation. Schwann cells (left) myelinate the axons in the *PNS,* while oligodendrocytes (right) form the myelin in the *CNS* (**Fig. 2.33**).

Note: In the *CNS,* one oligodendrocyte *always* wraps around *multiple* axons. In the *PNS,* one Schwann cell *may* ensheath *multiple* axons if the peripheral nerve is *unmyelinated.* If the peripheral nerve is *myelinated,* one Schwann cell *always* wraps around *one* axon. Owing to this improved insulation, the nerve conduction velocity is higher in myelinated nerves than in unmyelinated nerves. Myelinated fibers occur in areas where fast reaction speeds are needed (muscular contractions), while unmyelinated fibers occur in areas that do not require rapid information transfer, as in the transmission of visceral pain.

Because of the different cell types, myelin has a different composition in the CNS and PNS. This difference in myelination is also important clinically. An example is multiple sclerosis, in which the oligodendrocytes are damaged but the Schwann cells are not, so that the central myelin sheaths are disrupted while the peripheral myelin sheaths remain intact. Multiple sclerosis (MS) is a potentially debilitating disease in which your body's immune system eats away at the protective sheath (myelin) that covers axons. This interferes with neural transmission and hence the communication between your brain and the rest of your body. Ultimately, this may result in deterioration of the nerves themselves, a process that is not reversible.

Signs and symptoms vary widely, depending on the amount of damage and which nerves are affected. People with severe cases of MS may lose the ability to walk or speak. MS can be difficult to diagnose early in the course of the disease because signs and symptoms often come and go—sometimes disappearing for months.

2.8.2 Structure of a Node of Ranvier in the PNS

In the PNS, the *node of Ranvier* is the site where two Schwann cells come together. That site is marked by a small gap in the myelin sheath, which forms the morphological basis for *saltatory nerve conduction,* allowing impulses to be transmitted at a higher velocity (**Fig. 2.34**).

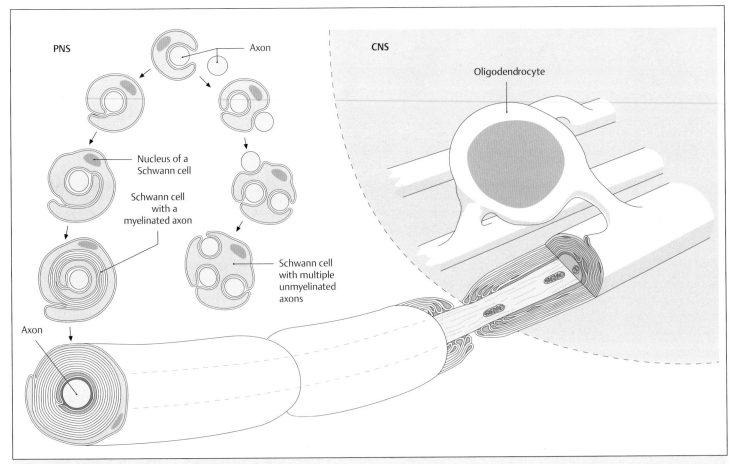

Fig. 2.33 Myelination differences in the PNS and CNS.

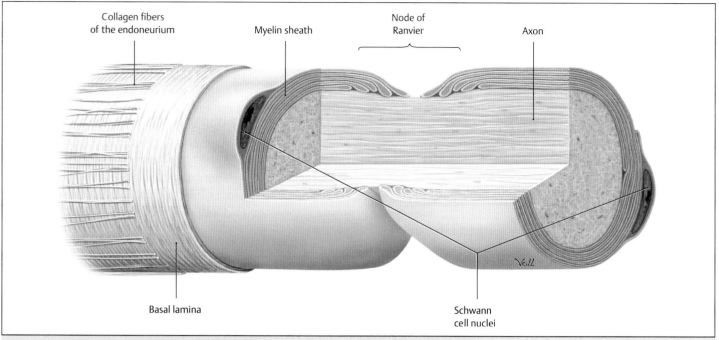

Fig. 2.34 Structure of a node of Ranvier in the PNS.

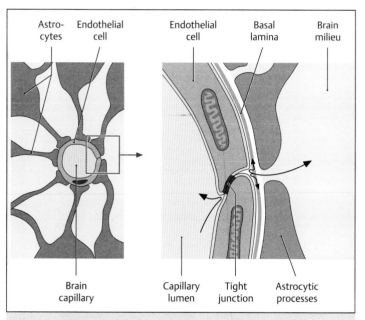

Fig. 2.35 Structure of the blood–brain barrier in the CNS.

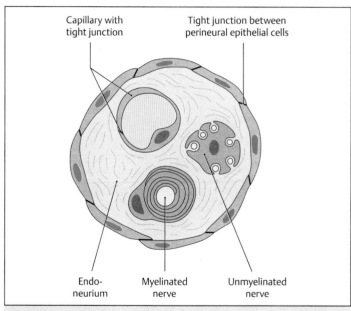

Fig. 2.36 Structure of the perineurial sheath in the PNS.

2.8.3 Structure of the Blood–Brain Barrier in the CNS

Besides the type of myelination, there is also a difference in tissue barriers between the CNS and PNS. The CNS is isolated from surrounding tissues by the blood–brain barrier. The components of the blood–brain barrier include (1) most importantly, a continuous capillary endothelial cell layer, sealed by tight junctions; (2) a continuous basal lamina surrounding the endothelial cells; and (3) enveloping astrocytic processes surrounding the brain capillary. This barrier serves to exclude macromolecules, as well as many small molecules that are not actively transported by the endothelial cells, thus protecting the delicate environment of the CNS. The barrier is vulnerable, however, to lipid-soluble molecules that can traverse the endothelial cell membranes. The perineurial sheath creates a similar barrier in the PNS (see Chapter 2.8.4). The blood–brain barrier helps protect the brain

from "foreign substances" in the blood that may damage the brain or hinder nerve transmission. It helps maintain a relatively constant environment for the brain (**Fig. 2.35**).

2.8.4 Structure of the Perineurial Sheath in the PNS

The perineurial sheath, like the blood–brain barrier, is formed by tight junctions between the epithelium-like fibroblasts. It isolates the milieu of the axon from that of the surrounding endoneural space (endoneurium), thereby preventing harmful substances from invading the axon. This tissue barrier must be surmounted by drugs that are designed to act on the axon, such as local anesthetic agents. Many extrinsic factors can open the blood–brain barrier and make the nervous system more susceptible to damage including exposure to radiation, microwaves, infectious agents, trauma, ischemia (reduced blood flow), or inflammation (**Fig. 2.36**).

3 Head, Skull, Neck Anatomy

3.1 Skull, Lateral View

3.1.1 Lateral View of the Skull (Cranium)

Left lateral view (**Fig. 3.1**). This view was selected as an introduction to the skull because it displays the greatest number of cranial bones (indicated by different colors in Chapter 3.1.2). The individual bones and their salient features as well as the cranial sutures and apertures are described in the units that follow. This unit reviews the principal structures of the lateral aspect of the skull. The chapter as a whole is intended to familiarize the reader with the names of the cranial bones before proceeding to finer anatomical details and the relationships of the bones to one another. The skull provides a degree of protection for the brain, particularly against injurious trauma, but as with protective helmets and headgear, only a degree of protection is afforded. The bones of the skull can be fractured or penetrated with subsequent direct injury to brain tissue.

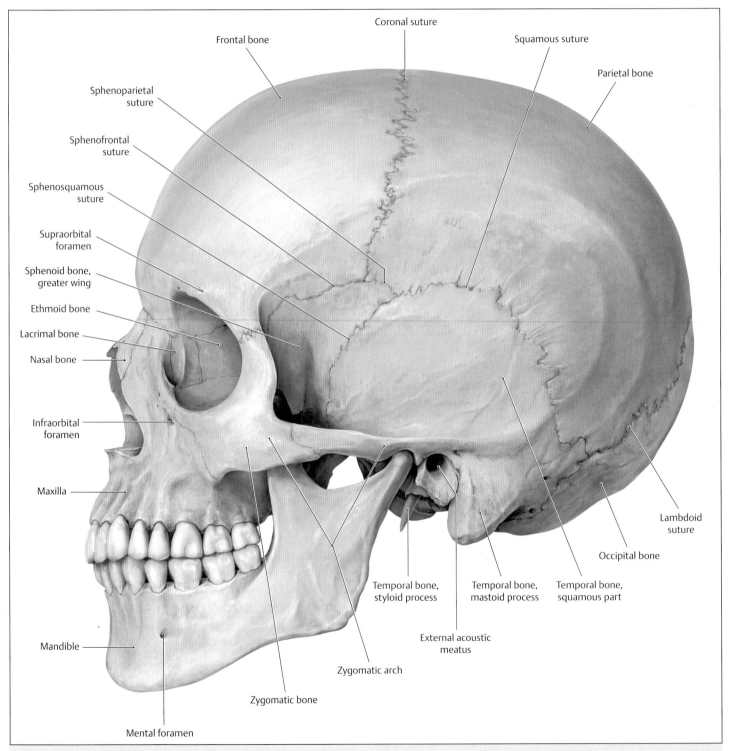

Fig. 3.1 Lateral view of the skull (cranium).

3.1.2 Lateral View of the Cranial Bones

Left lateral view (**Fig. 3.2**). The bones are shown in different colors to demonstrate more clearly their extents and boundaries.

3.1.3 Bones of the Neurocranium and Viscerocranium

Left lateral view (**Fig. 3.3**). The skull forms a bony capsule that encloses the brain, sensory organs, and viscera of the head. The greater size of the neurocranium (cranial vault) relative to the viscerocranium (facial skeleton) is a typical primate feature directly correlated with the larger primate brain. Does a bigger brain relate to greater intelligence? Scientists have been divided about what to measure and how to measure it. Anthropologists, including the great brain scientist Paul Broca, have used cephalometrics to address the issue. Perhaps improvements in measurement techniques will allow agreement about the relationship between brain size and intelligence, but for now no consensus exists. See **Table 3.1**.

3.1.4 Ossification of the Cranial Bones

Left lateral view (**Fig. 3.4**). The bones of the skull either develop directly from mesenchymal connective tissue (intramembranous ossification, gray) or form indirectly by the ossification of a cartilaginous model (endochondral ossification, blue). Elements derived from intramembranous and endochondral ossification (desmocranium, chondrocranium) may fuse together to form a single bone (e.g., the occipital bone, temporal bone, and sphenoid bone).

The clavicle is the only tubular bone that undergoes membranous ossification. This explains why congenital defects of *intramembranous* ossification affect both the skull and clavicle (*cleidocranial dysostosis*).

Table 3.1 Bones of the neurocranium and viscerocranium

Neurocranium (gray)	Viscerocranium (orange)
• Frontal bone	• Nasal bone
• Sphenoid bone (excluding the pterygoid process)	• Lacrimal bone
• Temporal bone (squamous part, petrous part)	• Ethmoid bone (excluding the cribriform plate)
• Parietal bone	• Sphenoid bone (pterygoid process)
• Occipital bone	• Maxilla
• Ethmoid bone (cribriform plate)	• Zygomatic bone
	• Temporal bone (tympanic part, styloid process)
	• Mandible
	• Vomer
	• Inferior nasal turbinate
	• Palatine bone
	• Hyoid bone

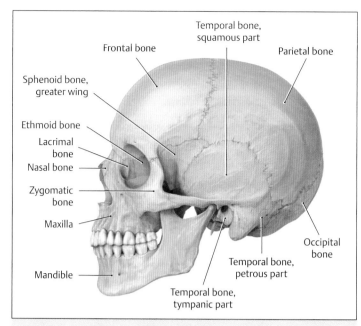

Fig. 3.2 Lateral view of the cranial bones.

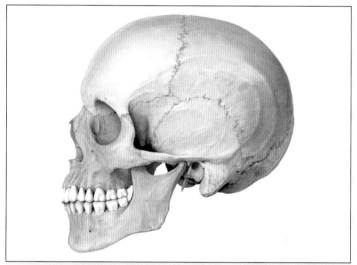

Fig. 3.3 Bones of the neurocranium (gray) and viscerocranium (orange).

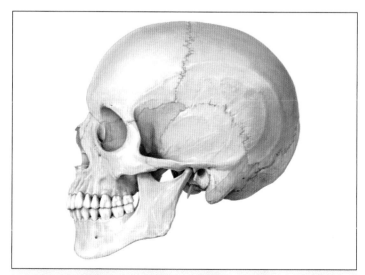

Fig. 3.4 Ossification of the cranial bones.

3.1.5 Bones of the Desmocranium and Chondrocranium

See **Table 3.2**.

Table 3.2 Bones of the desmocranium and chondrocranium

Desmocranium (gray)	Chondrocranium (blue)
• Nasal bone	• Ethmoid bone
• Lacrimal bone	• Sphenoid bone (excluding the medial plate of the pterygoid process)
• Maxilla	
• Mandible	
• Zygomatic bone	• Temporal bone (petrous and mastoid parts, styloid process)
• Frontal bone	
• Parietal bone	• Occipital bone (excluding the upper part of the squama)
• Occipital bone (upper part of the squama)	• Inferior nasal turbinate
• Temporal bone (squamous part, tympanic part)	• Hyoid bone
• Palatine bone	
• Vomer	

3.2 Skull, Anterior View

3.2.1 Anterior View of the Skull

See **Fig. 3.5**. The boundaries of the facial skeleton (viscerocranium) can be clearly appreciated in this view (the individual bones are shown in **Fig. 3.6**). The bony margins of the anterior nasal aperture mark the start of the respiratory tract in the skull. The nasal cavity, like the orbits, contains a sensory organ (the olfactory mucosa). The *paranasal sinuses* are shown schematically in **Fig. 3.7**. The anterior view of the skull also displays the three clinically important openings through which sensory nerves pass to supply the face: the supraorbital foramen, infraorbital foramen, and mental foramen. These openings will come into play when the sensory and motor functions of the cranial nerves that supply the head and neck are discussed.

3.2.2 Cranial Bones, Anterior View

See **Fig. 3.6**.

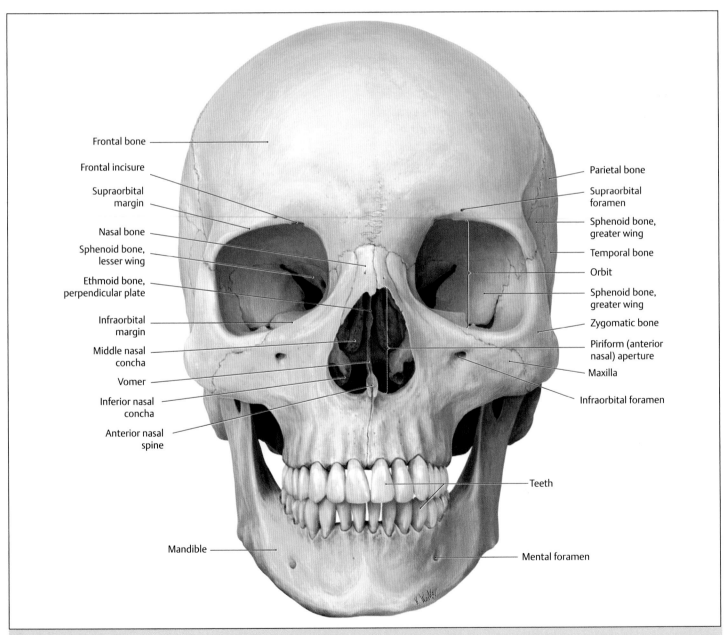

Fig. 3.5 Anterior view of the skull.

3.2.3 Paranasal Sinuses: Pneumatization Lightens the Bone

Anterior view (**Fig. 3.7**). Some of the bones of the facial skeleton are pneumatized, that is, they contain air-filled cavities that reduce the total weight of the bone. These cavities, called the paranasal sinuses, communicate with the nasal cavity and, like it, are lined by ciliated respiratory epithelium. Inflammations of the paranasal sinuses (sinusitis) and associated complaints are very common. Because some of the pain of sinusitis is projected to the skin overlying the sinuses, it is helpful to know the projections of the sinuses onto the surface of the skull.

3.2.4 Principal Lines of Force (Blue) in the Facial Skeleton

The pneumatized paranasal sinuses (Chapter 3.2.3) have a mechanical counterpart in the thickened bony "pillars" of the facial

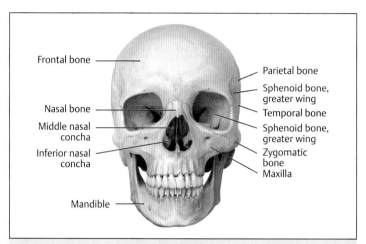

Fig. 3.6 Cranial bones (anterior view).

Frontal bone
Parietal bone
Sphenoid bone, greater wing
Nasal bone
Temporal bone
Middle nasal concha
Sphenoid bone, greater wing
Inferior nasal concha
Zygomatic bone
Maxilla
Mandible

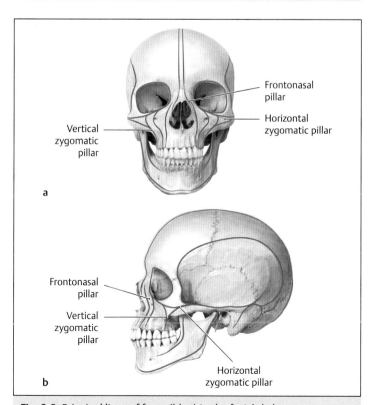

Fig. 3.8 Principal lines of force (blue) in the facial skeleton. (a) Anterior view. (b) Lateral view.

Frontonasal pillar
Horizontal zygomatic pillar
Vertical zygomatic pillar

a

Frontonasal pillar
Vertical zygomatic pillar
Horizontal zygomatic pillar

b

skeleton, which partially bound the sinuses. These pillars develop along the principal lines of force in response to local mechanical stresses (e.g., masticatory pressures). In visual terms, the frame-like construction of the facial skeleton may be likened to that of a frame house. The paranasal sinuses represent the rooms while the pillars (placed along major lines of force) represent the supporting columns (**Fig. 3.8**).

3.2.5 LeFort's Classification of Midfacial Fractures

The frame-like construction of the facial skeleton leads to characteristic patterns of fracture lines in the midfacial region (LeFort I, II, and III).

LeFort I: This fracture line runs across the maxilla and above the hard palate. The maxilla is separated from the upper facial skeleton, disrupting the integrity of the maxillary sinus (*low transverse fracture*).

LeFort II: The fracture line passes across the nasal root, ethmoid bone, maxilla, and zygomatic bone, creating a *pyramid fracture* that disrupts the integrity of the orbit.

LeFort III: The facial skeleton is separated from the base of the skull. The main fracture line passes through the orbits, and the fracture may additionally involve the ethmoid bones, frontal sinuses, sphenoid sinuses, and zygomatic bones. These fracture lines may become important in cases of traumatic head injury or the polytrauma related to blast injuries (**Fig. 3.9**).

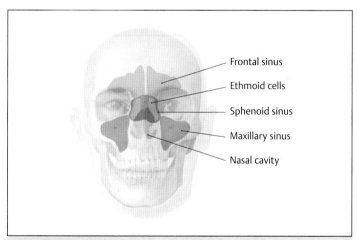

Frontal sinus
Ethmoid cells
Sphenoid sinus
Maxillary sinus
Nasal cavity

Fig. 3.7 Paranasal sinuses.

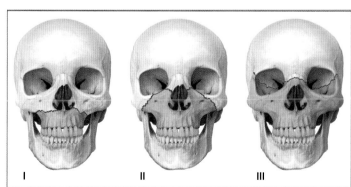

I II III

Fig. 3.9 LeFort's classification of midfacial fractures.

3.3 Skull, Posterior View and Cranial Sutures

3.3.1 Posterior View of the Skull

The occipital bone, which is dominant in this view, articulates with the parietal bones, to which it is connected by the lambdoid suture. The cranial sutures are a special type of syndesmosis (= ligamentous attachments that ossify with age, see **Table 3.3**). The outer surface of the occipital bone is contoured by muscular origins and insertions: the inferior, superior, and supreme nuchal lines (**Fig. 3.10**).

3.3.2 Posterior View of the Cranial Bones

Note: The temporal bone consists of two main parts based on its embryonic development: a squamous part and a petrous part (**Fig. 3.11**).

3.3.3 The Neonatal Skull

The flat cranial bones must grow as the brain expands, and so the sutures between them must remain open for some time (see Chapter 3.3.6). In the neonate, there are areas between the still-growing cranial bones that are not occupied by bone: the fontanelles. They close at different times (the sphenoid fontanelle in about the 6th month of life, the mastoid fontanelle in the 18th month, the anterior fontanelle in the 36th month). The *posterior fontanelle* provides a reference point for describing the position of the fetal head during childbirth, and the *anterior fontanelle* provides a possible access site for drawing a cerebrospinal fluid sample in infants (e.g., in suspected meningitis). Meningitis is an infection of the meninges or coverings of the brain (**Fig. 3.12**). The pia mater, arachnoid, and dura mater (the meninges) will be discussed later.

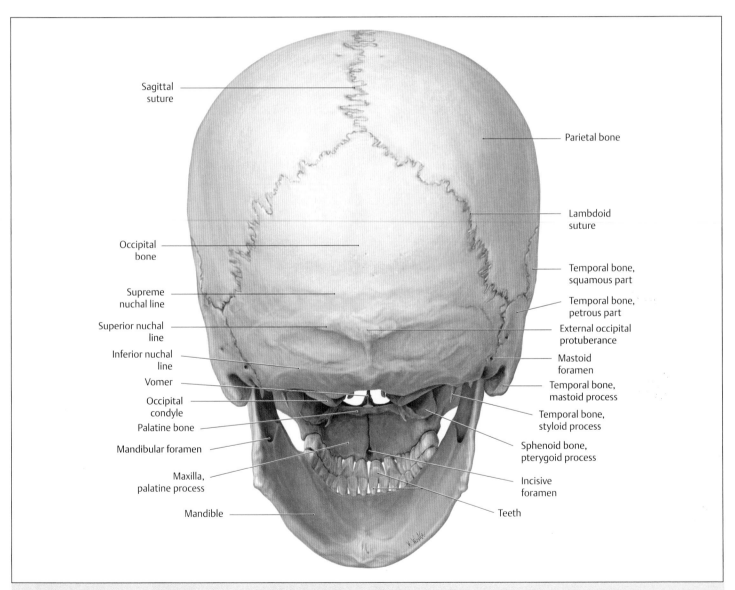

Fig. 3.10 Posterior view of the skull.

3.3.4 Cranial Deformities due to the Premature Closure of Cranial Sutures

The premature closure of a cranial suture (craniosynostosis) may lead to characteristic cranial deformities. The following sutures may close prematurely, resulting in various cranial shapes: (a) sagittal suture: scaphocephaly (long, narrow skull) (b) coronal suture: oxycephaly (pointed skull), (c) frontal suture: trigonocephaly (triangular skull), (d) Asymmetrical suture closure, usually involving the coronal suture: plagiocephaly (asymmetrical skull) (**Fig. 3.13**).

3.3.5 Hydrocephalus and Microcephaly

(a) Characteristic cranial morphology in *hydrocephalus.* When the brain becomes dilated due to cerebrospinal fluid accumulation *before* the cranial sutures ossify (hydrocephalus, "water on the brain"), the neurocranium will expand while the facial skeleton

remains unchanged. (b) *Microcephaly* results from premature closure of the cranial sutures. It is characterized by a small neurocranium with relatively large orbits (**Fig. 3.14**).

3.3.6 Age at Which the Principal Sutures Ossify

See **Table 3.3**.

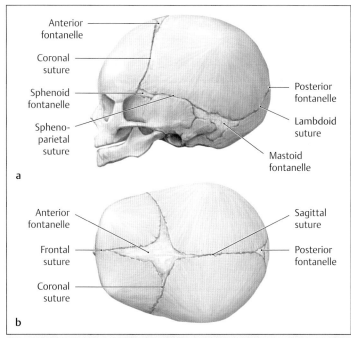

Fig. 3.12 Neonatal skull. **(a)** Left lateral view. **(b)** Superior view.

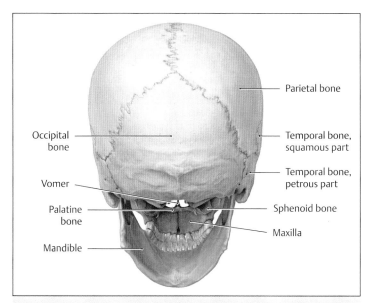

Fig. 3.11 Posterior view of the cranial bones.

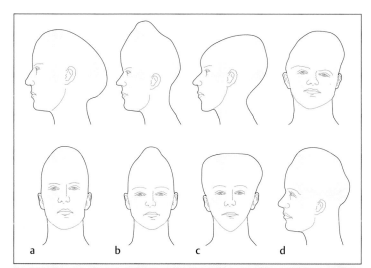

Fig. 3.13 Cranial deformities. **(a)** Sagittal suture (long, narrow skull). **(b)** Coronal suture (pointed skull). **(c)** Frontal suture (triangular skull). **(d)** Asymmetrical suture (asymmetrical skull).

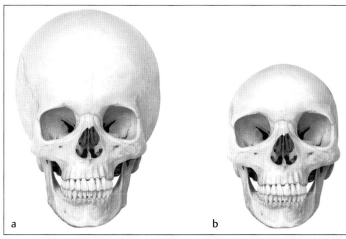

Fig. 3.14 **(a)** Hydrocephalus. **(b)** Microcephaly.

Table 3.3 Age at which principal sutures ossify

Suture	Age at ossification
Frontal suture	Childhood
Sagittal suture	20–30 years of age
Coronal suture	30–40 years of age
Lambdoid suture	40–50 years of age

3.4 Base of the Skull, External View

3.4.1 Bones of the Base of the Skull

Inferior view (**Fig. 3.15**). The base of the skull is composed of a mosaic-like assembly of various bones. It is helpful to review the shape and location of these bones before studying further details.

3.4.2 Relationship of the Foramen Lacerum to the Carotid Canal and Internal Carotid Artery

Left lateral view (**Fig. 3.16**). The foramen lacerum is not a true aperture, being occluded in life by a layer of fibrocartilage; it appears as an opening only in the dried skull. The foramen lacerum is closely related to the carotid canal and to the internal carotid artery that traverses the canal. The greater petrosal nerve and deep petrosal nerve pass through the foramen lacerum. The carotid canal

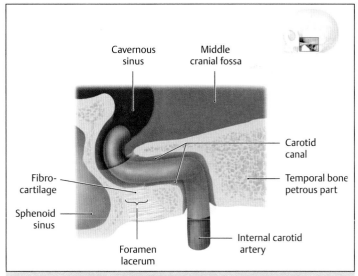

Fig. 3.16 Relationship of the foramen lacerum to the carotid canal and internal carotid artery.

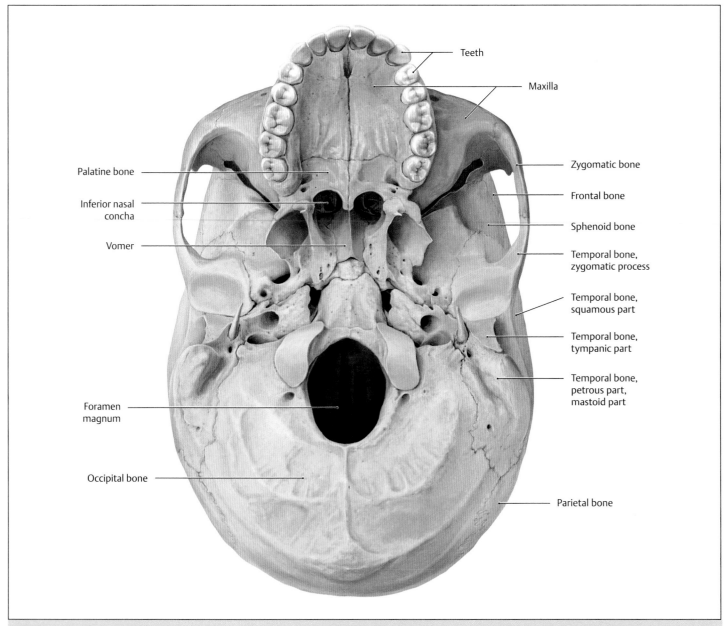

Fig. 3.15 Bones of the base of the skull.

allows passage of the internal carotid artery, one of the two principal sources of blood and nourishment to brain tissue.

3.4.3 The Basal Aspect of the Skull

Inferior view (**Fig. 3.17**). The principal external features of the base of the skull are labeled. Note particularly the openings that transmit nerves and vessels. With abnormalities of bone growth, these openings may remain too small or may become narrowed, compressing the neurovascular structures that pass through them. If the optic canal fails to grow normally, it may compress and damage the optic nerve, resulting in visual field defects. The symptoms associated with these lesions depend on the affected opening. The foramen magnum is the major skull opening that allows the spinal cord and brain stem to pass through the bony skull and connect with the brain. All of the structures depicted here will be considered in more detail in subsequent pages.

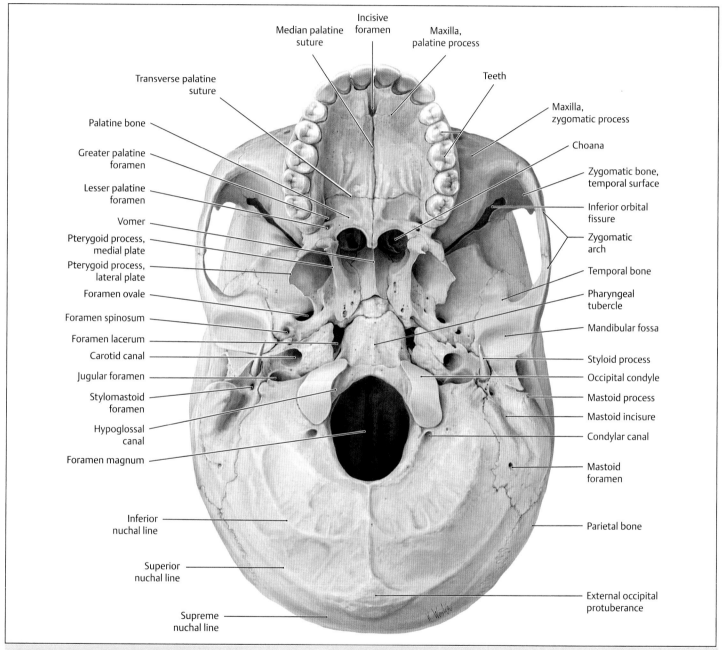

Fig. 3.17 Basal aspect of the skull.

3.5 Overview of the Entire Nervous System: Morphology and Spatial Orientation

3.5.1 Morphology of the Central Nervous System

A general morphological overview of the entire nervous system is necessary to help with understanding the material that follows (**Fig. 3.18**). The central nervous system (CNS) is divided into the brain and the spinal cord with the **brain (encephalon)** subdivided into the following regions:

- Cerebral hemispheres (telencephalon or endbrain).
- Interbrain (diencephalon).
- Cerebellum.
- Brainstem composed of the midbrain (mesencephalon), pons (bridge), and medulla oblongata.

In contrast, the other part of the CNS, the **spinal cord (medulla spinalis)** appears morphologically rather as one homogenous structure. In terms of its functions, however, the spinal cord, can also be divided into segments. The division of gray and white matter is clearly visible:

- Gray matter: centrally located, butterfly shaped structure.
- White matter: substance that surrounds the "butterfly".

3.5.2 Axes of the Nervous System and Directional Terms

The same planes, axes, and directional terms apply for both the entire body and the peripheral nervous system (PNS) (**Fig. 3.19**). However, with the CNS, one differentiates between two axes:

- Axis No. 1: Meynert's axis. It corresponds to the axes of the body and is used to designate locations in the spinal cord, brainstem (truncus encephali), and cerebellum.
- Axis No. 2: Forel's axis. It runs horizontally through the diencephalon and telencephalon and forms an 80-degree angle to axis 1. As a result, the diencephalon and telencephalon lie "face down."

Note: In order to avoid topographical misunderstandings, the following directional terms for axis No. 2 (Forel's axis) are used:

- Basal instead of ventral.
- Parietal instead of dorsal.
- Frontal and oral/rostral, respectively, instead of cranial.
- Occipital instead of caudal.

3.5.3 Morphology of the Peripheral Nervous System

See **Fig. 3.20**.

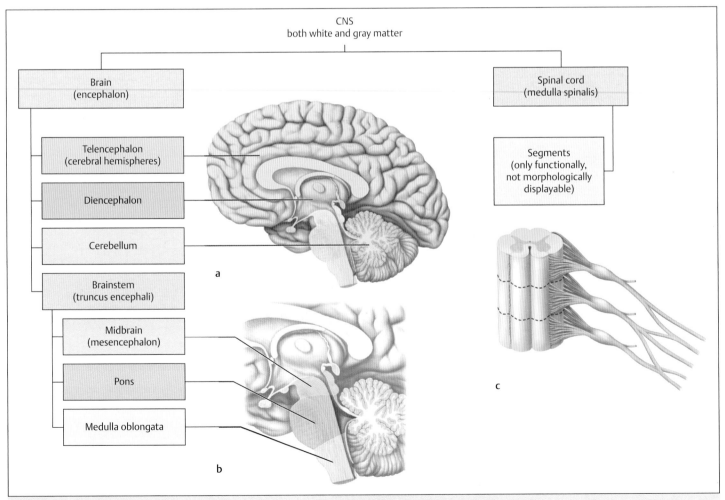

Fig. 3.18 Morphology of the CNS. (**a, b**) Right side of the brain, medial view. (**c**) Ventral view of a section of the spinal cord.

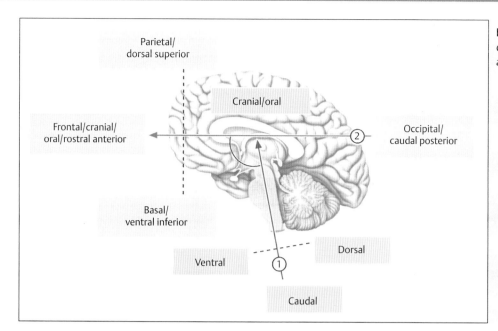

Fig. 3.19 Axes of the nervous system and directional terms. (1) Meynert axis. (2) Forel axis.

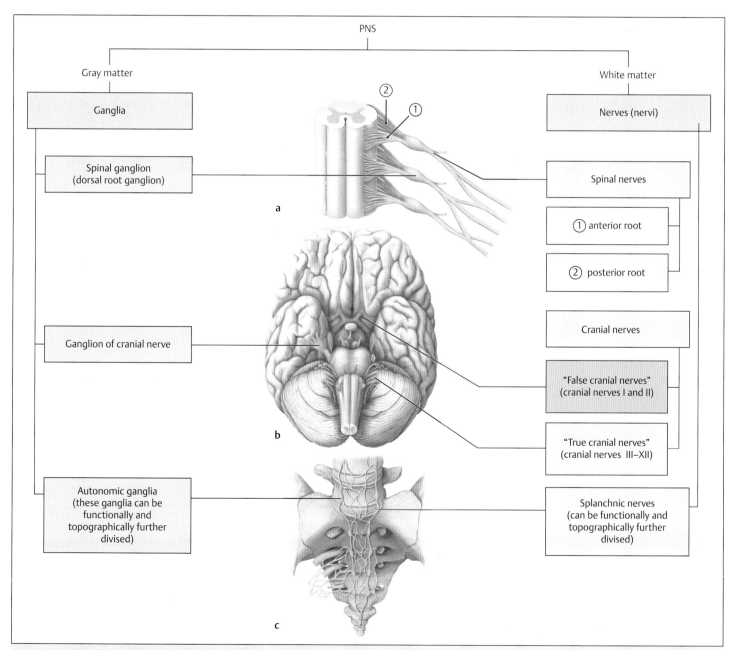

Fig. 3.20 **(a)** Ventral view of a segment of the spinal cord. **(b)** View of base of the brain. **(c)** View of sympathetic ganglia and nerves located anteriorly to the sacrum.

The nerves and ganglia forming the PNS and are generally named for the part of the CNS with which they communicate:

- Spinal nerves (connect the periphery of the body with the spinal cord. Usually 31 or 32 pairs. Spinal nerves (except those related to vertebral levels T1 to T11 or T12) generally have their ventral rami form plexuses for reasons of functionality.
- Cranial nerves (connect the periphery of the body to the brain), 12 pairs.

Nerve cells found within ganglia (in the PNS) can be classified based on their affiliation with a particular functional division of the nervous system:

- Sensory neurons can be found within either division of nervous system. In the PNS, sensory neurons are found within the sensory (dorsal root) ganglia on the posterior (dorsal) root of the spinal nerve. In the CNS, sensory neurons are found within the sensory nuclei associated with the appropriate cranial nerves that contain sensory fibers.

- Ganglia of the autonomic nervous system contain postganglionic sympathetic and parasympathetic neurons that control the organs of the body. Autonomic ganglia are associated with splanchnic nerves that take vasomotor fibers to the viscera. The autonomic nervous system also demonstrates characteristic plexus formation.

Note: The distinction of sensory nerves in the CNS applies except for a few special cases. For instance, cranial nerves I (olfactory) and II (optic) are not true nerves but parts of the telencephalon or diencephalon, which clearly make them part of the CNS. For historical reasons, they have been called "nerves," which is systemically false. These "bogus" cranial nerves (colored red on the brain in the figure above) are often contrasted with the 10 true cranial nerves (colored yellow on this figure), which are clearly part of the PNS. In the interest of clarity, further details are omitted at this point. For our purposes, we will consider the cranial nerves to be the traditional 12, including the olfactory and optic "nerves."

4 Anatomy of the Brain and Nervous Systems

4.1 Brain, Macroscopic Organization

4.1.1 Left Lateral View of the Brain

See **Fig. 4.1.**

The cerebrum is divided macroscopically into four lobes:

- Frontal lobe
- Parietal lobe
- Temporal lobe
- Occipital lobe

The surface contours of the cerebrum are defined by convolutions (gyri) and depressions (sulci). An example is the central sulcus, which separates the precentral gyrus from the postcentral gyrus (sometimes labeled the fissure of Rolando). These two gyri are functionally important because the *precentral gyrus* is concerned with voluntary motor activity while the *postcentral gyrus* is concerned with the conscious perception of body sensation. Deep within the lateral sulcus is the *insular lobe,* often called simply the insula. The lateral sulcus is sometimes labeled the Sylvian fissure and is another major landmark on the lateral cerebrum. The sulci are narrowed and compressed in *brain edema* (excessive fluid accumulation in the brain), but they are enlarged in *brain atrophy* (e.g., Alzheimer's disease) because of tissue loss from the gyri. The brains that are available for dissection in medical school courses frequently manifest signs of brain atrophy. Often the atrophy is predominantly frontal in males and predominantly occipital in females, but the reason for this disparity is unknown.

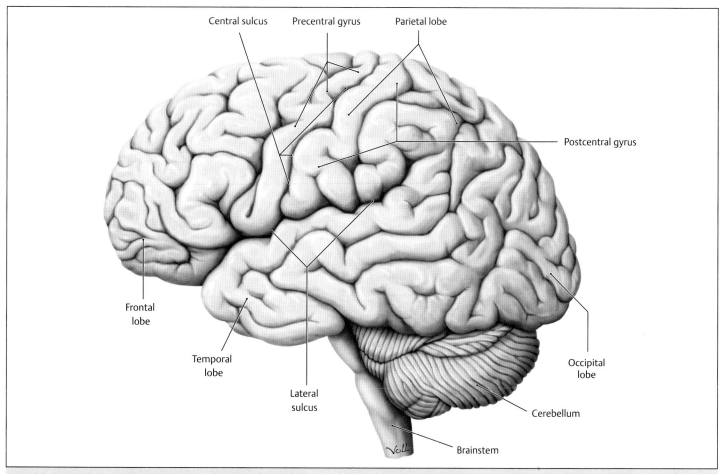

Fig. 4.1 Left lateral view of the brain.

4.1.2 Basal View of the Brain

The spinal cord is seen in its upper cervical portion. This view demonstrates the sites of emergence of most of the cranial nerves (yellow) from the brainstem. The frontal lobes, temporal lobes, pons, medulla oblongata, and cerebellum are the principal structures that can be identified on the base of the brain. This view clearly displays the two hemispheres and the *longitudinal cerebral fissure* between them. The gyri vary considerably in different individuals, and even the convolutions of a single brain may show marked side-to-side differences, perhaps due to the specialization of the hemispheres (**Fig. 4.2**).

4.1.3 Midsagittal Section of the Brain Showing the Medial Surface of the Right Hemisphere

The brain has been split along the longitudinal cerebral fissure (**Fig. 4.3**). Developmentally, the brain can be divided into several major parts, all of which are visible in this section:

- Telencephalon (cerebrum)
- Diencephalon
- Mesencephalon (midbrain)
- Pons
- Medulla oblongata
- Cerebellum

The medulla oblongata is continuous inferiorly with the spinal cord, with no definite anatomical boundary between them. The mesencephalon (midbrain), pons, and medulla oblongata are collectively referred to as the *brainstem* based on their common embryological and functional features. The brainstem lies near the anterior surface of the cerebellum.

4.1.4 Terms of Location and Direction in the Central Nervous System

Midsagittal section viewed from the left side (**Fig. 4.4**). Repeated references are made in subsequent units to two different axes of the brain: the *Meynert axis,* which is used to designate locations in the brainstem, and the *Forel axis,* which describes the topography of the diencephalon and telencephalon.

- The **Meynert axis** (1) passes through the brainstem and corresponds roughly to the longitudinal body axis.
- The **Forel axis** (2) runs horizontally through the diencephalon and telencephalon.

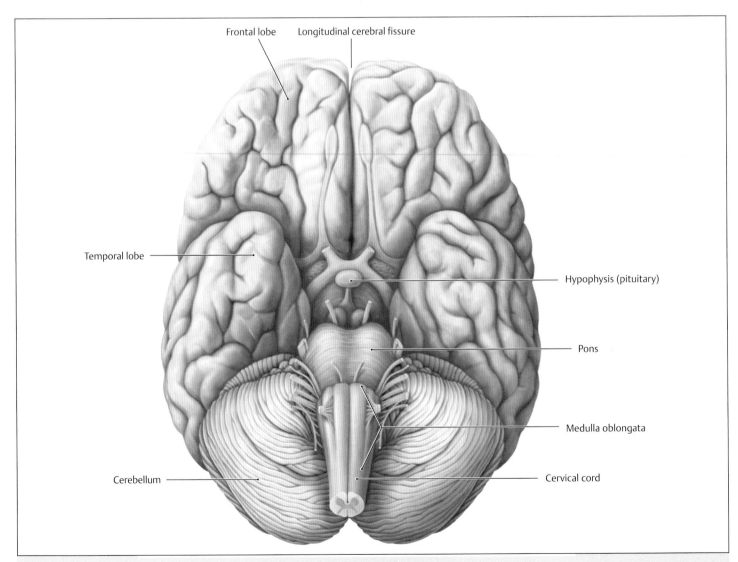

Frontal lobe   Longitudinal cerebral fissure

Temporal lobe

Hypophysis (pituitary)

Pons

Medulla oblongata

Cerebellum   Cervical cord

Fig. 4.2 Basal view of the brain.

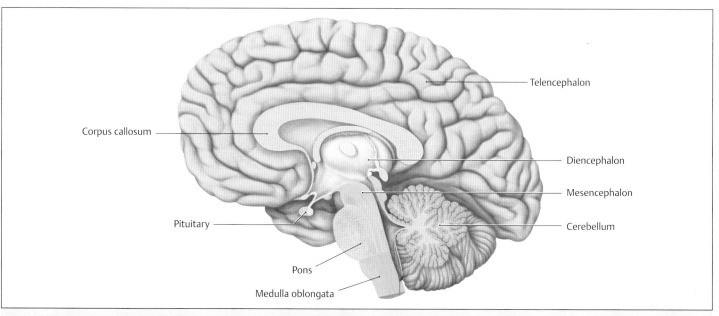

Fig. 4.3 Midsagittal section of the brain showing the medial surface of the right hemisphere.

Corpus callosum

Telencephalon

Diencephalon

Mesencephalon

Cerebellum

Pituitary

Pons

Medulla oblongata

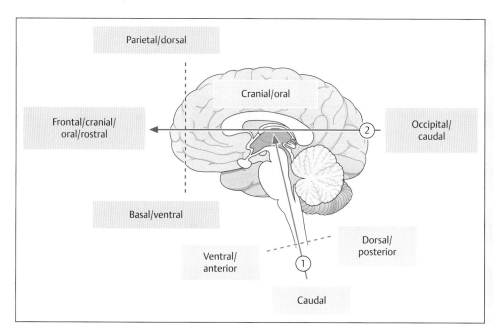

Fig. 4.4 Midsagittal section viewed from the left side. (1) Meynert axis. (2) Forel axis.

Parietal/dorsal

Cranial/oral

Frontal/cranial/oral/rostral

Occipital/caudal

Basal/ventral

Dorsal/posterior

Ventral/anterior

Caudal

The following chapters on the central nervous system (CNS) begin with the cerebrum and proceed downward to other brain structures and the spinal cord. Our approach to CNS topography also proceeds from outside to inside, following the order in which the structures are encountered in a dissection. Neuroanatomy is particularly challenging because we cannot directly infer the function of a structure from its appearance as we can with muscle tissue, for example. This presentation of the CNS therefore ends with a chapter on functional systems. In describing the functional systems, we will use a peripheral-to-central approach (i.e., from the simple to the complex) so that the reader may better understand the path followed by a stimulus from its source to its various relay stations in the CNS.

4.2 Coronal Sections: III and IV

4.2.1 Coronal Section III

The inferior (temporal) horn of the lateral ventricle appears somewhat larger in the plane of this section. In the ventricular system, we can now see the floor of the *third ventricle* (see Chapter 4.2.2) and the surrounding hypothalamus. The thalamus cannot yet be seen, as it lies slightly above and behind the hypothalamus. The *anterior commissure* appears in this plane as does the *globus pallidus*, which consists of a medial and a lateral segment. The large descending pathway, the corticospinal tract, passes through the *internal capsule*, which has a somatotopic organization. The genu of the internal capsule transmits axons for the pharynx, larynx, and jaw (**Fig. 4.5**). The course of these axons is shown schematically in chapter 4.2.3 (the fornix appears in chapter 4.2.4).

4.2.2 Ventricular System

Left lateral view (**Fig. 4.6**).

4.2.3 Course of the Pyramidal Tract in the Internal Capsule

Left anterior view (**Fig. 4.7**).

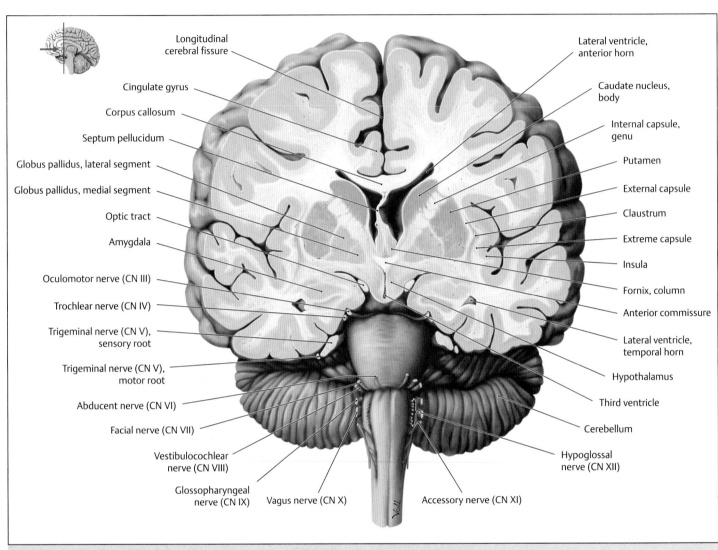

Fig. 4.5 Coronal section III.

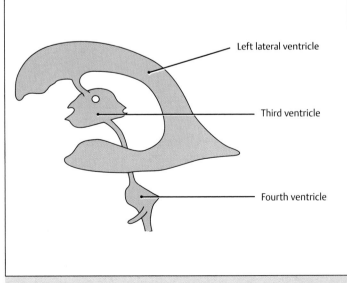

Fig. 4.6 Ventricular system.

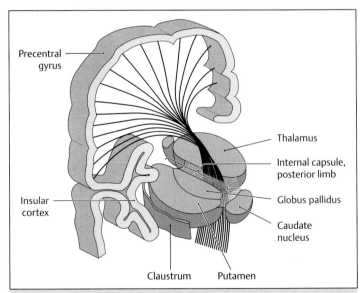

Fig. 4.7 Course of the pyramidal tract in the internal capsule.

4.2.4 Coronal Section IV

The division of the globus pallidus into medial and lateral segments can now be seen clearly (**Fig. 4.8**). This section displays the full width of both the inferior horn of the lateral ventricle and the *claustrum* (believed to be important in the regulation of sexual behavior). While the plane in A passed through the anterior commissure, this more occipital plane slices the mammillary bodies (see chapter 4.2.5). Pathological changes in the mammillary bodies can be found during autopsy of chronic alcoholics. The mammillary bodies are flanked on each side by the *foot of the hippocampus*. An important part of the limbic system, the mammillary bodies are connected to the hippocampus by the *fornix* (see chapter 4.2.6). Because of the anatomical curvature of the fornix, its *column* is visible in more frontal sections (see chapter 4.2.1), while its *crura* appear as widely separated structures in more occipital sections. The *septum pellucidum* stretches between the fornix and corpus callosum, forming the medial boundary of the lateral ventricles (see Chapters 4.2.1 and 4.2.4).

The first structure of the brainstem, the *pons*, can also be identified in this section.

4.2.5 Midsagittal Section through the Diencephalon and Brainstem

Lateral view (**Fig. 4.9**).

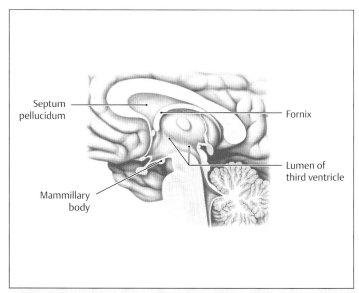

Fig. 4.9 Midsagittal section through the diencephalon and brainstem.

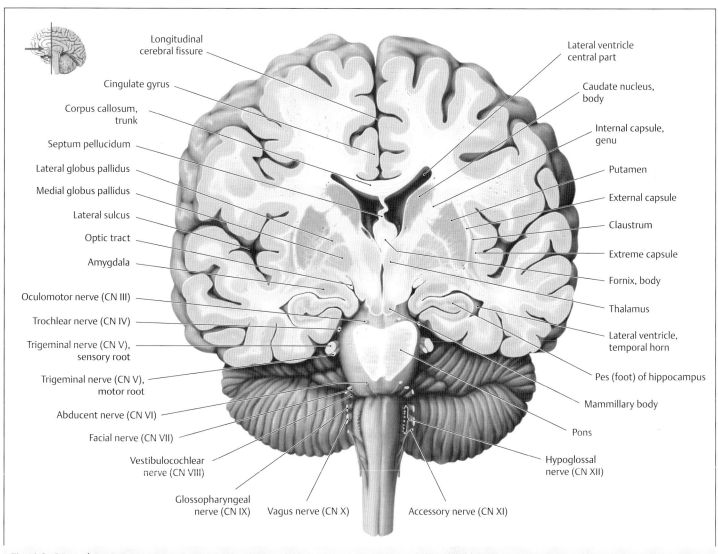

Fig. 4.8 Coronal section IV.

4.2.6 Mammillary Bodies and Fornix

See **Fig. 4.10**.

4.3 Transverse Sections: III and IV

4.3.1 Transverse Section III

The lateral ventricles communicate with the third ventricle through the *interventricular foramina* (of Monro). They are located directly anterior to the thalamus. The nuclei of the telencephalon make up the deep gray matter (unmyelinated cell bodies) of the cerebrum (**Fig. 4.11**). The spatial relationship between the caudate nucleus and thalamus is illustrated in **Fig. 4.12**. The caudate nucleus is larger frontally, and the thalamus larger occipitally. While the caudate nucleus and putamen of the motor system belong to the telencephalon, the thalamus of the sensory system belongs to the diencephalon. This transverse section passes through the caudate nucleus twice due to the anatomical curvature of the nucleus. This is the first transverse section that displays the globus pallidus, part of the motor system. The insular cortex is seen with the *claustrum* medial to it. The *crura of the fornix* are seen as posterior to the thalamus.

They unite at a slightly higher level to form the *body of the fornix,* which lies just below the corpus callosum and was visible in the previous section. The course of the internal capsule is visible in both this section and the last.

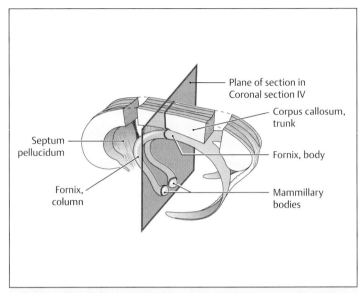

Fig. 4.10 Mammillary bodies and fornix.

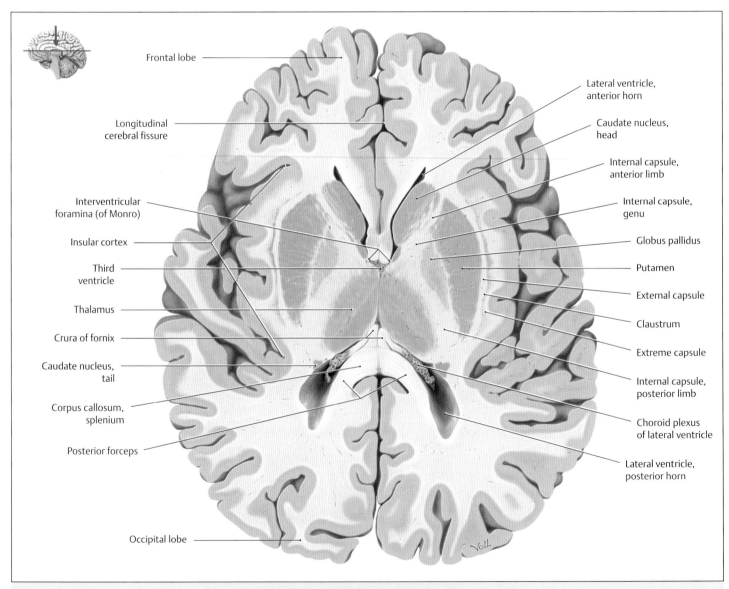

Fig. 4.11 Transverse section III.

4.3.2 Spatial Relationships of the Caudate Nucleus, Putamen, Thalamus, and Lateral Ventricles

Left anterior oblique view (**Fig. 4.12**).

4.3.3 Transverse Section IV

The nuclei shown in the previous section appear here as a roughly circular mass at the center of the brain, surrounded by the gray matter of the cerebral cortex, also called the *pallium* ("cloak") for obvious reasons. The choroid plexus is here visible in both lateral ventricles. This section cuts the occipital part of the corpus callosum, the *splenium,* as well as the basal portion of the *insular cortex.* The insula is a cortical region that lies below the surface and is covered by the opercula (**Fig. 4.13**).

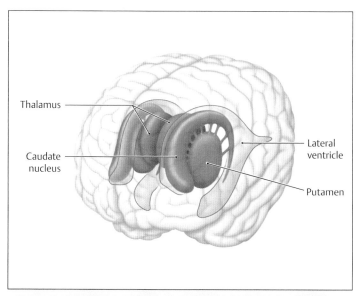

Fig. 4.12 Spatial relationships of the caudate nucleus, putamen, thalamus, and lateral ventricles.

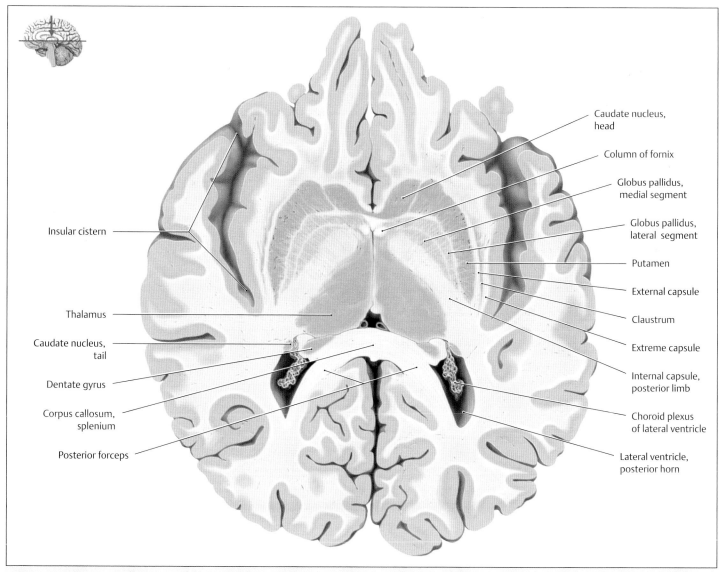

Fig. 4.13 Transverse section IV.

4.3.4 Left Insular Region

Lateral view (**Fig. 4.14**).

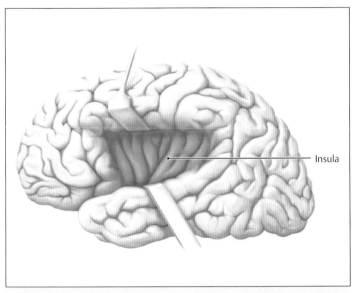

Insula

Fig. 4.14 Left insular region.

4.4 Sagittal Sections: IV to VI

Left lateral view (**Fig. 4.15**). The dominant ventricular structures in all three of these sections are the anterior horn and central part of the *lateral ventricle* (the junction with the laterally situated posterior horn appears only in **Fig. 4.15a**). The *corpus callosum*, which connects functionally related areas of the two cerebral hemispheres (commissural tract), can be identified in the cerebral white matter although it is not sharply delineated (**Fig. 4.15a–c**). As the sections move closer to the cerebral midline, the putamen grows smaller while the caudate nucleus becomes increasingly prominent (**Fig. 4.15a–c**). These two bodies are known collectively as the *corpus striatum*, and their characteristic striations are seen particularly well in **Fig. 4.15a** (the white matter that separates the gray-matter streaks of the corpus striatum is the *internal capsule*). The previous sagittal sections showed only the lateral segment of the *globus pallidus*, but its medial segment is displayed in both **Fig. 4.15a** and **Fig. 4.15b**. As the globus pallidus disappears and the putamen becomes less prominent, the nuclei of the medially situated thalamus become visible below the lateral ventricle (**Fig. 4.15c**; the subthalamic nuclei include the anterior, posterior, and lateral ventral nuclei of the diencephalon). The location of the thalamus explains why

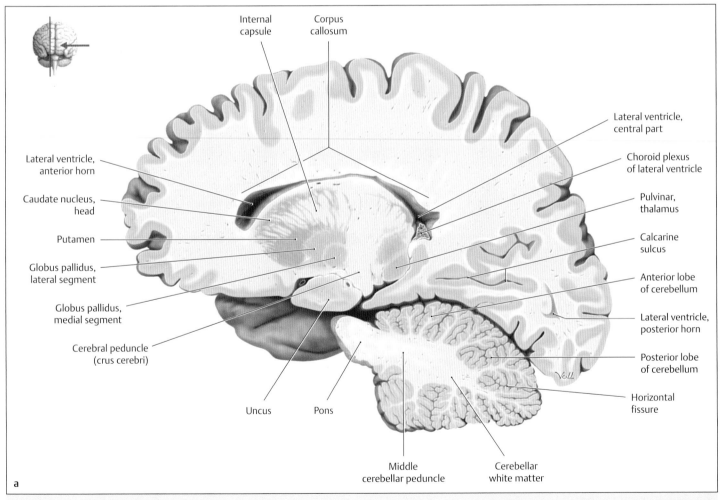

Internal capsule

Corpus callosum

Lateral ventricle, central part

Choroid plexus of lateral ventricle

Lateral ventricle, anterior horn

Pulvinar, thalamus

Caudate nucleus, head

Calcarine sulcus

Putamen

Anterior lobe of cerebellum

Globus pallidus, lateral segment

Lateral ventricle, posterior horn

Globus pallidus, medial segment

Posterior lobe of cerebellum

Cerebral peduncle (crus cerebri)

Horizontal fissure

Uncus   Pons

Middle cerebellar peduncle

Cerebellar white matter

a

Fig. 4.15 (**a**) Sagittal sections IV–VI.

(Continued)

it is sometimes referred to as the *dorsal thalamus*. **Fig. 4.15c** also shows the *substantia nigra* in the mesencephalon (below the diencephalon), the inferior olivary nucleus in the underlying medulla oblongata, and the *dentate nucleus* of the cerebellum. The ascending and descending tracts previously visible only in the internal capsule can now be seen in the pons, part of the

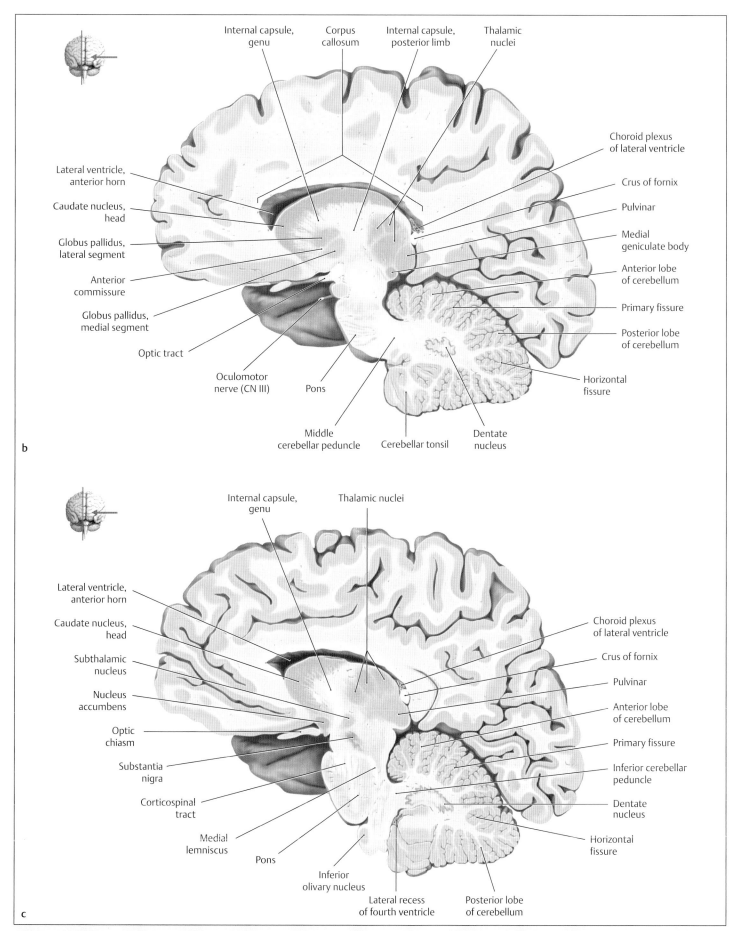

Internal capsule, genu
Corpus callosum
Internal capsule, posterior limb
Thalamic nuclei
Choroid plexus of lateral ventricle
Crus of fornix
Pulvinar
Medial geniculate body
Anterior lobe of cerebellum
Primary fissure
Posterior lobe of cerebellum
Horizontal fissure
Lateral ventricle, anterior horn
Caudate nucleus, head
Globus pallidus, lateral segment
Anterior commissure
Globus pallidus, medial segment
Optic tract
Oculomotor nerve (CN III)
Pons
Middle cerebellar peduncle
Cerebellar tonsil
Dentate nucleus

b

Internal capsule, genu
Thalamic nuclei
Choroid plexus of lateral ventricle
Crus of fornix
Pulvinar
Anterior lobe of cerebellum
Primary fissure
Inferior cerebellar peduncle
Dentate nucleus
Horizontal fissure
Lateral ventricle, anterior horn
Caudate nucleus, head
Subthalamic nucleus
Nucleus accumbens
Optic chiasm
Substantia nigra
Corticospinal tract
Medial lemniscus
Pons
Inferior olivary nucleus
Lateral recess of fourth ventricle
Posterior lobe of cerebellum

c

Fig. 4.15 *(Continued)* (**b, c**) Sagittal sections IV–VI.

brainstem (**Fig. 4.15c**, corticospinal tract). The only visible portion of the fourth ventricle, barely sectioned in **Fig. 4.15c**, is its lateral recess.

4.5 Brain and Meninges In Situ*

Superior view (**Fig. 4.16**). The calvaria (domed skull bone) has been removed, and the superior sagittal sinus and its

*In situ is a Latin phrase meaning "exactly in the place where it occurs or is found."

lateral lacunae have been opened (**Fig. 4.16a**). The dura mater has been removed from the left hemisphere, and the dura and arachnoid have been removed from the right hemisphere (**Fig. 4.16b**). The brain and spinal cord are covered by membranes called meninges, which form a sac filled with cerebrospinal fluid (CSF). The meninges are composed of the following three layers:

- Outer layer: The *dura mater* ("tough mother," often shortened to "dura") is a tough layer of collagenous connective tissue. It consists of two layers, an inner meningeal layer and an outer

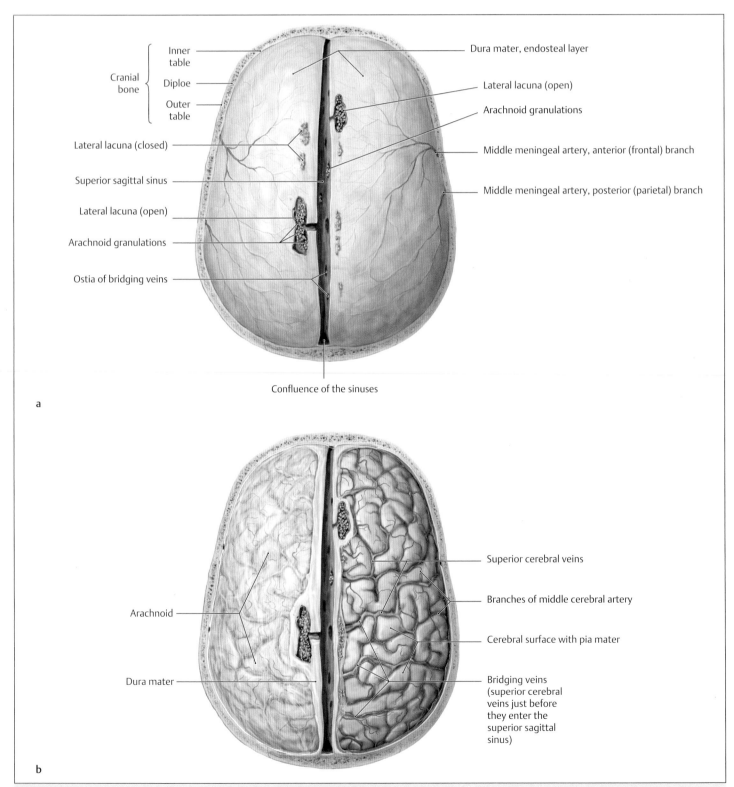

Fig. 4.16 (a, b) Brain and meninges in situ (superior view).

endosteal layer. The periosteal layer adheres firmly to the periosteum of the calvaria within the cranial cavity, but it is easy to separate the inner layer from the bone in this region, leaving it on the cerebrum as illustrated here (**Fig. 4.16a**).

- Middle layer: The *arachnoid* ("spider or web-like" arachnoid membrane) is a translucent membrane through which the cerebrum and the blood vessels in the subarachnoid space can be seen (**Fig. 4.16b**).
- Inner layer: The *pia mater* directly invests the cerebrum and lines its fissures (**Fig. 4.16b**).

The arachnoid and pia are collectively called the *leptomeninges*. The space between them, called the subarachnoid space, is filled with CSF and envelops the brain. It contains the major cerebral arteries and the superficial cerebral veins, which drain chiefly through "bridging veins" into the superior sagittal sinus. The dura mater in the midline forms a double fold between the periosteal and meningeal layers that encloses the endothelium-lined superior sagittal sinus, which has been opened in the illustration. Inspection of the opened sinus reveals the arachnoid granulations. These protrusions of the arachnoid are sites for the reabsorption

of CSF. Arachnoid granulations are particularly abundant in the lateral lacunae (gaps or empty spaces) of the superior sagittal sinus. The dissection in (**Fig. 4.16a**) shows how the middle meningeal artery is situated between the dura and calvaria. Rupture of this vessel causes blood to accumulate between the bone and dura, forming an epidural hematoma.

4.5.1 Projection of Important Brain Structures onto the Skull (Anterior View)

See **Fig. 4.17**. The largest structures of the cerebrum (telencephalon) are the frontal and temporal lobes. The falx cerebri separates the two cerebral hemispheres in the midline (not visible here). In the brainstem, we can identify the pons and medulla oblongata on both sides of the midline below the telencephalon. The superior sagittal sinus and the paired sigmoid sinuses can also be seen. The anterior horns of the two lateral ventricles are projected onto the forehead.

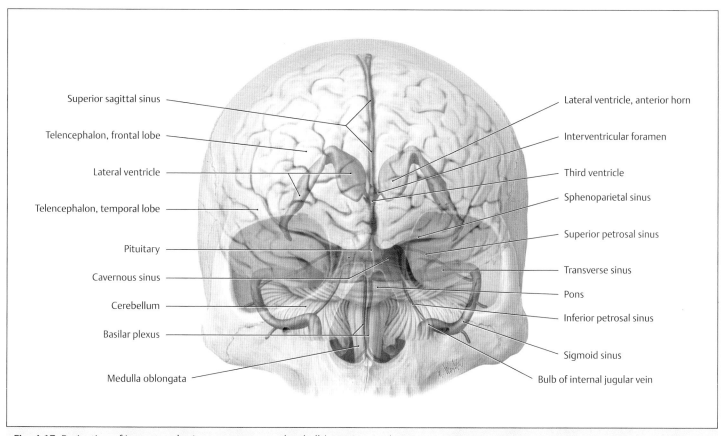

Fig. 4.17 Projection of important brain structures onto the skull (anterior view).

4.5.2 Projection of Important Brain Structures onto the Skull (Lateral View)

See **Fig. 4.18**. The relationship of specific lobes of the cerebrum to the cranial fossae (small cavities or depressions) can be appreciated in this view. The frontal lobe lies in the anterior cranial fossa, the temporal lobe in the middle cranial fossa, and the cerebellum in the posterior cranial fossa. The following dural venous sinuses can be identified: the superior and inferior sagittal sinus, straight sinus, transverse sinus, sigmoid sinus, cavernous sinus, superior and inferior petrosal sinus, and occipital sinus.

4.6 Meninges of the Brain and Spinal Cord

4.6.1 Blood Supply of the Dura Mater

Midsagittal section, left lateral view with branches of the middle meningeal artery exposed at several sites (**Fig. 4.19**). Most of the dura mater in the cranial cavity receives its blood supply from the middle meningeal artery, a terminal branch of the maxillary artery. The other vessels shown here are of minor clinical importance. The essential function of the middle meningeal artery is, however, not to supply the meninges (as its name might suggest) but to supply the calvaria (dome-like superior portion of the skull). Head injuries may cause the middle meningeal artery to rupture, leading to life-threatening complications (epidural hematoma).

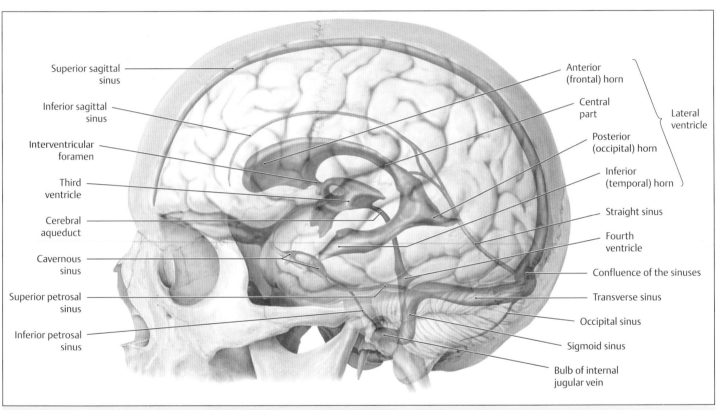

Fig. 4.18 Projection of important brain structures onto the skull (left lateral view).

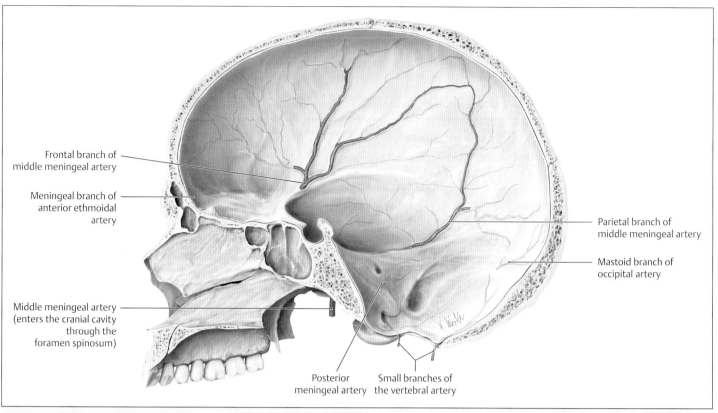

Frontal branch of middle meningeal artery

Meningeal branch of anterior ethmoidal artery

Middle meningeal artery (enters the cranial cavity through the foramen spinosum)

Parietal branch of middle meningeal artery

Mastoid branch of occipital artery

Posterior meningeal artery

Small branches of the vertebral artery

Fig. 4.19 Blood supply of the dura mater (midsagittal section).

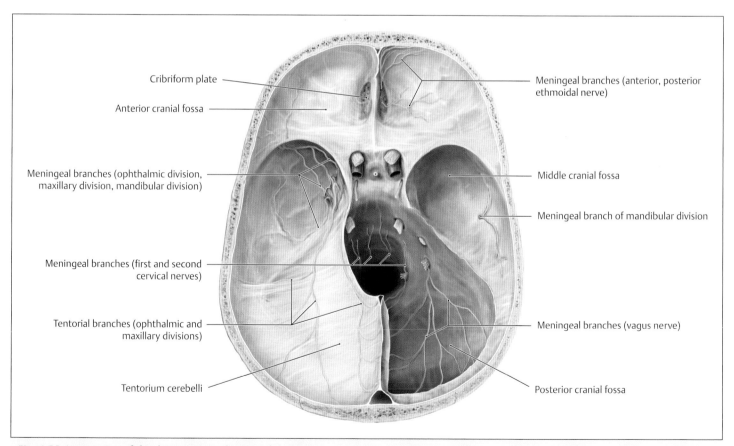

Cribriform plate

Anterior cranial fossa

Meningeal branches (ophthalmic division, maxillary division, mandibular division)

Meningeal branches (first and second cervical nerves)

Tentorial branches (ophthalmic and maxillary divisions)

Tentorium cerebelli

Meningeal branches (anterior, posterior ethmoidal nerve)

Middle cranial fossa

Meningeal branch of mandibular division

Meningeal branches (vagus nerve)

Posterior cranial fossa

Fig. 4.20 Innervation of the dura mater in the cranial cavity.

4.6.2 Innervation of the Dura Mater in the Cranial Cavity

Superior view with the tentorium cerebelli removed on the right side (**Fig. 4.20**). The intracranial meninges are supplied by meningeal branches from all three divisions of the trigeminal nerve and also by branches of the vagus nerve and the first two cervical nerves. Irritation of these sensory fibers due to meningitis is manifested clinically by headache and reflex nuchal stiffness (the neck is hyperextended in an attempt to relieve tension on the inflamed meninges). The brain itself is insensitive to pain.

4.6.3 Meninges and Their Spaces

Transverse section through the calvaria (schematic) (**Fig. 4.21**). The meninges have two spaces that do not exist under normal conditions, as well as one physiological space:

- Epidural space: This space is not normally present in the brain (contrast with chapter 4.6.5, which shows the physiological epidural space in the spinal canal). It develops in response to bleeding from the middle meningeal artery or one of its branches (arterial bleeding). The extravasated (extravasation = bleeding) blood separates the dura mater from the bone, dissecting an epidural space between the inner table of the calvaria and the dura (epidural hematoma).
- Subdural space: Bleeding from the bridging veins artificially opens the subdural space between the meningeal layer of the dura mater and upper layer of the arachnoid membrane (subdural hematoma). The cells of the uppermost layer of the arachnoid (neurothelium) are interconnected by a dense network of tight junctions, creating a tissue barrier (blood–CSF barrier).

- Subarachnoid space: This physiologically normal space lies just beneath the arachnoid. It is filled with CSF and is traversed by blood vessels. Bleeding into this space (subarachnoid hemorrhage) is usually arterial bleeding from an aneurysm (abnormal circumscribed dilation) of the basal cerebral arteries.

4.6.4 Transverse Section through the Spinal Cord and Its Meninges

Cervical vertebra viewed from above (**Fig. 4.22**). Caudal to the foramen magnum (below the hole at the base of the skull), the dura mater separates from the periosteum; that is, the meningeal and periosteal layers of the dura mater separate from each other to define a physiological space, the epidural space. This space is occupied by fatty tissue and venous plexuses. The dorsal and ventral roots of the spinal nerves course within the dural sac of the spinal cord and collectively form the cauda equina ("horse's tail") in the lower part of the sac (not shown here). The dorsal and ventral roots unite within a dural sleeve at the intervertebral

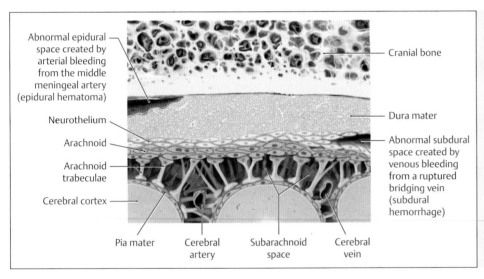

Labels: Abnormal epidural space created by arterial bleeding from the middle meningeal artery (epidural hematoma); Neurothelium; Arachnoid; Arachnoid trabeculae; Cerebral cortex; Cranial bone; Dura mater; Abnormal subdural space created by venous bleeding from a ruptured bridging vein (subdural hemorrhage); Pia mater; Cerebral artery; Subarachnoid space; Cerebral vein

Fig. 4.21 Meninges and their spaces (transverse section).

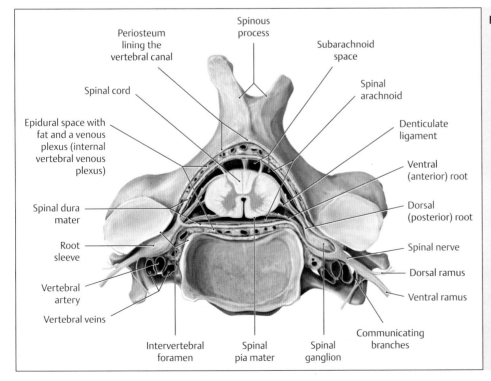

Labels: Periosteum lining the vertebral canal; Spinous process; Subarachnoid space; Spinal cord; Spinal arachnoid; Epidural space with fat and a venous plexus (internal vertebral venous plexus); Denticulate ligament; Ventral (anterior) root; Spinal dura mater; Dorsal (posterior) root; Root sleeve; Spinal nerve; Vertebral artery; Dorsal ramus; Vertebral veins; Ventral ramus; Intervertebral foramen; Spinal pia mater; Spinal ganglion; Communicating branches

Fig. 4.22 Cervical vertebra viewed from above.

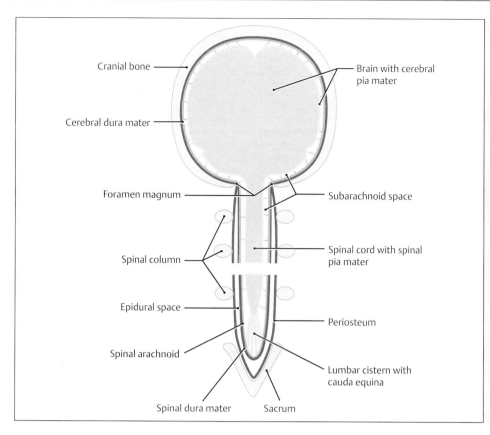

Cranial bone

Cerebral dura mater

Foramen magnum

Spinal column

Epidural space

Spinal arachnoid

Spinal dura mater

Sacrum

Brain with cerebral pia mater

Subarachnoid space

Spinal cord with spinal pia mater

Periosteum

Lumbar cistern with cauda equina

Fig. 4.23 Meninges in the cranial cavity and spinal canal.

foramina to form the spinal nerves. After the two roots have fused lateral to the spinal ganglion, the spinal nerve emerges from the dural sac. The *pia mater* invests the surfaces of the brain and spinal cord in the same fashion. The denticulate ligaments are sheets of pial connective tissue that pass from the spinal cord to the dura and are oriented in the coronal plane.

4.6.5 Meninges in the Cranial Cavity and Spinal Canal

The periosteum of the bones and the meningeal layer of the dura mater are fused together inside the cranial cavity (**Fig. 4.23**). Caudal to the foramen magnum, however, these two layers of collagenous connective tissue separate from each other to form the epidural space. Because of the mobility of the spinal column, the periosteum of the vertebrae must be free to move relative to the dural sac. This is accomplished by the presence of the epidural space, which exists physiologically only within the spinal canal. It contains fat and venous plexuses (see Chapter 4.6.4). This space has major clinical importance, as it is the compartment into which epidural anesthetics are injected, for example, for chronic back pain.

4.7 Ventricular System, Overview

4.7.1 Overview of the Ventricular System and Important Neighboring Structures

Left lateral view (**Fig. 4.24**). The ventricular system is a greatly expanded and convoluted tube that represents an upward prolongation of the central spinal canal into the brain. There are *four cerebral ventricles*, or cavities, filled with CSF and lined by a specialized epithelium, the ependyma. The four ventricles are as follows:

- The *two* lateral ventricles, each of which communicates through an interventricular foramen with the
- Third ventricle, which in turn communicates through the cerebral aqueduct with the
- Fourth ventricle. This ventricle communicates with the subarachnoid space (see Chapter 4.7.2).

The largest ventricles are the lateral ventricles, each of which consists of an anterior, inferior, and posterior horn and a central part. Certain portions of the ventricular system can be assigned to specific parts of the brain: the anterior (frontal) horn to the frontal lobe of the cerebrum, the inferior (temporal) horn to the temporal lobe, the posterior (occipital) horn to the occipital lobe, the third ventricle to the diencephalon, the aqueduct to the midbrain (mesencephalon), and the fourth ventricle to the hindbrain (rhombencephalon).

CSF is formed mainly by the choroid plexus, a network of vessels that is present to some degree in each of the four ventricles. Another site of CSF production is the ependyma. Certain diseases (e.g., atrophy or shrinkage of brain tissue in Alzheimer's disease and internal hydrocephalus) are characterized by abnormal enlargement of the ventricular system and are diagnosed from the size of the ventricles in sectional images of the brain.

This unit deals with the ventricular system and neighboring structures. The next unit will trace the path of the CSF from its production to its reabsorption. The last unit on the CSF spaces will deal with the specialized functions of the ependyma, the circumventricular organs, and the physiological tissue barriers in the brain.

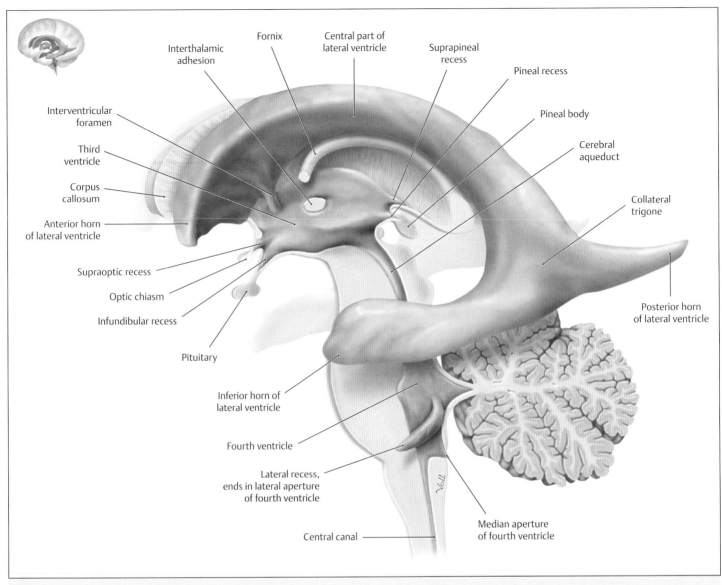

Fornix

Central part of
lateral ventricle

Suprapineal
recess

Interthalamic
adhesion

Pineal recess

Pineal body

Interventricular
foramen

Cerebral
aqueduct

Third
ventricle

Corpus
callosum

Collateral
trigone

Anterior horn
of lateral ventricle

Supraoptic recess

Optic chiasm

Infundibular recess

Posterior horn
of lateral ventricle

Pituitary

Inferior horn of
lateral ventricle

Fourth ventricle

Lateral recess,
ends in lateral aperture
of fourth ventricle

Median aperture
of fourth ventricle

Central canal

Fig. 4.24 Ventricular system (left lateral view).

4.7.2 Cast of the Ventricular System

Cast specimens are used to demonstrate the connections between the ventricular cavities (**Fig. 4.25**). Each lateral ventricle communicates with the third ventricle through an interventricular foramen. The third ventricle communicates through the cerebral aqueduct with the fourth ventricle in the rhombencephalon. The ventricular system has a fluid capacity of approximately 30 mL, about 1 fluid ounce or 1.5 tablespoons, while the subarachnoid space has a capacity of approximately 120 mL (about 4 fluid ounces).

Note the three apertures (paired lateral apertures [foramina of Luschka] and an unpaired median aperture [foramen of Magendie]), through which CSF flows from the deeper ventricular system into the more superficial subarachnoid space.

4.7.3 Important Structures Neighboring the Lateral Ventricles

View of the brain from upper left (**Fig. 4.26a**).
    The following brain structures border on the lateral ventricles:

- The caudate nucleus (anterolateral wall of the anterior horn)
- The thalamus (posterolateral wall of the anterior horn)
- The putamen, which is lateral to the lateral ventricle and does not border it directly.

View of the inferior horn of the left lateral ventricle in the opened temporal lobe (**Fig. 4.26b**).
    The hippocampus is visible in the anterior part of the floor of the inferior horn. Its anterior portions with the hippocampal digitations protrude into the ventricular cavity.

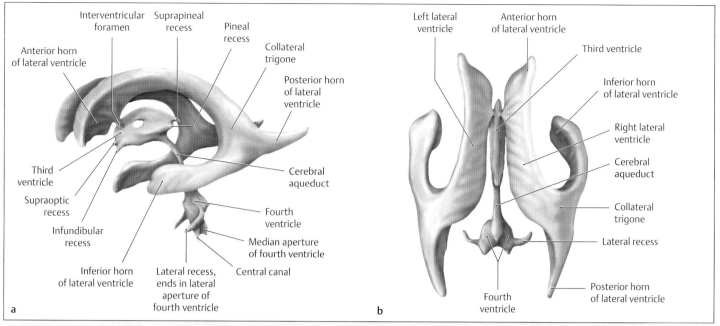

Fig. 4.25 Cast of the ventricular system. **(a)** Left lateral view. **(b)** Superior view.

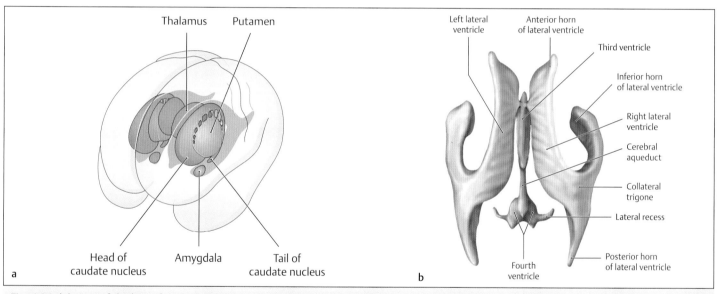

Fig. 4.26 (a) View of the brain from upper left. **(b)** View of the inferior horn of the left lateral ventricle.

4.7.4 Lateral Wall of the Third Ventricle

The lateral wall of the third ventricle is formed by structures of the diencephalon (epithalamus, thalamus, hypothalamus). Protrusions of the thalami on both sides may touch each other (interthalamic adhesion) but are not functionally or anatomically connected and thus do not constitute a commissural or connecting tract (**Fig. 4.27**).

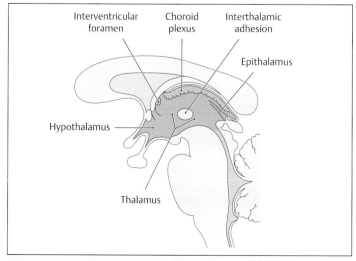

Fig. 4.27 Lateral wall of the third ventricle (midsagittal section, left lateral view).

4.8 Cerebrospinal Fluid, Circulation and Cisterns

CSF is produced in the choroid plexus, which is present to some extent in each of the four cerebral ventricles. It flows through the median aperture and paired lateral apertures into the subarachnoid space, which contains expansions called cisterns. Most of the CSF drains from the subarachnoid space through the arachnoid granulations, and smaller amounts drain along the proximal portions of the spinal nerves into venous plexuses or lymphatic pathways (see Chapter 4.8.6). The cerebral ventricles and subarachnoid space have a combined capacity of approximately 150 mL (about 5 fluid ounces) of CSF (20% in the ventricles and 80% in the subarachnoid space). This volume is completely replaced two to four times daily, so that approximately 500 mL (2 cups or about the size of a Starbucks Venti) of CSF must be produced each day. Obstruction of CSF drainage will therefore cause a rise in intracranial pressure (**Fig. 4.28**).

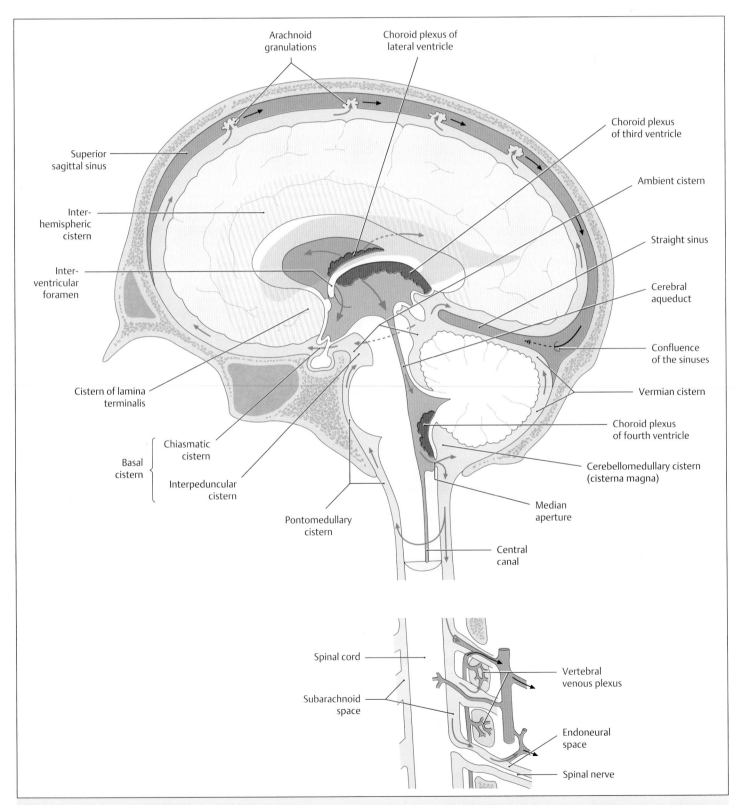

Fig. 4.28 Cerebrospinal fluid circulation and the cisterns.

4.8.1 Choroid Plexus in the Lateral Ventricles

Surrounding brain tissue has been removed down to the floor of the lateral ventricles, where the choroid plexus originates. The plexus is adherent to the ventricular wall at only one site (see Chapter 4.8.4) and can thus float freely in the ventricular system (**Fig. 4.29**).

4.8.2 Choroid Plexus in the Fourth Ventricle

Portions of the choroid plexus are attached to the roof of the fourth ventricle and run along the lateral aperture (**Fig. 4.30**). Free ends of the choroid plexus may extend through the lateral apertures into the subarachnoid space on both sides ("Bochdalek's flower basket").

4.8.3 Taeniae of the Choroid Plexus

The choroid plexus is formed by the ingrowth of vascular loops into the ependyma, which firmly attach it to the wall of the associated ventricle (see Chapter 4.8.6). When the plexus tissue is removed with forceps, its lines of attachment, called taeniae, can be seen (**Fig. 4.31**).

4.8.4 Histological (Thin Slice of Tissue Applied to a Microscopic Slide) Section of the Choroid Plexus, with a Detail Showing the Structure of the Plexus Epithelium

The choroid plexus is a protrusion of the ventricular wall. It is often likened to a cauliflower because of its extensive surface folds. Unlike cauliflower, it is not edible. The epithelium of the choroid plexus consists of a single layer of cuboidal cells and has a brush border on its apical surface (to increase the surface area further) (**Fig. 4.32**).

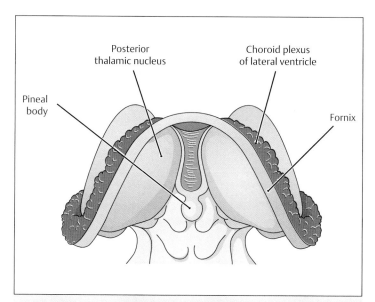

Fig. 4.29 Rear view of the thalamus.

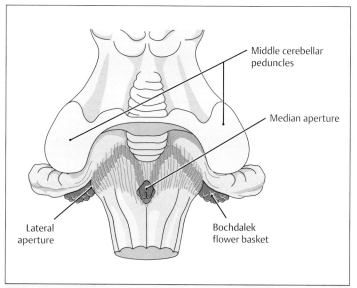

Fig. 4.30 Posterior view of the partially opened rhomboid fossa (with the cerebellum removed).

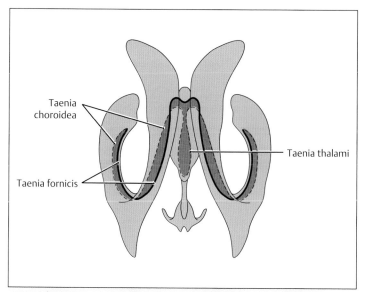

Fig. 4.31 Superior view of the ventricular system.

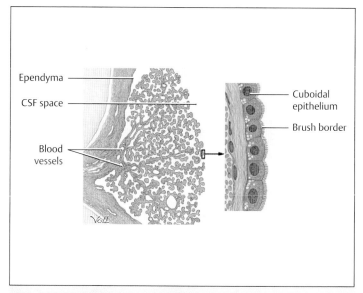

Fig. 4.32 Histological section of the choroid plexus.

4.8.5 Schematic Diagram of Cerebrospinal Fluid Circulation

As noted earlier, the choroid plexus is present to some extent in each of the four cerebral ventricles. It produces CSF, which flows through the two lateral apertures (not shown) and median aperture into the subarachnoid space. From there, most of the CSF drains through the arachnoid granulations into the dural venous sinuses (**Fig. 4.33**).

4.8.6 Subarachnoid Cisterns

The cisterns are CSF-filled expansions of the subarachnoid space (**Fig. 4.34**). They contain the proximal portions of some cranial nerves and basal cerebral arteries (veins are not shown). When arterial bleeding occurs (as from a ruptured aneurysm), blood will seep into the subarachnoid space and enter the CSF. A ruptured intracranial aneurysm is a frequent cause of blood in the CSF (methods of sampling the CSF are described subsequently).

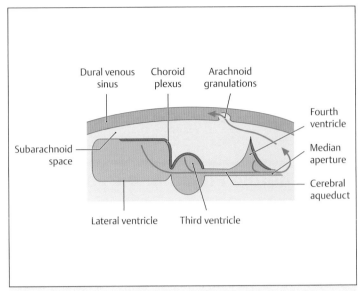

Fig. 4.33 Schematic diagram of cerebrospinal fluid circulation.

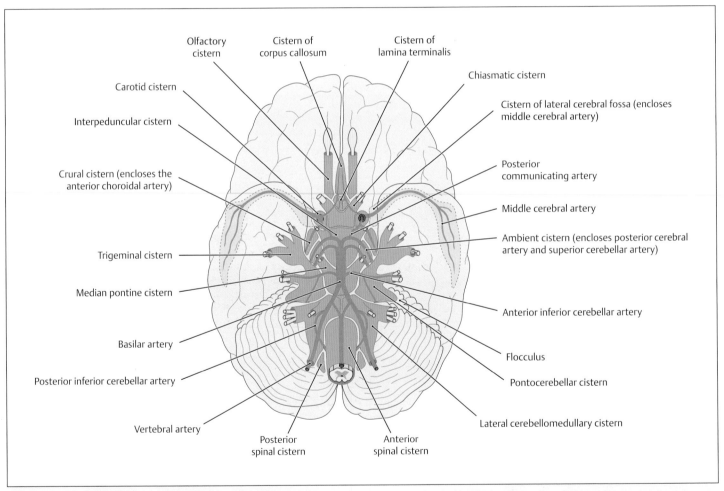

Fig. 4.34 Subarachnoid cisterns (basal view).

4.9 Telencephalon, Development and External Structure

4.9.1 Terms of Location and Direction

See **Fig. 4.35**. Terms of location and direction in the telencephalon and diencephalon are based on the Forel axis (2), which runs horizontally through the forebrain. (1) Brainstem axis (Meynert's axis).

4.9.2 Development of the Cerebral Cortex

The cerebral hemispheres can be divided into phylogenetically ancient ("paleo"), old ("archi"), and new ("neo") parts (see Chapter 4.9.4). The cerebral cortex together with associated areas of underlying white matter is called the pallium, a term sometimes used interchangeably, but not commonly, with cortex (**Fig. 4.36**).

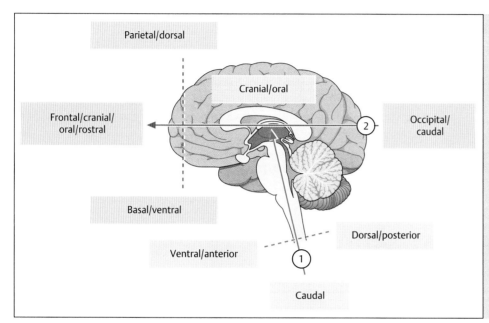

Parietal/dorsal

Cranial/oral

Frontal/cranial/ oral/rostral

Occipital/ caudal

2

Basal/ventral

Dorsal/posterior

Ventral/anterior

1

Caudal

Fig. 4.35 Midsagittal section viewed from the left side. (1) Meynert axis. (2) Forel axis.

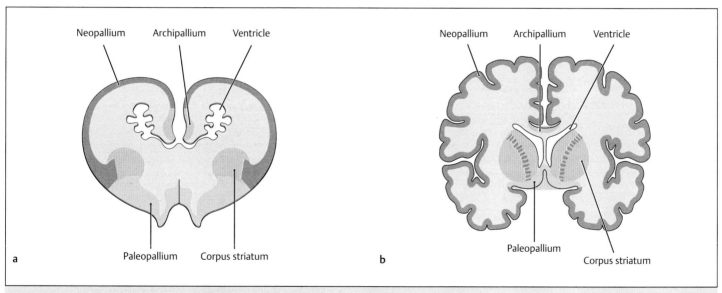

Neopallium Archipallium Ventricle

Neopallium Archipallium Ventricle

Paleopallium Corpus striatum

a

Paleopallium

Corpus striatum

b

Fig. 4.36 (a) Embryonic brain. **(b)** Adult brain.

4.9.3 Gray and White Matter in the Telencephalon

See **Fig. 4.37a**.

Gray Matter:

- Cerebral cortex: Contains most of the gray matter of the telencephalon. It is divided on histological grounds into two parts:
  - Isocortex: Corresponds to the neocortex (see Chapter 4.9.2); largest part of the cerebral cortex, consisting of six layers.
  - Allocortex: Corresponds to the paleo- and archicortex (see Chapter 4.9.2); consists of *three* or *four* layers.
- Subcortical nuclei: Basal ganglia: the caudate nucleus and putamen (collectively called the corpus striatum), and the globus pallidus. *Note:* The basal ganglia are often called the basal nuclei. Because they are located in the CNS, however, the term "ganglia" is more common, if imprecise, than "nuclei." Another of life's little contradictions and exceptions to the rule keeps us on our toes.
- Other gray-matter nuclei that are not included among the basal ganglia of the telencephalon:
  - Amygdala: Often considered a transitional form between the two types of gray matter—cortex and basal ganglia—based on its location
  - Claustrum

White matter:

Tissue below the cerebral cortex and surrounding the subcortical nuclei. *Note:* The white matter also contains nuclei of the diencephalon.

See **Fig. 4.37b**. Part of the cerebral cortex sinks below the surface during development, forming the insula. The insula has been postulated by some as an important area for motor speech plans and the disorder of apraxia of speech. The portions of the cerebral cortex that overlie deeper cortical areas are called opercula ("little lids").

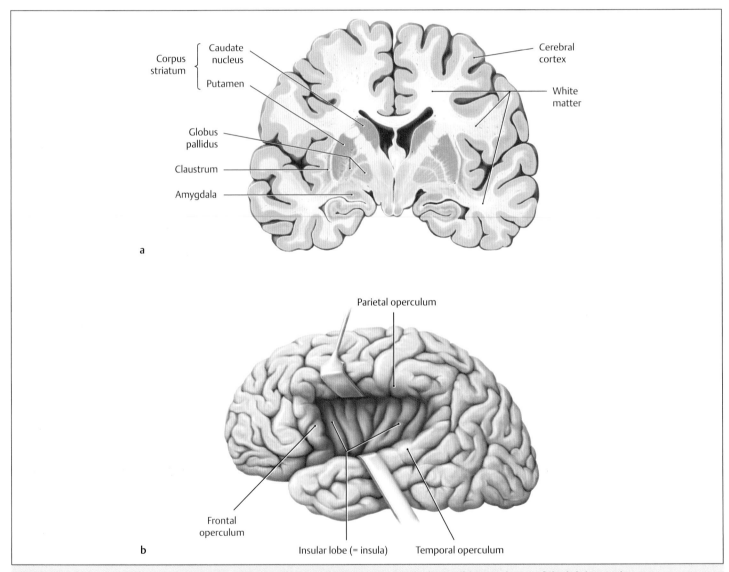

Fig. 4.37 (a) Coronal section showing the distribution of gray and white matter in the brain. (b) Lateral view of the left hemisphere.

4.9.4 Phylogenetic Origins of Major Components of the Telencephalon

See **Table 4.1**.

4.9.5 Division of the Cerebral Hemispheres into Lobes

The two cerebral hemispheres are the externally visible part of the telencephalon (**Fig. 4.38**). They are separated from each other by the longitudinal cerebral fissure and each one is subdivided into six lobes:

- Frontal lobe
- Parietal lobe
- Temporal lobe
- Occipital lobe
- Insular lobe (insula)
- Limbic lobe (limbus)

The surface contours of the cerebral hemispheres are highly variable between individuals. A histological subdivision into cortical areas is more meaningful in terms of functional brain organization than a macroscopic subdivision into gyri and sulci.

Table 4.1 Terms and descriptions of brain areas

Phylogenetic term	Structure in the embryonic brain	Structure(s) in the adult brain	Cortical structure
Paleopallium (oldest part)	Floor of the hemispheres	• Rhinencephalon (= olfactory bulb plus surrounding region)	Allocortex
Archipallium (old part)	Medial portion of hemispheric wall	• Ammon's horn (largest part, not shown here) ∘ Indusium griseum • Fornix	Allocortex
Neopallium (newest part)	Most of the brain surface plus the deeper corpus striatum	• Neocortex (= cortex), largest part of the cerebral cortex ∘ Insula • Corpus striatum	Isocortex

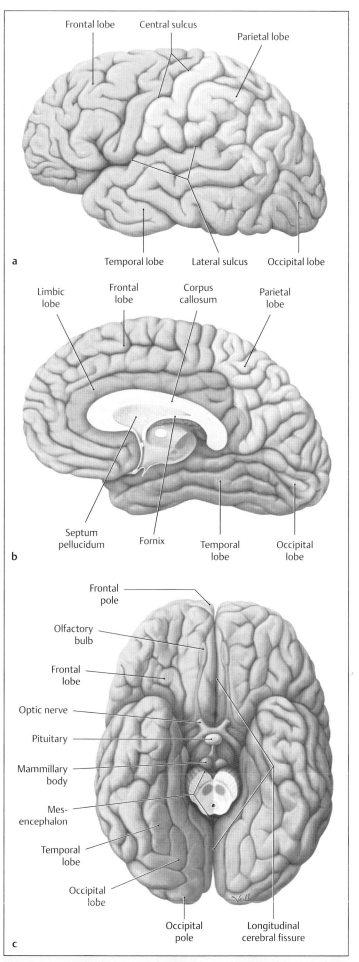

Fig. 4.38 **(a)** Left lateral view of the left hemisphere. **(b)** Left lateral view of the right hemisphere. **(c)** Basal view with the brainstem removed, showing the cut surface of the midbrain (mesencephalon).

4.10 Neocortex, Cortical Areas

4.10.1 Brodmann's Areas in the Neocortex

As noted earlier, the surface of the brain consists macroscopically of lobes, gyri, and sulci (**Fig. 4.39**). Microscopically, however, subtle differences can be found in the distribution of the cortical neurons, and some of these differences do not conform to the gross surface anatomy of the brain. Portions of the cerebral cortex that have the same basic microscopic features are called *cortical areas* or *cortical fields*. This organization into cortical areas is based on the distribution of neurons in the different layers of the cortex *(cytoarchitectonics)*. In the brain map shown at left, these areas are indicated by different colors. Although the size of the cortical areas may vary between individuals, the

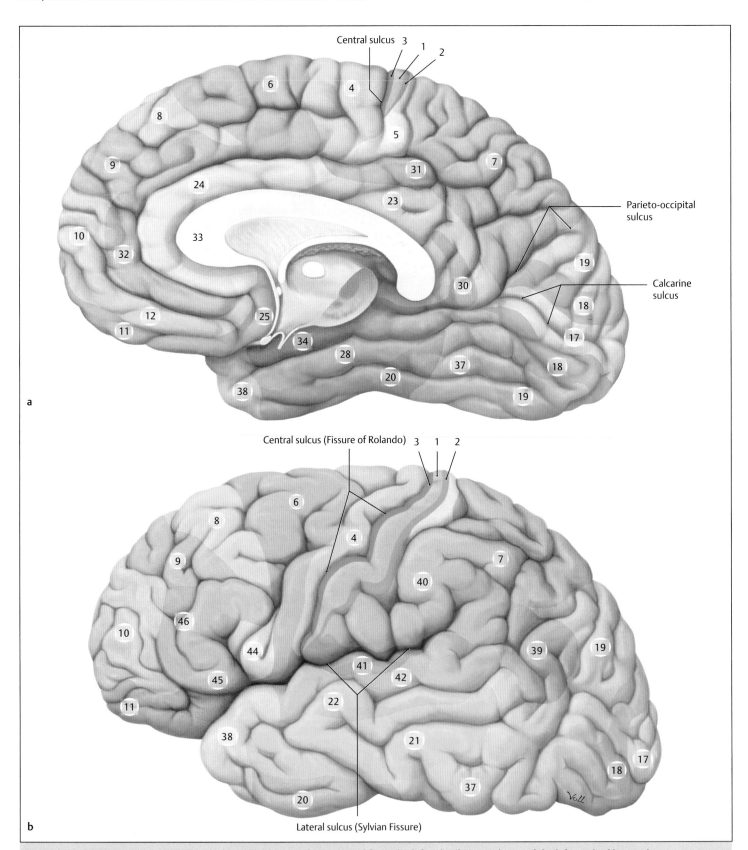

Fig. 4.39 **(a)** Midsagittal section of the right cerebral hemisphere, viewed from the left side. **(b)** Lateral view of the left cerebral hemisphere.

brain map pictured here is still used today as a standard reference chart. It was developed in the early 20th century by the anatomist Korbinian Brodmann (1868–1918), who spent years painstakingly examining the cellular architecture of the cortex in a single brain. It has long been thought that the map created by Brodmann accurately reflects the functional organization of the cortex, and indeed, modern imaging techniques have shown that many of the cytologically defined areas are associated with specific functions. There is no need, of course, to memorize the location of all the cortical areas, but the following areas are of special interest:

- Areas 1, 2, and 3: Primary somatosensory cortex
- Area 4: Primary motor cortex
- Area 17: Primary visual cortex (striate area, the extent of which is best appreciated in the midsagittal section)
- Areas 41 and 42: Auditory cortex
- Areas 44 and 45: Broca's area
- Area 22: Wernicke's area
- Area 39: Angular gyrus (important for reading and dyslexia)
- Areas 39 and 19: Parietal–temporal–occipital (PTO) cortex (important as one of three primary speech areas along with Broca's and Wernicke's areas)

- Areas 11, 12, and 25: Frontal cortex areas involved in cognition, inhibition and self-regulation, and "executive function" (the cognitive processes that regulate an individual's ability to organize thoughts and activities, prioritize tasks, manage time efficiently, and make decisions; impairment of executive function is seen in a range of disorders, including traumatic brain injury [TBI], stroke, dementias, and frontal lobe tumors).

4.10.2 Visual Cortex (Striate Area)

The primary visual cortex (striate area, shaded yellow) is the only cortical area that can be clearly recognized by its macroscopic appearance (**Fig. 4.40a**). It extends along both sides of the calcarine sulcus at the occipital pole. In an unstained coronal section (**Fig. 4.40b**), the *stria of Gennari* can be identified as a prominent white stripe within the gray cortical area. This stripe contains cortical association fibers that synapse with the neurons of the internal granular layer (IV). The pyramidal cell layers (efferent fibers) are attennated in the visual cortex, while the granular cell layers where the afferent fibers from the lateral geniculate nucleus terminate are markedly enlarged.

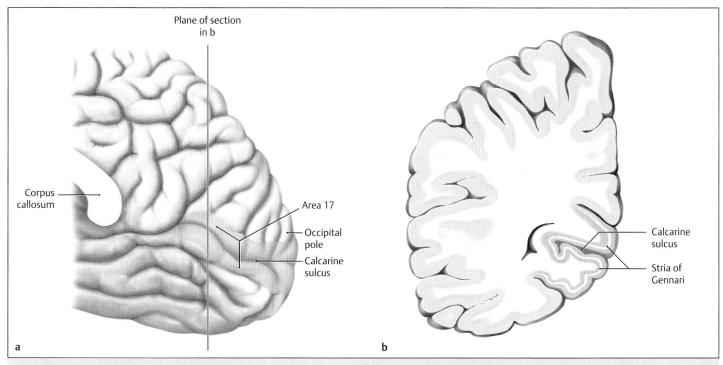

Fig. 4.40 Visual Cortex. **(a)** Right hemisphere viewed from the left side. **(b)** Coronal section (anterior view).

4.11 Allocortex, Overview

4.11.1 Overview of the Allocortex

Structures belonging to the allocortex are indicated by colored shading (**Fig. 4.41**). The allocortex consists of the phylogenetically old part of the cerebral cortex. It is very small in relation to the cortex as a whole. Unlike the isocortex, which has a six-layered structure, the allocortex (*allo* = "other") usually consists of *three* layers that encompass the paleo- and archicortexes. Additionally, there exist four-layered transitional areas between the allocortex and isocortex: the *peri*paleocortex (not indicated separately in the drawing) and the *peri*arehicortex (indicated by pink shading). An important part of the allocortex is the *rhinencephalon* ("olfactory brain"). Olfactory impulses that are perceived by the olfactory bulb are the only sensory afferent impulses that do not reach the cerebral cortex by way of the dorsal thalamus. Another important part of the allocortex is the hippocampus and its associated nuclei. As in the isocortex,

the gyral patterns of the allocortex do not always conform to its histological organization. The allocortex along with other parts of the brain that are evolutionarily older are sometimes referred to as the reptilian or "triune" brain since they are associated with more primitive drives and behaviors.

4.11.2 Organization of the Archipallium: Deeper Parts

The archicortex described in Chapter 4.11.1 is the *only* part of the archipallium that is located on the brain surface (**Fig. 4.42**). The deeper parts of the archipallium, which lie within the white matter, are the hippocampus ("sea horse"), indusium griseum ("gray covering"), and fornix ("arch"). All three structures are part of the *limbic system*, and together form a border ("limbus") around the corpus callosum as a result of their migration during development. The limbic system is highly related to emotions. The limbic system is a complex set of structures that lies on

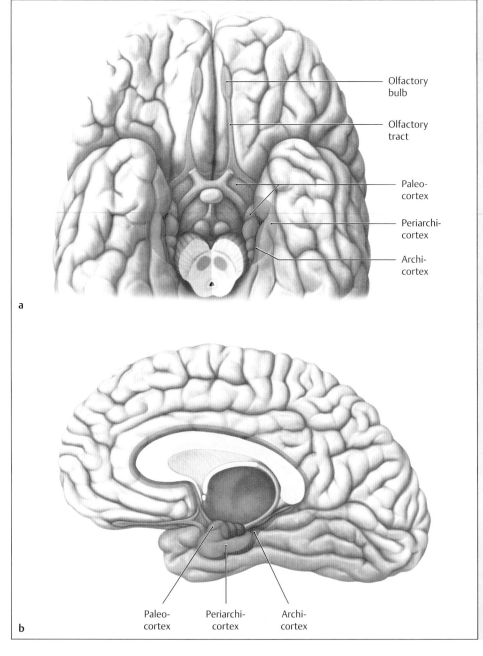

Fig. 4.41 Allocortex. **(a)** View of the base of the brain. **(b)** Median surface of the right hemisphere.

Olfactory bulb

Olfactory tract

Paleo-cortex

Periarchi-cortex

Archi-cortex

a

Paleo-cortex   Periarchi-cortex   Archi-cortex

b

both sides of the thalamus, just under the cerebrum. It includes the hypothalamus, the hippocampus, the amygdala, and several other nearby areas. It appears to be primarily responsible for our emotional life, and has a role in the formation of memories. The limbic system is the ruler of our emotional life and connected to our hormonal life. It helps us cry, yearn, enjoy, love, laugh, wonder, fear the bogeyman, frustrate others, be flooded with insecurity, express anger or apathy, or feel stupid and worthless.

4.11.3 Topography of the Fornix, Corpus Callosum, and Septum Pellucidum

Occipital view from upper left (**Fig. 4.43**). The fornix is a tract of the archicortex that is closely apposed but functionally

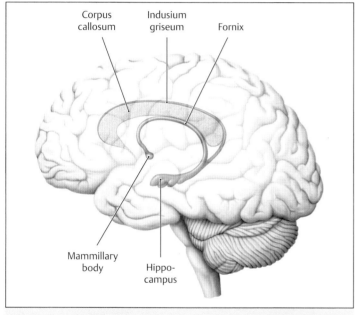

Fig. 4.42 Archipallium. Lateral view of the left hemisphere.

unrelated to the corpus callosum. The corpus callosum is the largest neocortical commissural tract between the hemispheres, serving to interconnect cortical areas of similar function in the two hemispheres. The septum pellucidum is a thin plate that stretches between the corpus callosum and fornix, forming the medial boundary of the lateral ventricles. Between the two septa is a cavity of variable size, the *cavum septi pellucidi.* The cholinergic nuclei in the septa, which are involved in the organization of memory, are connected to the hippocampus by the fornix.

4.11.4 Topography of the Hippocampus, Fornix, and Corpus Callosum

Viewed from the upper left and oral aspect (**Fig. 4.44**). This drawing shows the hippocampus on the floor of the inferior horn of the lateral ventricle. The left and right *crura of the fornix* unite to form the *commissure of the fornix* (see Chapter 4.11.3) and the *body of the fornix*, which divides anteriorly into left and right bundles, the *columns of the fornix*. The fornix is a white-matter tract connecting the hippocampus to the mammillary bodies in the diencephalon. Contained within the fornix are hippocampal neurons whose axons project to the septum, mammillary bodies, contralateral hippocampus, and other structures. This important pathway is part of the *limbic system*. The paired structure of the hippocampus has a major role in the consolidation and coordination of memories and has been implicated in very famous case studies (H.M., a classic case with bilateral hippocampal injury) with severe anterograde amnesia (memory impairment characterized by the impairment in laying down new memories).

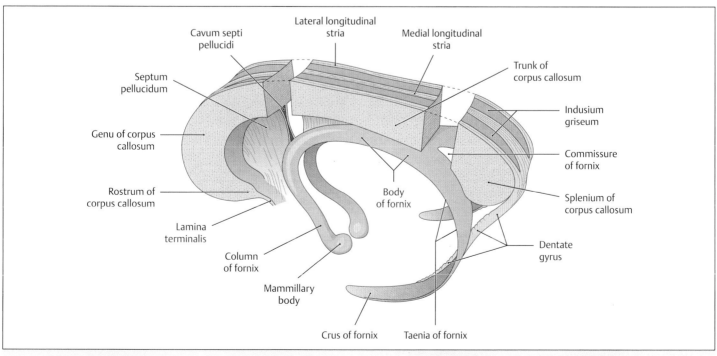

Fig. 4.43 Topography of the fornix, corpus callosum, and septum pellucidum.

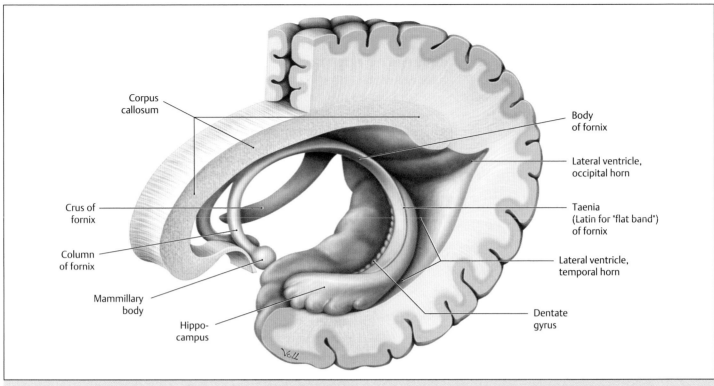

Fig. 4.44 Topography of the hippocampus, fornix, and corpus callosum.

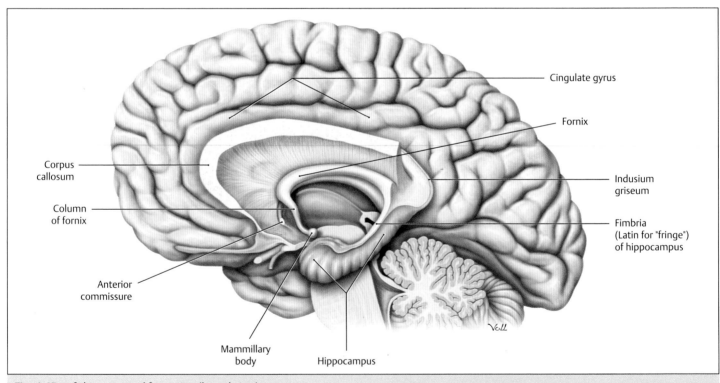

Fig. 4.45 Left hippocampal formation (lateral view).

4.12 Allocortex: Hippocampus and Amygdala

4.12.1 Left Hippocampal Formation

Most of the left hemisphere has been dissected away, leaving only the corpus callosum, fornix, and hippocampus (**Fig. 4.45**). The intact right hemisphere is visible in the background.

The hippocampal formation is an important component of the *limbic system*.

The fiber tract of the fornix connects the hippocampus to the mammillary body. The hippocampus integrates information from various brain areas and influences endocrine, visceral, and emotional processes via its efferent output. As noted, it is particularly associated with the consolidation of memory and implicated in types of amnesias (memory loss). Lesions of the hippocampus can therefore cause specific defects in memory formation (anterograde amnesia).

Besides the hippocampus, which is the largest part of the archicortex, we can recognize another component of the archicortex, the indusium griseum.

4.12.2 Right Hippocampal Formation and the Caudal Part of the Fornix

Left medial view (**Fig. 4.46**). Compare this medial view of the right hippocampal formation with the lateral view in Chapter 4.12.1. A useful landmark is the calcarine sulcus, which leads to the occipital pole. The cortical areas that border the hippocampus (e.g., the parahippocampal gyrus) are particularly apparent in this view.

4.12.3 Left Temporal Lobe with the Inferior Horn of the Lateral Ventricle Exposed

Transverse section, posterior view of the hippocampus on the floor of the inferior (temporal) horn (**Fig. 4.47a**). The following structures can be identified from lateral to medial: hippocampus, fimbria, dentate gyrus, hippocampal sulcus, and parahippocampal gyrus. Coronal sections of the left hippocampus (**Fig. 4.47b**). The hippocampus appears here as a curled band (Ammon's horn = the hippocampus proper), which shows considerable structural diversity in its different portions. The junction between the entorhinal cortex (entorhinal region) in the parahippocampal gyrus and Ammon's horn is formed by a transitional area, the

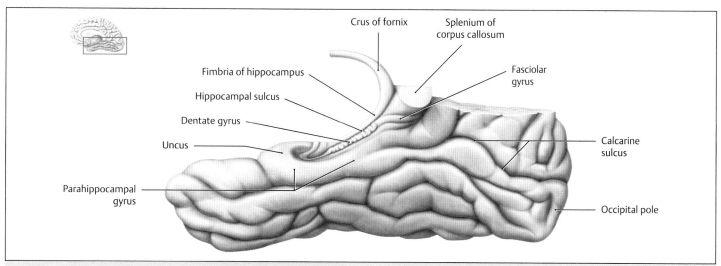

Fig. 4.46 Right hippocampal formation and the caudal part of the fornix.

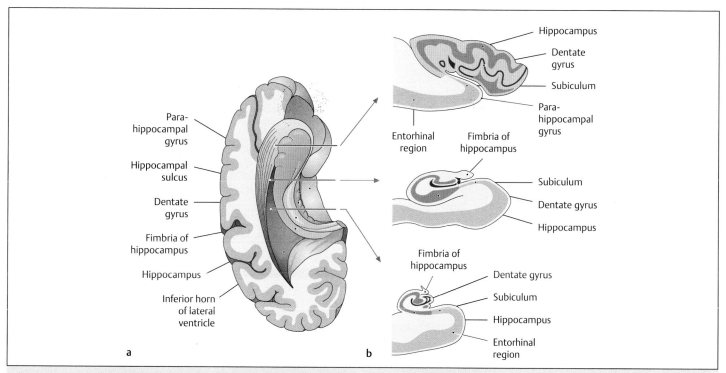

Fig. 4.47 Left temporal lobe. **(a)** Transverse section. **(b)** Coronal sections of the left hippocampus.

subiculum. The entorhinal region is the "gateway" to the hippocampus, through which the hippocampus receives most of its afferent fibers.

4.12.4 Relationship of the Amygdala to Internal Brain Structures

Lateral view of the left hemisphere (**Fig. 4.48**). The amygdala (amygdaloid body) is located below the putamen and anterior to the tail of the caudate nucleus. The fibers of the pyramidal tract run posterior and medial to the amygdala.

4.12.5 Amygdala

Coronal section at the level of the interventricular foramen (**Fig. 4.49a**). The amygdala extends medially to the inferior surface of the cortex of the temporal lobe. For this reason, it is considered to be part of the cortex as well as a nuclear complex that has migrated into the white matter. Stimulation of the amygdala in humans leads to changes in mood, ranging from rage and fear to rest and relaxation depending on the emotional state of the patient immediately prior to stimulation. Since the amygdala functions as an "emotional amplifier," lesions affect the patient's evaluation of events' emotional significance. The surrounding periamygdaline cortex and the corticomedial half of the amygdala are part of the primary olfactory cortex. Hence, these portions of the amygdala are considered part of the paleocortex, while the deeper portion is characterized as "nuclear."

Fig. 4.49b shows the two main groups of nuclei in the amygdala:

- Phylogenetically old corticomedial group:
  - Cortical nucleus
  - Central nucleus
- Phylogenetically new basolateral group:
  - Basal nucleus
  - Lateral nucleus

The basal nucleus can be subdivided into a parvocellular medial part and a macrocellular lateral part.

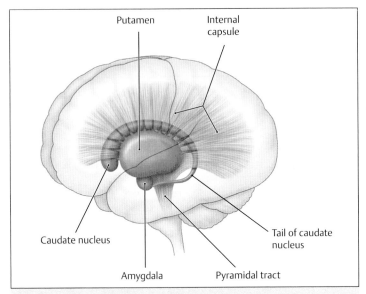

Fig. 4.48 Relationship of the amygdala to internal brain structures.

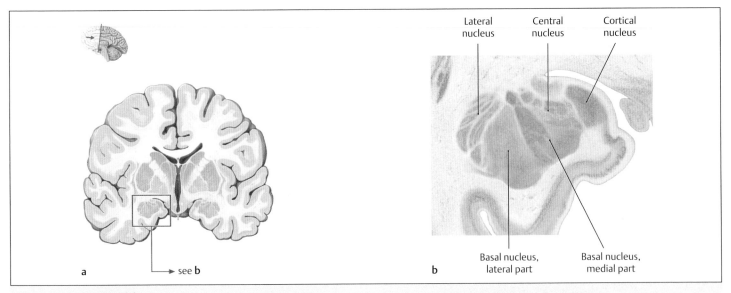

Fig. 4.49 (a, b) Amygdala.

4.13 Telencephalon: White Matter and Basal Ganglia

4.13.1 Teased Fiber Preparation of the White Matter of the Telencephalon

Lateral view of the left hemisphere (**Fig. 4.50**). This dissection shows the superficial layer of white matter (myelinated neuron axons) located between the basal ganglia and the gray matter (unmyelinated neuronal cell bodies) of the cerebral cortex. A special preparation technique was used to display the fiber structure of the white matter, which normally has a uniform white appearance. The fiber structure is defined by the tracts (bundles of myelinated axons) that interconnect different areas of the gray matter. For example, we can identify the short cerebral arcuate fibers (U fibers) that run between two adjacent gyri as well as the association fibers that span multiple gyri (e.g., the superior longitudinal and frontotemporal fasciculi). When these tracts are damaged (e.g., in multiple sclerosis), the communication pathways within the brain cease to function normally. This may lead to central paralysis, visual disturbances (optic nerve damage), and behavioral changes (damage to the frontal cortex).

4.13.2 Projection of the Basal Ganglia onto the Brain Surface and Ventricular System

View from the upper left anterior aspect (**Fig. 4.51a**). The basal ganglia are masses of gray matter deep within the brain that contain the cell bodies of neurons. Further details on the basal ganglia are shown in Chapter 4.13.3. Left lateral view (**Fig. 4.51b**). The caudate nucleus is closely applied to the concave lateral wall of the lateral ventricle. It is connected to the putamen by numerous streak-like bands of gray matter (corpus striatum).

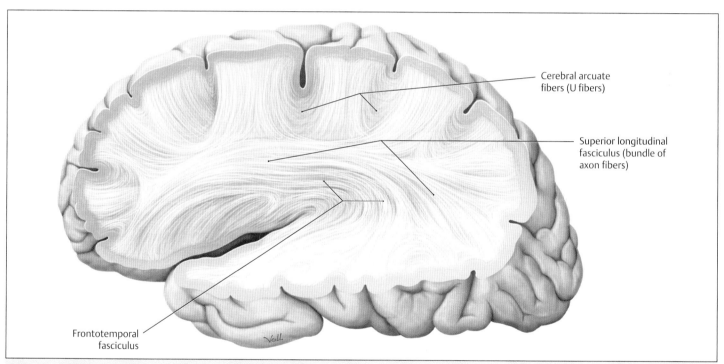

Fig. 4.50 Teased fiber preparation of the white matter of the telencephalon.

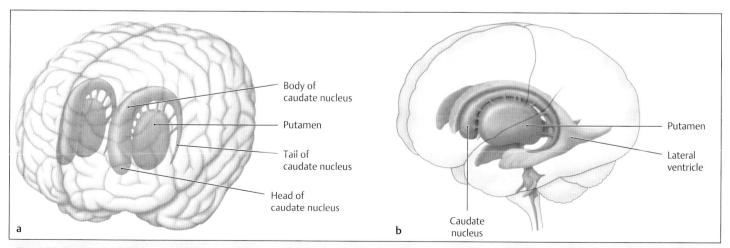

Fig. 4.51 Projection of the basal ganglia onto the brain surface and ventricular system. (a) View from the upper left anterior aspect. (b) Left lateral view.

4.13.3 Basal Ganglia

Transverse section through the cerebrum at the level of the corpus striatum, viewed from above (**Fig. 4.52a**). In a strict anatomical sense, the basal ganglia consist of the caudate nucleus, putamen, and globus pallidus. Developed mentally, the globus pallidus is a part of the diencephalon that has migrated into the telencephalon, but it is still counted among the basal ganglia. The basal ganglia are an essential component of the extrapyramidal motor system. The extrapyramidal system is composed of motor fibers that do not pass through the pyramidal tracts of the medulla, but that nevertheless exert a measure of control over bodily movements. The system comprises a complexity of pathways and feedback loops that compose it. Nevertheless, the extrapyramidal system can be divided into three controlling systems: the cortically originating indirect pathways, the feedback loops, and the auditory-visual-vestibular descending pathways. The basal ganglia and extrapyramidal system are important in fine tuning and coordinating movements and in neurological movement disorders, such as Parkinson's disease and dystonia, and can greatly affect motor control of speech and other movements. The claustrum ("barrier") is a strip of gray matter lateral to the putamen. It is not part of the basal ganglia but instead has reciprocal connections with sensory areas of the cerebral cortex.

Coronal section through the cerebrum at the level of the olfactory tract, anterior view (**Fig. 4.52b**). This section demonstrates

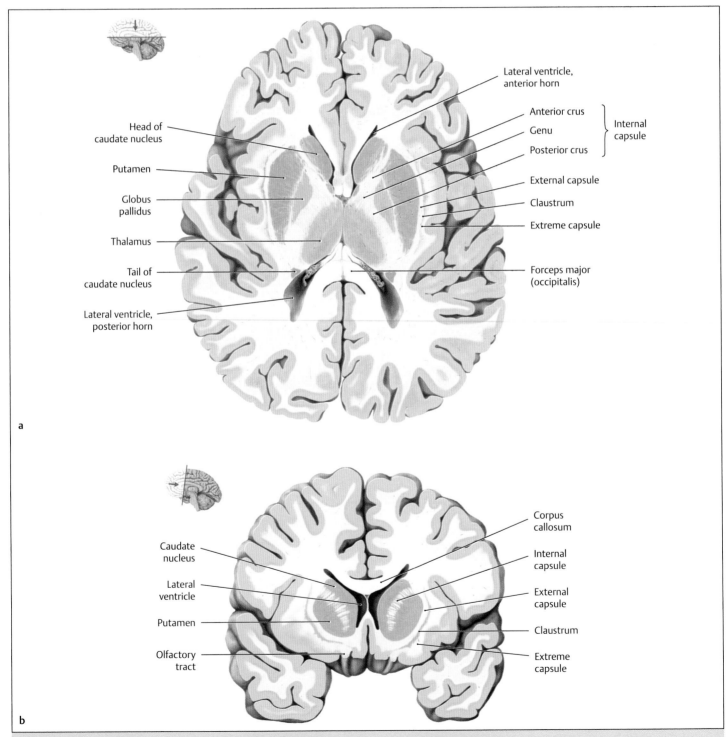

Fig. 4.52 Basal ganglia. **(a)** Transverse section. **(b)** Coronal section.

how the caudate nucleus and putamen are separated from each other by the fibrous white matter of the internal capsule. The caudate nucleus and putamen together constitute the corpus striatum (often shortened to "striatum"). The globus pallidus is not visible because it is occipital to this plane of section.

4.13.4 Relationship between the Corpus Striatum and Lentiform Nucleus

The caudate nucleus and putamen together constitute the corpus striatum, while the putamen and globus pallidus make up the lentiform ("lens-shaped") nucleus (**Fig. 4.53**). Although the globus pallidus and the putamen are anatomically juxtaposed, the putamen is functionally associated instead with the caudate nucleus. Developmentally, the putamen is part of the telencephalon and the globus pallidus is part of the diencephalon. Role of subcortical structures in speech and language: Not only are the basal ganglia important to the control and fine tuning of motor speech, but contemporary models propose to explain the possible contribution of various subcortical structures to language processing in the context of evidence gained from observation of the effects of circumscribed surgically induced lesions in the basal ganglia and thalamus on language function. A theory of subcortical (thalamic and basal ganglia) participation in language and linguistic processing awaits accumulating evidence. Who knows where every speck of language resides? Further research will tell us.

4.14 Diencephalon, External Structure

4.14.1 The Diencephalon and Brainstem

The telencephalon (cerebrum) has been removed from around the thalamus, and the cerebellum has also been removed (**Fig. 4.54**). The parts of the diencephalon visible in this dissection are the thalamus, the lateral geniculate body, and the optic tract. The lateral geniculate body and optic tract are components of the visual pathway. *Note:* The retina and associated optic nerve

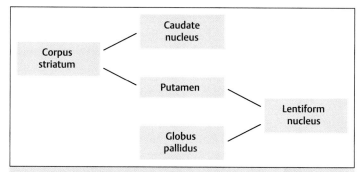

Fig. 4.53 Relationship between the corpus striatum and lentiform nucleus.

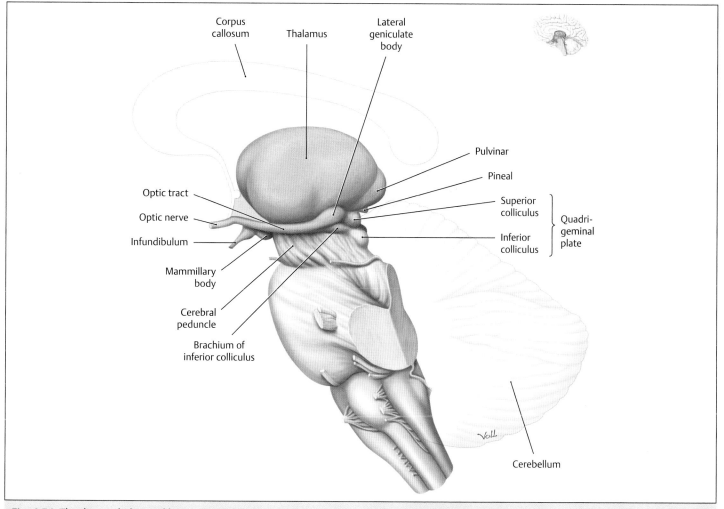

Fig. 4.54 The diencephalon and brainstem (left lateral view).

form an anterior extension of the diencephalon. The paired optic nerves, of course, are also cranial nerves. Departing from the convention of yellow for nerves, we have colored the optic nerve blue to emphasize this relationship.

4.14.2 Arrangement of the Diencephalon around the Third Ventricle

Posterior view of an oblique transverse section through the telencephalon with the corpus callosum, fornix, and choroid plexus removed (**Fig. 4.55**). Removal of the choroid plexus leaves behind its line of attachment, the *taenia ("flat band") choroidea*. The thin wall of the third ventricle has been removed with the choroid plexus to expose the thalamic surface medial to the boundary line of the taenia choroidea. The thin ventricular wall has been left on the thalamus lateral to the taenia choroidea. This thin layer of telencephalon, called the *lamina affixa*, is colored brown in the drawing and covers the thalamus (part of the diencephalon), shown in blue. Because the thalamostriate vein marks this boundary between the diencephalon and telencephalon, it is featured prominently in the drawing.

Lateral to the vein is the caudate nucleus, which is part of the telencephalon.

4.14.3 Views of the Diencephalon and Brainstem

Anterior view (**Fig. 4.56a**). The optic tract marks the lateral boundary of the diencephalon. It winds around the cerebral peduncles (crura cerebri), which are part of the adjacent midbrain (mesencephalon).

Posterior view with the cerebellum and telencephalon removed (**Fig. 4.56b**). The epithalamus, which is formed by the pineal and the two habenulae ("reins"), is well displayed in this posterior view. The epithalamus is associated with smell, emotional associations of smell, the hormone melatonin, and its relationship to sleep and circadian rhythm. The lateral geniculate body is an important relay station in the visual pathway, just as the medial geniculate body is an important relay station in the auditory pathway. Both are counted among the thalamic nuclei, and together they constitute the *metathalamus*, an extension of the thalamus proper. The pulvinar ("pillow"), which encompasses the posterior thalamic nuclei, is seen particularly well in this section.

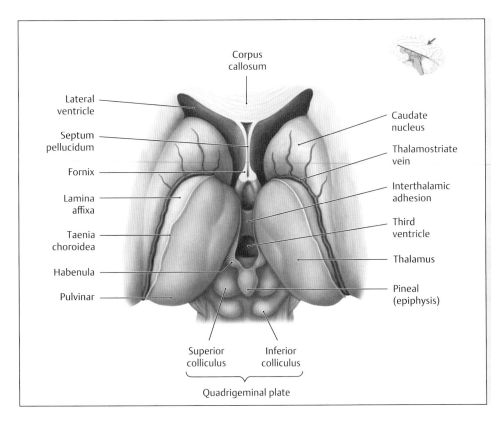

Corpus callosum

Lateral ventricle

Septum pellucidum

Fornix

Lamina affixa

Taenia choroidea

Habenula

Pulvinar

Caudate nucleus

Thalamostriate vein

Interthalamic adhesion

Third ventricle

Thalamus

Pineal (epiphysis)

Superior colliculus   Inferior colliculus

Quadrigeminal plate

Fig. 4.55 Posterior view of an oblique transverse section through the telencephalon.

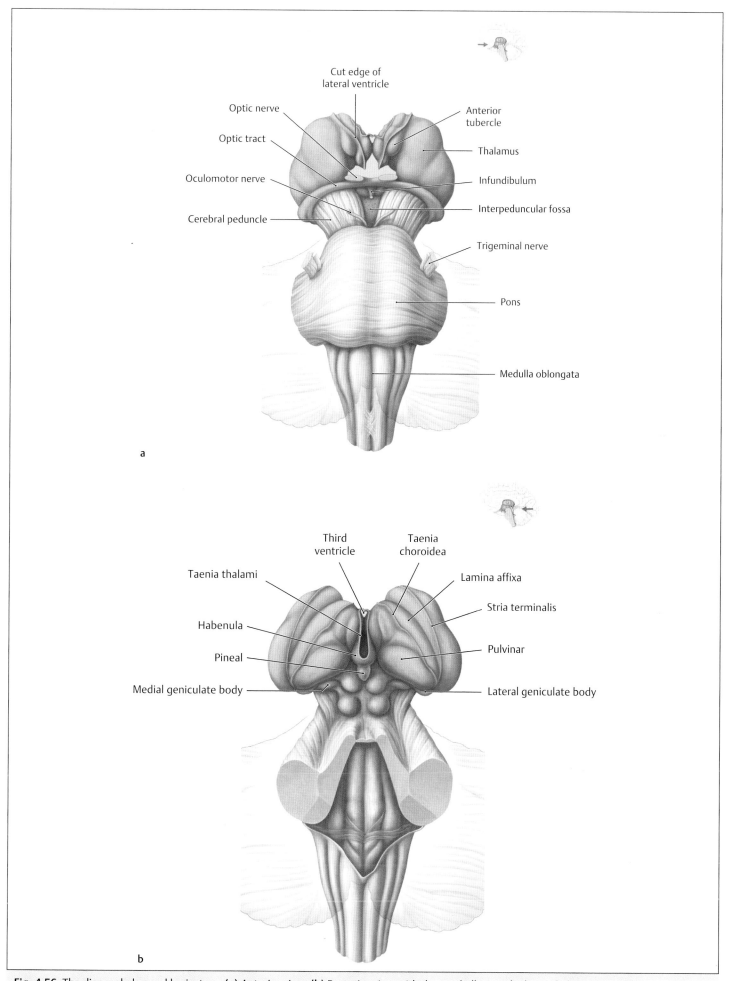

Cut edge of
lateral ventricle

Optic nerve

Anterior
tubercle

Optic tract

Thalamus

Oculomotor nerve

Infundibulum

Interpeduncular fossa

Cerebral peduncle

Trigeminal nerve

Pons

Medulla oblongata

a

Third
ventricle

Taenia
choroidea

Taenia thalami

Lamina affixa

Stria terminalis

Habenula

Pineal

Pulvinar

Medial geniculate body

Lateral geniculate body

b

Fig. 4.56 The diencephalon and brainstem. **(a)** Anterior view. **(b)** Posterior view with the cerebellum and telencephalon removed.

4.14.4 Location of the Diencephalon in the Adult Brain

Basal view of the brain (the brainstem has been sectioned at the level of the midbrain or mesencephalon) (**Fig. 4.57**). The structures that can be identified in this view represent the parts of the diencephalon situated on the basal surface of the brain. This view also demonstrates how the optic tract, which is part of the diencephalon, winds around the cerebral peduncles of the mesencephalon. Because of the expansion of the telencephalon, only a few structures of the diencephalon can be seen on the undersurface of the brain:

- Optic nerve
- Optic chiasm
- Optic tract
- Tuber cinereum with the infundibulum
- Mammillary bodies
- Medial geniculate body: The neural structure that serves as the last of a series of processing centers along the auditory pathway from the cochlea
- Lateral geniculate body
- Posterior lobe of the pituitary gland

4.15 Diencephalon, Internal Structure

See **Fig. 4.58**.

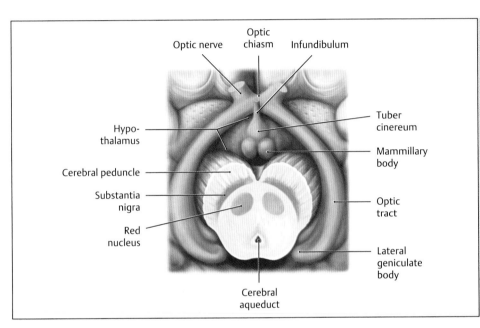

Optic nerve

Optic chiasm

Infundibulum

Hypo-thalamus

Cerebral peduncle

Substantia nigra

Red nucleus

Tuber cinereum

Mammillary body

Optic tract

Lateral geniculate body

Cerebral aqueduct

Fig. 4.57 Basal view of the brain.

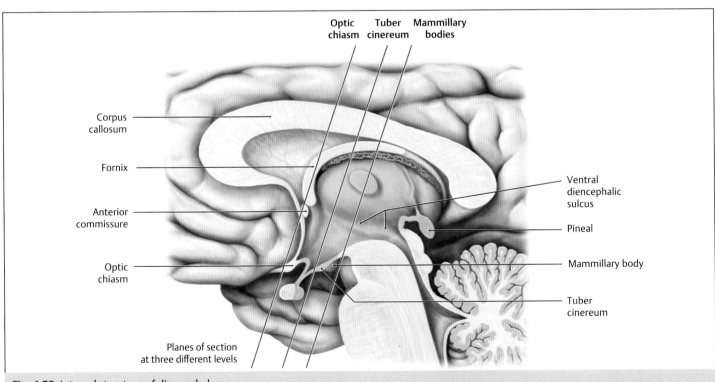

Optic chiasm

Tuber cinereum

Mammillary bodies

Corpus callosum

Fornix

Anterior commissure

Optic chiasm

Ventral diencephalic sulcus

Pineal

Mammillary body

Tuber cinereum

Planes of section at three different levels

Fig. 4.58 Internal structure of diencephalon.

Table 4.2 Four parts of the diencephalon

Part	Boundary line	Structure	Function
Epithalamus		• Pineal gland • Habenulae	Regulation of circadian rhythms; linking of olfactory system to brainstem
	Dorsal diencephalic sulcus		
Thalamus		• Thalamus	Relay of sensory information; assistance in regulation of motor function; perhaps some subcortical language functions
	Middle diencephalic sulcus		
Subthalamus		• Subthalamic nucleus • Zona incerta • Globus pallidus	Relay of sensory information (somatomotor zone of diencephalon); an important site, along with the globus pallidus internus, for deep brain implant stimulation for modification of Parkinson's disease and other movement disorders
	Ventral diencephalic sulcus (= hypothalamic sulcus)[a]		
Hypothalamus		• Optic chiasm, optic tract • Tuber cinereum, neurohypophysis • Mammillary bodies	Coordination of autonomic nervous system with endocrine system; participation in visual pathway

[a]This is the only sulcus shown in the table.

4.15.1 The Four Parts of the Diencephalon

See **Table 4.2**.

4.15.2 Coronal Sections through the Diencephalon at Three Different Levels

Level of the optic chiasm (Fig. 4.59a): Portions of the diencephalon and telencephalon appear in this section, which clearly shows the position of the diencephalon on both sides of the third ventricle. An outpouching of the third ventricle, the preoptic recess, is located above the optic chiasm. Its connection to the third ventricle lies outside this plane of section.

Level of the tuber cinereum (Fig. 4.59b), just behind the interventricular foramen: The boundary between the diencephalon and telencephalon is clearly defined only in the region about the ventricles; the underlying nuclear areas blend together with no apparent boundary. Along the lateral ventricles, the boundary between the diencephalon and telencephalon is marked by the lamina affixa, a narrow strip of telencephalon that overlies the thalamus. It can be seen that layers of gray matter permeate the internal capsule in its dorsal portion.

Level of the mammillary bodies (Fig. 4.59c): This section displays the thalamic nuclei. More than 120 separate nuclei may be counted, depending on the system of nomenclature used. Most of these nuclei cannot be grossly identified in anatomical specimens.

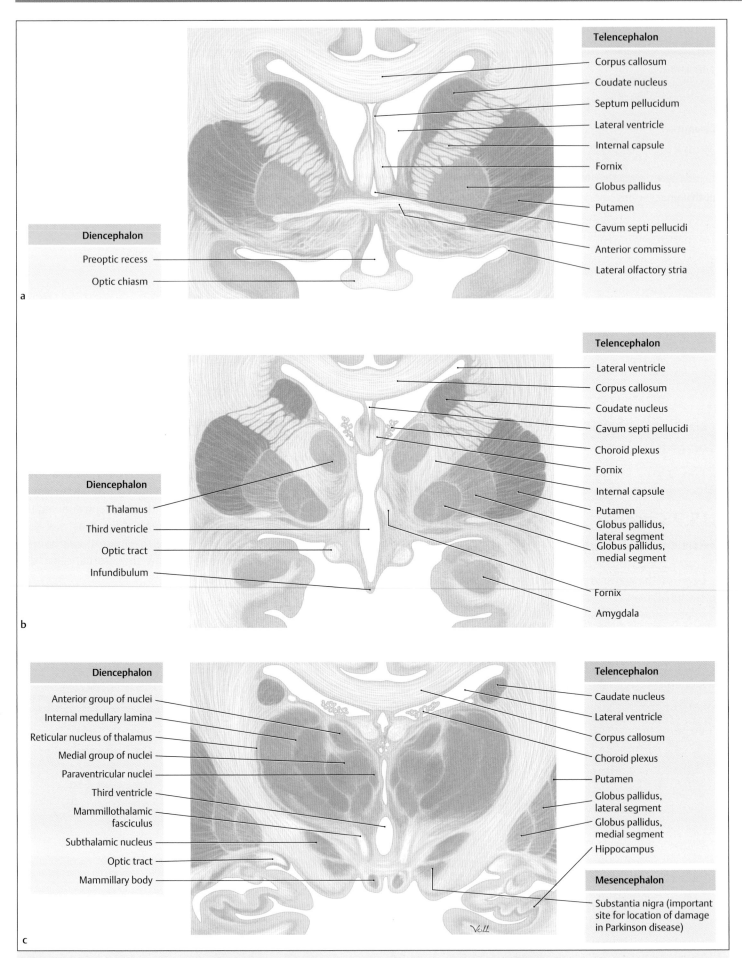

Telencephalon

- Corpus callosum
- Coudate nucleus
- Septum pellucidum
- Lateral ventricle
- Internal capsule
- Fornix
- Globus pallidus
- Putamen
- Cavum septi pellucidi
- Anterior commissure
- Lateral olfactory stria

Diencephalon

- Preoptic recess
- Optic chiasm

a

Telencephalon

- Lateral ventricle
- Corpus callosum
- Coudate nucleus
- Cavum septi pellucidi
- Choroid plexus
- Fornix
- Internal capsule
- Putamen
- Globus pallidus, lateral segment
- Globus pallidus, medial segment
- Fornix
- Amygdala

Diencephalon

- Thalamus
- Third ventricle
- Optic tract
- Infundibulum

b

Diencephalon

- Anterior group of nuclei
- Internal medullary lamina
- Reticular nucleus of thalamus
- Medial group of nuclei
- Paraventricular nuclei
- Third ventricle
- Mammillothalamic fasciculus
- Subthalamic nucleus
- Optic tract
- Mammillary body

Telencephalon

- Caudate nucleus
- Lateral ventricle
- Corpus callosum
- Choroid plexus
- Putamen
- Globus pallidus, lateral segment
- Globus pallidus, medial segment
- Hippocampus

Mesencephalon

- Substantia nigra (important site for location of damage in Parkinson disease)

c

Fig. 4.59 Coronal sections through the diencephalon. **(a)** Optic chiasm. **(b)** Tuber cinereum. **(c)** Mammillary bodies.

4.16 Thalamus: Thalamic Nuclei

4.16.1 Functional Organization of the Thalamus

Almost all of the sensory pathways are relayed via the thalamus and project to the cerebral cortex (see Chapter 4.16.7, thalamic radiation) (**Fig. 4.60**). Consequently, a lesion of the thalamus or its cortical projection fibers caused by a stroke or other disease leads to sensory disturbances. Although a diffuse kind of sensory perception may take place at the thalamic level (especially pain perception), cortical processing (by the telencephalon) is necessary in order to transform unconscious perception into conscious perception. The olfactory system is an exception to this rule, although its olfactory bulb is still an extension of the telencephalon. *Note:* Centers in the thalami direct neural impulses both upstream and downstream (sensory and motor but major descending motor tracts from the cerebral cortex generally bypass the thalamus.

4.16.2 Spatial Arrangement of the Thalamic Nuclear Groups

The thalamus is a collection of approximately 120 nuclei that process sensory information (**Fig. 4.61**). They are broadly classified as specific or nonspecific:

- Specific nuclei and the fibers arising from them (thalamic radiation, see Chapter 4.16.7) have direct connections with specific areas of the *cerebral cortex*. The specific thalamic nuclei are subdivided into four groups:
  - Anterior nuclei (yellow)
  - Medial nuclei (red)
  - Ventrolateral nuclei (green)
  - Dorsal nuclei (blue)

The dorsal nuclei are in contact with the medial and lateral geniculate bodies. Located beneath the pulvinar, these two nuclear bodies contain the *nuclei of the medial and lateral geniculate bodies (auditory and visual pathways)*, and are collectively called the *metathalamus*. Like the pulvinar, they belong to the category of specific thalamic nuclei.

- *Nonspecific nuclei* have no direct connections with the cerebral cortex. Part of a general arousal system, they are connected directly to the brainstem. The only nonspecific nuclei shown in this diagram (orange, see Chapter 4.16.6 for further details) are the centromedian nucleus and the intralaminar nuclei.

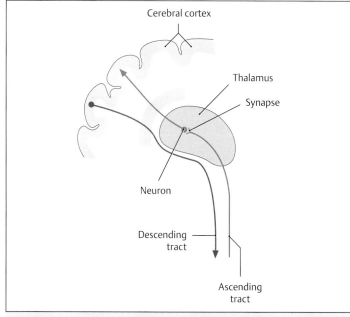

Fig. 4.60 Functional organization of the thalamus.

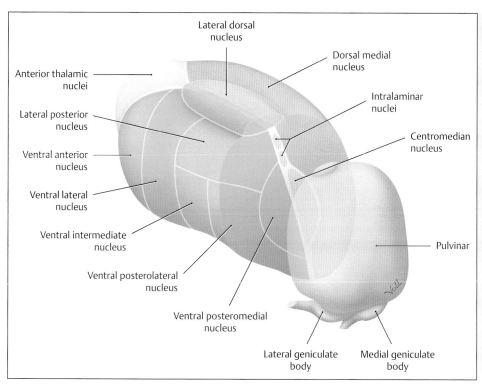

Fig. 4.61 Left thalamus viewed from the lateral and occipital aspect.

4.16.3 Thalamic Nuclei

See **Table 4.3.**

4.16.4 Division of the Thalamic Nuclei by the Medullary Laminae (Thin Sheets or Layers)

Coronal section at the level of the mammillary bodies. Several groups of thalamic nuclei are grossly separated into larger nuclear complexes by fibrous sheets called medullary laminae. The following laminae are shown in the diagram (**Fig. 4.62**):

- Internal medullary lamina between the medial and ventrolateral thalamic nuclei
- External medullary lamina between the lateral nuclei and the reticular nucleus of the thalamus

4.16.5 Somatotopic (Related to Specific Areas of the Body) Organization of the Specific Thalamic Nuclei

Transverse section (**Fig. 4.63**). The specific thalamic nuclei (defined in Chapters 4.16.2 and 4.16.3) are topographically arranged according to their functional relation to specific regions of the body. Afferent fibers from the spinal cord, brainstem, and cerebellum are localized to specific areas of the thalamus, where the corresponding thalamic nuclei are clustered. This pattern of somatotopic arrangement, a recurring theme in neural organization, is here illustrated for the ventrolateral thalamic nuclei (green in **Fig. 4.61**, **Fig. 4.62**, **Fig. 4.63**). Axons from the crossed superior cerebellar peduncle terminate in the ventral lateral nucleus of the thalamus (2); information on body position, coordination, and muscle tone travels by this pathway to the motor cortex, which also shows a pattern of somatotopic organization. The *lateral* part of the ventral lateral nucleus relays impulses from the extremities, while the *medial* part relays impulses from the head. The ventral intermediate nucleus (3) receives afferent input from the vestibular nuclei concerning the coordination of gaze toward the ipsilateral side. The large sensory pathways of the spinal cord (the tracts of the posterior funiculus) are relayed to the nuclei cuneatus and gracilus, which send their axons through the medial lemniscus to terminate in the ventral posterolateral nucleus (4), while the trigeminal sensory pathways from the head terminate in the ventral posteromedial nucleus (5, trigeminal lemniscus). Topographical localization according to function is a basic principle of neural organization.

Table 4.3 Nomenclature of the thalamic nuclei

Name	Alternative name	Properties
Specific thalamic nuclei (cortically dependent)	Palliothalamus	Project to the cerebral cortex (pallium)
Nonspecific thalamic nuclei (cortically independent)	Truncothalamus	Project to the brainstem, diencephalon, and corpus striatum
Integration nuclei		Project to other nuclei within the thalamus (classified as nonspecific thalamic nuclei)
Intralaminar nuclei		Nuclei in the white matter of the internal medullary lamina (classified as nonspecific thalamic nuclei)

Ventrolateral thalamic nuclei — Medial thalamic nuclei — Anterior thalamic nuclei

Reticular nucleus of thalamus

External medullary lamina

Internal medullary lamina

Mammillary body

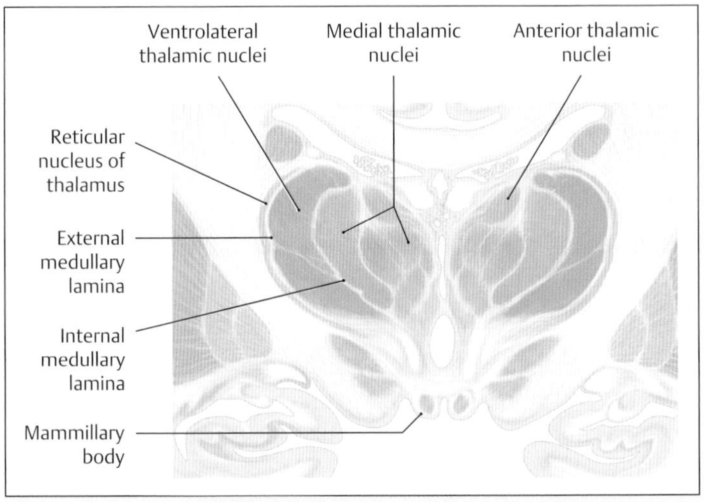

Fig. 4.62 Coronal section at the level of the mammillary bodies.

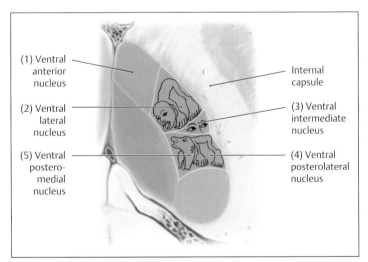

(1) Ventral anterior nucleus

(2) Ventral lateral nucleus

(5) Ventral posteromedial nucleus

Internal capsule

(3) Ventral intermediate nucleus

(4) Ventral posterolateral nucleus

Fig. 4.63 Somatotopic organization of the specific thalamic nuclei (transverse section).

4.16.6 Nonspecific Thalamic Nuclei

The nonspecific thalamic nuclei project to the brainstem, to other nuclei in the diencephalon (including other thalamic nuclei), and to the corpus striatum. They have no direct connections with the cerebral cortex, acting only indirectly on the cortex (**Fig. 4.64**). The medial *nonspecific* thalamic nuclei are subdivided into two groups:

- Nuclei of the central thalamic gray matter (median nucleus): Small groups of cells distributed along the wall of the third ventricle.
- Intralaminar nuclei, located in the internal medullary lamina. The largest nucleus of this group is the centromedian nucleus.
- The lateral *specific* thalamic nucleus shown in the diagram is the reticular nucleus of the thalamus, which is situated lateral to the other specific thalamic nuclei. The reticular nucleus is the source of the electrical impulses recorded in an electroencephalogram (EEG).

4.16.7 Thalamic Radiations

The axons of the specific thalamic nuclei (so called because their fibers project to specific cortical areas) are collected into tracts that form the thalamic radiations (**Fig. 4.65**). The arrangement of the fibers shows that the specific thalamic nuclei have connections with all areas of the cortex. The anterior thalamic radiation projects to the frontal lobe, the central thalamic radiation to the parietal lobe, the posterior thalamic radiation to the occipital lobe, and the inferior thalamic radiation to the temporal lobe.

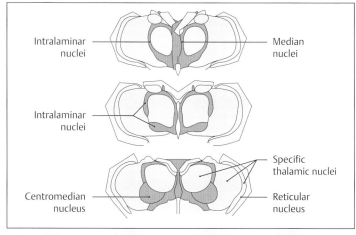

Fig. 4.64 Coronal sections presented in an oral-to-caudal series.

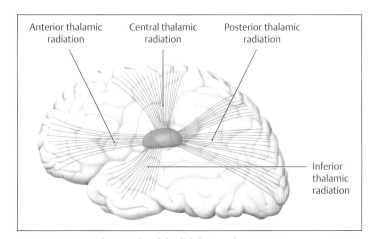

Fig. 4.65 Lateral ventricle of the left hemisphere.

4.17 Thalamus: Projections of the Thalamic Nuclei

4.17.1 Ventrolateral Thalamic Nuclei: Afferent and Efferent Connections

The ventral posterolateral nucleus (VPL) and ventral posteromedial nucleus (VPM) are the major thalamic relay centers for somatosensory information (**Fig. 4.66**).

- The *medial lemniscus* ends in the *VPL*. It contains sensory fibers for position sense, vibration, pressure, discrimination, and touch that are relayed from the nucleus gracilis and nucleus cuneatus.
- Pain and temperature fibers from the trunk and limbs travel through the lateral *spinothalamic tract* to lateral portions of the *VPL*. These sensations are relayed from this nucleus to the somatosensory cortex.
- Pain and temperature information from the head region is conveyed by the *trigeminal system* (= trigeminothalamic tract) to

the *VPM*. As in the ventrolateral nucleus (VL), they synapse with third-order thalamic neurons that project to the postcentral gyrus.

A *lesion of the VPL* leads to contralateral disturbances of superficial and deep sensation with dysesthesia and an abnormal feeling of heaviness in the limbs (lesion of the medial lemniscus). Because the pain fibers of the spinothalamic tract terminate in the basal portions of the VPL, lesions in that region may additionally cause severe pain ("thalamic pain"). The VL projects to somatomotor cortical areas (6aα and 6aβ). The VL nuclei form a feedback loop with the motor areas of the cortex, and so lesions of these nuclei are characterized by motor deficits.

4.17.2 Anterior Nucleus and Centromedian Nucleus: Afferent and Efferent Connections

The anterior nucleus receives *afferent fibers* from the mammillary body by way of the mammillothalamic (**Fig. 4.67**). The anterior nucleus establishes both afferent and efferent connections with

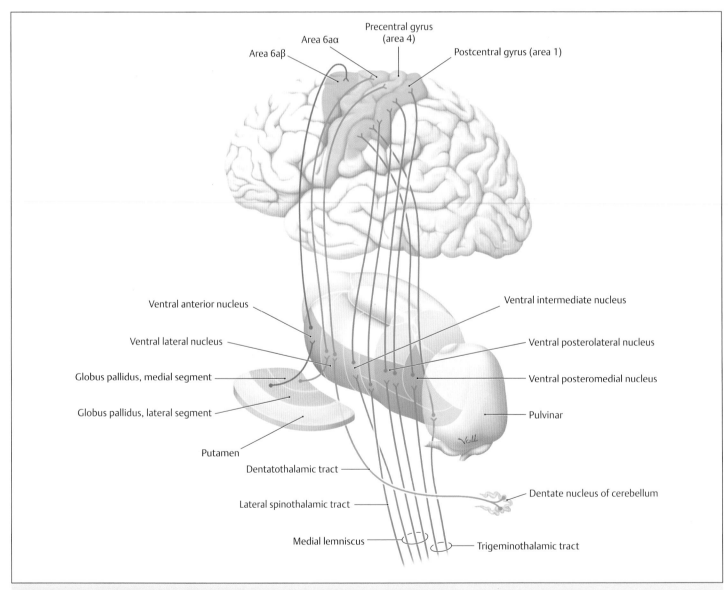

Fig. 4.66 Ventrolateral thalamic nuclei.

the cingulate gyrus of the telencephalon. The largest nonspecific thalamic nucleus is the centromedian nucleus, which is one of the intralaminar nuclei. It receives *afferent fibers* from the cerebellum, reticular formation, and medial pallidus. Its *efferent fibers* project to the head of the caudate nucleus and the putamen. The centromedian nucleus is an important component of the ascending reticular activation system (ARAS, arousal system). Essential for maintaining the waking state, the ARAS begins in the reticular formation of the brainstem and is relayed in the centromedian nucleus.

4.17.3 Medial, Dorsal, and Lateral Thalamic Nuclei: Afferent and Efferent Connections

The **medial thalamic nuclei** receive their afferent input from ventral and intralaminar thalamic nuclei (not shown), the hypothalamus, the mesencephalon, and the globus/pallidus (**Fig. 4.68**). Their efferent fibers project to the frontal lobe and

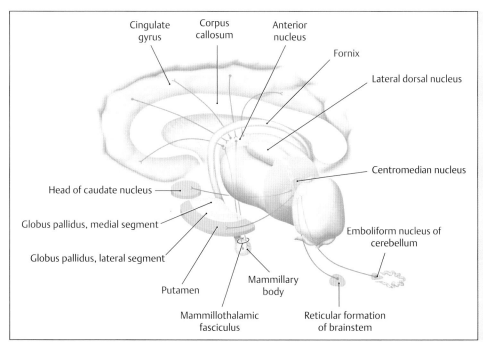

Fig. 4.67 Anterior nucleus and centromedian nucleus.

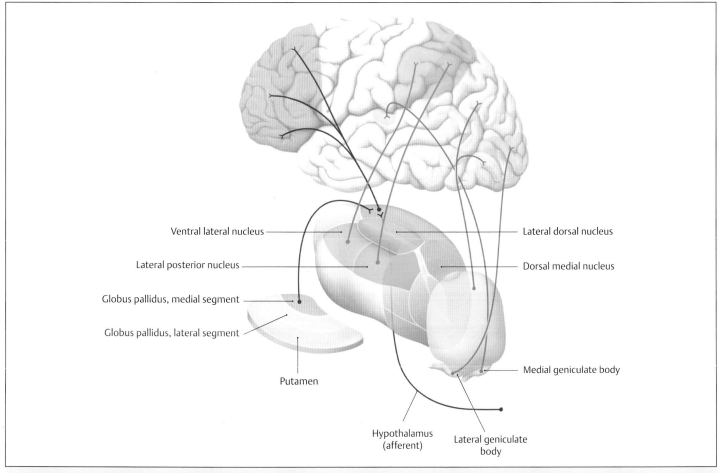

Fig. 4.68 Medial, dorsal, and lateral thalamic nuclei.

premotor cortex, and afferent fibers from these regions return to the nuclei. The destruction of these tracts leads to *frontal lobe syndrome*, which is characterized by a loss of self-control (episodes of childish jocularity alternating with suspicion and becoming rude in speech or behavior). Frontal lobe syndrome may be caused by damage to these tracts as well as direct injury to the frontal lobes. As with the classic case of Phineas Gage who survived a horrible injury to the frontal lobes that drastically altered his personality, an individual who is previously capable of judgment and sustained application and organization of his life becomes aimless and socially disinhibited, and may lose tact, sensitivity, and self-control. Additionally, the individual affected by these pathologies in the prefrontal cortex may demonstrate impulsiveness and a failure to appreciate the consequences of his or her reckless behavior. Think of the behaviors portrayed in the Jackass American films. Recklessness leads to injury. Frontal lobe syndrome can be caused by head trauma or may be the consequence of brain tumor, cerebrovascular accident, infection, or a degenerative cortical disease such as Alzheimer's disease. The **dorsal nuclei** are formed by the pulvinar, which is the largest nuclear complex of the thalamus. The pulvinar receives afferent fibers from other thalamic nuclei, particularly the intralaminar nuclei (not shown). Its efferent fibers terminate in the association areas of the parietal and occipital lobes, which have reciprocal connections with the pulvinar. The lateral geniculate body (part of the visual pathway) projects to the visual cortex, while the medial geniculate body (part of the auditory pathway) projects to the auditory cortex. The **lateral nuclei** consist of the lateral dorsal nucleus and lateral posterior nucleus. They represent the dorsal portion of the ventrolateral group and receive their input from other thalamic nuclei (hence the term "integration nuclei"). Their efferent fibers terminate in the parietal lobe of the brain.

4.17.4 Synopsis of Some Clinically Important Connections of the Specific Thalamic Nuclei

The specific thalamic nuclei project to the cerebral cortex. **Table 4.4** lists the origins of the tracts that terminate in the nuclei, the nuclei themselves, and the sites to which their afferent fibers project.

Table 4.4 Thalamic projections

Thalamic afferents (structures that project to the thalamus)	Thalamic nucleus (abbreviation)	Thalamic efferents (structure to which the thalamus projects)
Mammillary body (mammillothalamic fasciculus)	Anterior nucleus (NA)	Cingulate gyrus (limbic system)
Cerebellum, red nucleus	Ventral lateral nucleus (VL)	Premotor cortex (areas 6aα and 6aβ)
Posterior funiculus, lateral funiculus (somatosensory input, limbs, trunk)	Ventral posterolateral nucleus (VPL)	Postcentral gyrus (sensory cortex) = somatosensory cortex (see Chapter 4.17.1)
Trigeminothalamic tract (somatosensory input, head)	Ventral posteromedial nucleus (VPM)	Postcentral gyrus (sensory cortex) = somatosensory cortex (see Chapter 4.17.1)
Inferior brachium (part of the auditory pathway)	Medial geniculate nucleus (body) (MCB)	Transverse temporal gyri (auditory cortex)
Optic tract (part of the visual pathway)	Lateral geniculate nucleus (body) (LCB)	Striate area (visual cortex)

4.18 Hypothalamus

4.18.1 Location of the Hypothalamus

Coronal section (**Fig. 4.69**). The hypothalamus is the lowest level of the diencephalon, situated below the thalamus. It is the only externally visible portion of the diencephalon. Located on either side of the third ventricle, its size is most clearly appreciated in a midsagittal section that bisects the third ventricle (see **Fig. 4.70a**).

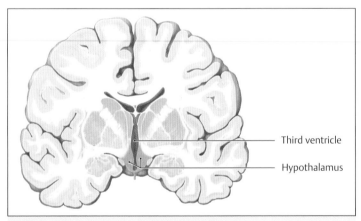

Third ventricle

Hypothalamus

Fig. 4.69 Hypothalamus (coronal section).

4.18.2 Nuclei in the Right Hypothalamus

The hypothalamus is a small nuclear complex located ventral to the thalamus and separated from it by the hypothalamic sulcus. Despite its small size, the hypothalamus is the command center for all autonomic functions in the body (**Fig. 4.70**). The autonomic nervous system is a part of the peripheral nervous system (PNS) that functions to regulate the basic visceral (organ) processes needed for the maintenance of normal bodily functions. It operates independent of voluntary control, although certain events, such as emotional stress, fear, sexual excitement, and alterations in the sleep–wakefulness cycle change the level of autonomic activity. The Terminologia Anatomica lists over 30 hypothalamic nuclei located in the lateral wall and floor of the third ventricle. Only a few of the larger, more clinically important nuclei are mentioned in this unit. Three groups of nuclei are listed below in an oral-to-caudal sequence, and their functions are briefly described:

- The anterior (rostral) group of nuclei (green) synthesizes the hormones released from the posterior lobe of the pituitary gland, and consists of the following:
  - Preoptic nucleus
  - Paraventricular nucleus
  - Supraoptic nucleus

- The middle (tuberal) group of nuclei (blue) controls hormone release from the anterior lobe of the pituitary gland, and consists of the following:
  - Dorsomedial nucleus
  - Ventromedial nucleus
  - Tuberal nuclei

- The posterior (mammillary) group of nuclei (red) activates the sympathetic nervous system when stimulated. It consists of the following:
  - Posterior nucleus
  - Mammillary nuclei located in the mammillary bodies

The coronal section (**Fig. 4.70c**) shows the further subdivision of the hypothalamus by the fornix into lateral and medial zones. The three nuclear groups described above are part of the *medial zone*, whereas the nuclei in the *lateral* zone are not subdivided into specific groups. Bilateral lesions of the mammillary bodies and their nuclei are manifested by *Korsakoff's syndrome*, which is frequently associated with alcoholism (cause: vitamin B_1 [thiamine] deficiency). The memory impairment that occurs in this syndrome mainly affects short-term memory, and the patient may fill in the memory gaps with fabricated information. This fabrication is sometimes known as "confabulation" and is a characteristic feature of alcohol-induced Korsakoff's syndrome. (My aunt was Helen Keller. I invented Mickey Mouse). A major neuropathological finding is the presence of hemorrhages in the mammillary bodies, which are sectioned at autopsy to confirm the diagnosis.

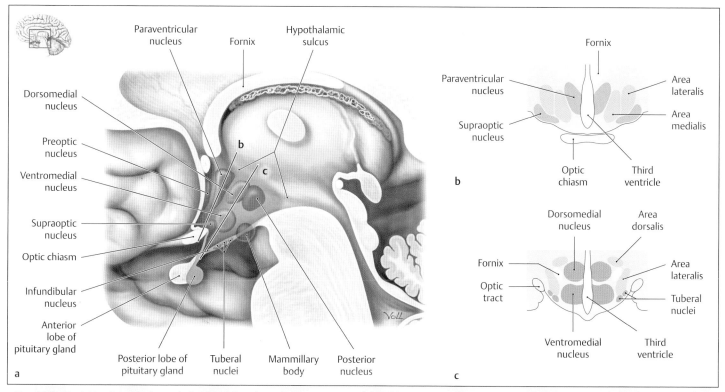

Fig. 4.70 Nuclei in the right hypothalamus. **(a)** Midsagittal section of the right hemisphere viewed from the medial side. **(b, c)** Coronal sections.

4.18.3 Important Afferent and Efferent Connections of the Hypothalamus

Midsagittal section of the right hemisphere viewed from the medial side (**Fig. 4.71**). Because the hypothalamus coordinates all the autonomic functions in the body, it establishes afferent (blue) and efferent (red) connections with many brain regions. The following are particularly important:

(a) Afferent connections (to the hypothalamus) (**Fig. 4.71a**):

- The fornix conveys afferent fibers from the hippocampus; it is an important fiber tract of the limbic system.
- The medial forebrain bundle transmits afferent fibers from the olfactory areas to the preoptic nuclei.
- The stria terminalis conveys afferent fibers from the amygdala.
- The peduncle of the mammillary bodies transmits visceral afferent fibers and impulses from erogenous zones (nipples, genitalia).

(b) Efferent connections (from the hypothalamus) (**Fig. 4.71b**):

- The dorsal longitudinal fasciculus passes to the brainstem where it is relayed several times before reaching the parasympathetic nuclei.
- The mammillotegmental tract distributes efferent fibers to the tegmentum of the midbrain; these are then relayed to the reticular formation. The fibers of this tract mediate the exchange of autonomic information between the hypothalamus, cranial nerve nuclei, and spinal cord.
- The mammillothalamic fasciculus conveys efferent fibers to the anterior thalamic nucleus, which is connected to the cingulate gyrus. This is part of the limbic system, which is so principal in the regulation, perception, and production of the spectrum of human emotions and basic human drives.
- The hypothalamic–hypophyseal and tuberohypophyseal tracts are efferent tracts to the pituitary gland.

4.18.4 Functions of the Hypothalamus

The hypothalamus is the coordinating center of the autonomic nervous system. There is no specific sympathetic or parasympathetic control center. Certain functions can be assigned to specific regions or nuclei in the hypothalamus, and these relationships are outlined in **Table 4.5**. Not all of the regions or nuclei listed in the table are shown in the drawings.

Table 4.5 Nuclei and functions of hypothalamus

Region or nucleus	Function
Anterior preoptic region	Maintain constant body temperature; **lesion:** central hypothermia
Posterior region	Respond to temperature changes, e.g., sweating; **lesion:** hypothermia
Midanterior and posterior regions	Activate sympathetic nervous system
Paraventricular and anterior regions	Activate parasympathetic nervous system
Supraoptic and paraventricular nuclei	Regulate water balance; **lesion:** diabetes insipidus, also lack of thirst response resulting in hyponatremia[a]
Anterior nuclei • Medial part ∘ Lateral part	Regulate appetite and food intake • **Lesion:** Obesity ∘ **Lesion:** Anorexia and emaciation

[a] Hyponatremia refers to a lower-than-normal level of sodium in the blood. Sodium is essential for many body functions, including the maintenance of fluid balance, regulation of blood pressure, and normal function of the nervous system. Hyponatremia has sometimes been referred to as "water intoxication," especially when it is due to the consumption of excess water, for example, during strenuous exercise, without adequate replacement of sodium. This condition can cause headaches, cramps, confusion and altered mental states, and seizures.

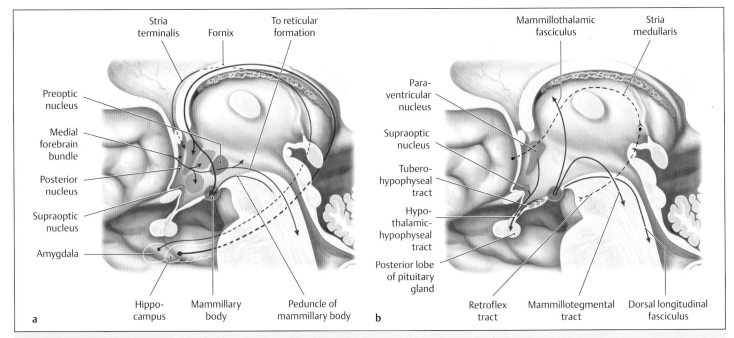

Fig. 4.71 (a) Afferent connections to the hypothalamus. (b) Efferent connections from the hypothalamus.

4.19 Brainstem, Organization and External Structure

4.19.1 Terms of Location and Direction in the Brainstem

These terms are based on the nearly vertical *Meynert's brainstem axis* (compare with the horizontal Forel's axis, which was used as a reference line in previous units). Just dorsal to the brainstem is the cerebellum (**Fig. 4.72**), which will be described in subsequently.

4.19.2 Relationship of the Brainstem to the Cerebral and Cerebellar Hemispheres

Basal view (**Fig. 4.73**). The brainstem is a midline structure flanked by the cerebrum and cerebellum. Its anatomical subdivisions are best appreciated in the midsagittal section (see Chapter 4.19.3). The third through twelfth pairs of cranial nerves (CN III–XII) enter or emerge from the brainstem (see Chapter 4.19.5).

4.19.3 Division of the Brainstem into Levels

Midsagittal section (**Fig. 4.74**). The brainstem is divided macroscopically into three levels, with the bulge of the pons marking the boundary lines between the parts:

- Mesencephalon (midbrain)
- Pons
- Medulla oblongata

The location and contents of these parts are summarized in Chapter 4.19.4. The three levels are easily distinguished from one another by gross visual inspection, although they are not differentiated in a functional sense. The *functional organization* of the brainstem (see Chapter 4.19.4) is determined chiefly by the arrangement of the cranial nerve nuclei. Given the close proximity of nuclei and large fiber tracts in this region, even a small lesion of the brainstem (e.g., hemorrhage, tumor) may lead to extensive and complex alterations of sensorimotor function.

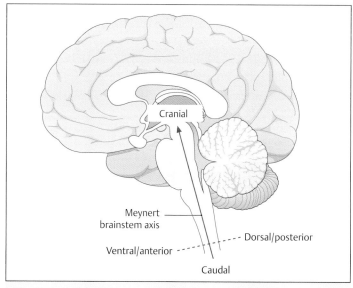

Fig. 4.72 Terms of location and direction in the brainstem.

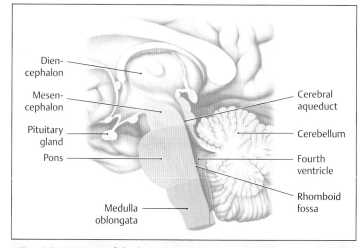

Fig. 4.73 Relationship of the brainstem to the cerebral and cerebellar hemispheres (basal view).

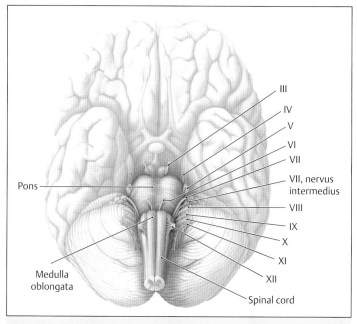

Fig. 4.74 Division of the brainstem.

4.19.4 Overview of the Brainstem

Topographical Organization

- *Craniocaudal direction:*
  - Mesencephalon (midbrain)
  - Pons
  - Medulla oblongata
- *Anteroposterior direction:*
  - Base (mesencephalon: cerebral peduncles; pons: basal part; medulla oblongata: pyramids)
  - Tegmentum (present as such in all three parts)
  - Section of ventricular system (upper part: cerebral aqueduct, fourth ventricle, central canal)
  - Tectum ("roof"; present only in the mesencephalon; quadrigeminal plate)
- The cerebellum adjoins the brainstem dorsally.

Functional Organization

- *Mediolaterally into four longitudinal nuclear columns:*
  - Somatic efferent (motor) column
  - Visceral efferent (motor) column
  - Visceral afferent (sensory) column
  - Somatic afferent (sensory) column
- *Organization into different structures:*
  - Nuclei of cranial nerves III–XII
  - Red nucleus, substantia nigra (motor coordination centers)
  - Reticular formation (diffuse nuclear aggregations for autonomic functions)
  - Ascending and descending tracts
  - Dorsal column nuclei (nucleus gracilis and nucleus cuneatus)
  - Pontine nuclei

4.19.5 Brainstem

(a) Anterior view (**Fig. 4.75a**). The sites of entry and emergence of the 10 pairs of cranial nerves (III–XII) are particularly well displayed in this view. *Note:* Cranial nerve II (optic nerve) is a derivative of the diencephalon. Note also the site below the pyramids where the pyramidal fibers cross over the midline from each side (decussation of the pyramids). Most of the axons of the large motor pathway for the trunk and limbs cross to the opposite side at this level.

(b) Posterior view (**Fig. 4.75b**). Since the cerebellum has been removed, we can see the rhomboid fossa, which forms the floor of the fourth ventricle. The surface of the fossa is raised by several cranial nerve nuclei, which bulge into the fourth ventricle. The cerebellum is connected to the brainstem by three cerebellar peduncles on each side:

- Superior cerebellar peduncle
- Middle cerebellar peduncle
- Inferior cerebellar peduncle

The superior and inferior cerebellar peduncles border portions of the rhomboid fossa and thus contribute to the boundaries of the fourth ventricle.

(c) Left lateral view (**Fig. 4.75c**). In addition to the cerebellar peduncles, this view displays the superior and inferior colliculi. Together with their counterparts on the right side, the colliculi form the quadrigeminal plate (see **Fig. 4.75b**), which is a prominent structure of the mesencephalon. The two superior colliculi are part of the visual pathway, while the inferior colliculi are part of the auditory pathway. The trochlear nerve (CN IV) runs forward below the inferior colliculus, and is the only cranial nerve that emerges from the dorsal side of the brainstem. The olive appears as a prominence on the side of the medulla oblongata. The olive is named after that little green accompaniment sometimes found in a martini. The nuclei within the olive function as a relay station for the motor system.

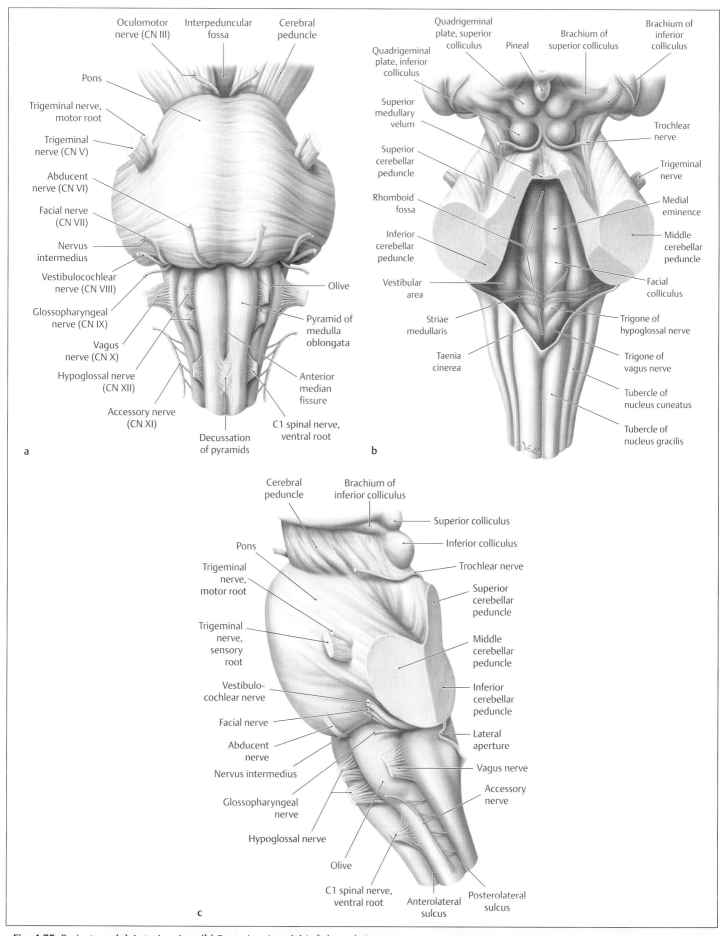

Oculomotor nerve (CN III)
Interpeduncular fossa
Cerebral peduncle
Pons
Trigeminal nerve, motor root
Trigeminal nerve (CN V)
Abducent nerve (CN VI)
Facial nerve (CN VII)
Nervus intermedius
Vestibulocochlear nerve (CN VIII)
Glossopharyngeal nerve (CN IX)
Vagus nerve (CN X)
Hypoglossal nerve (CN XII)
Accessory nerve (CN XI)
Decussation of pyramids
Olive
Pyramid of medulla oblongata
Anterior median fissure
C1 spinal nerve, ventral root

a

Quadrigeminal plate, superior colliculus
Quadrigeminal plate, inferior colliculus
Pineal
Brachium of superior colliculus
Brachium of inferior colliculus
Superior medullary velum
Trochlear nerve
Superior cerebellar peduncle
Trigeminal nerve
Rhomboid fossa
Medial eminence
Inferior cerebellar peduncle
Middle cerebellar peduncle
Vestibular area
Facial colliculus
Striae medullaris
Trigone of hypoglossal nerve
Taenia cinerea
Trigone of vagus nerve
Tubercle of nucleus cuneatus
Tubercle of nucleus gracilis

b

Cerebral peduncle
Brachium of inferior colliculus
Superior colliculus
Pons
Inferior colliculus
Trigeminal nerve, motor root
Trochlear nerve
Superior cerebellar peduncle
Trigeminal nerve, sensory root
Middle cerebellar peduncle
Vestibulo-cochlear nerve
Inferior cerebellar peduncle
Facial nerve
Abducent nerve
Lateral aperture
Nervus intermedius
Vagus nerve
Glossopharyngeal nerve
Accessory nerve
Hypoglossal nerve
Olive
C1 spinal nerve, ventral root
Anterolateral sulcus
Posterolateral sulcus

c

Fig. 4.75 Brainstem. **(a)** Anterior view. **(b)** Posterior view. **(c)** Left lateral view.

4.20 Brainstem: Cranial Nerve Nuclei, Red Nucleus, and Substantia Nigra

4.20.1 Cranial Nerve Nuclei in the Brainstem

Posterior view with the cerebellum removed, exposing the rhomboid fossa (**Fig. 4.76a**). Midsagittal section of the right half of the brainstem viewed from the left side (**Fig. 4.76b**).

The diagrams show the nuclei themselves and the course of the tracts leading to and away from them (the vestibular and cochlear nuclei are not shown).

The arrangement of the cranial nerve nuclei is easier to understand when we divide them into functional nuclear columns. The *motor nuclei*, which give rise to the efferent fibers, are shown on the left side of **Fig. 4.76a**, and the *sensory nuclei*, where the afferent fibers terminate, are shown in **Fig. 4.76b**. The arrangement of these nuclei can be derived from the arrangement of the nuclei in the spinal cord. The function and connections of some of these cranial nerves can be evaluated in a clinical neurological

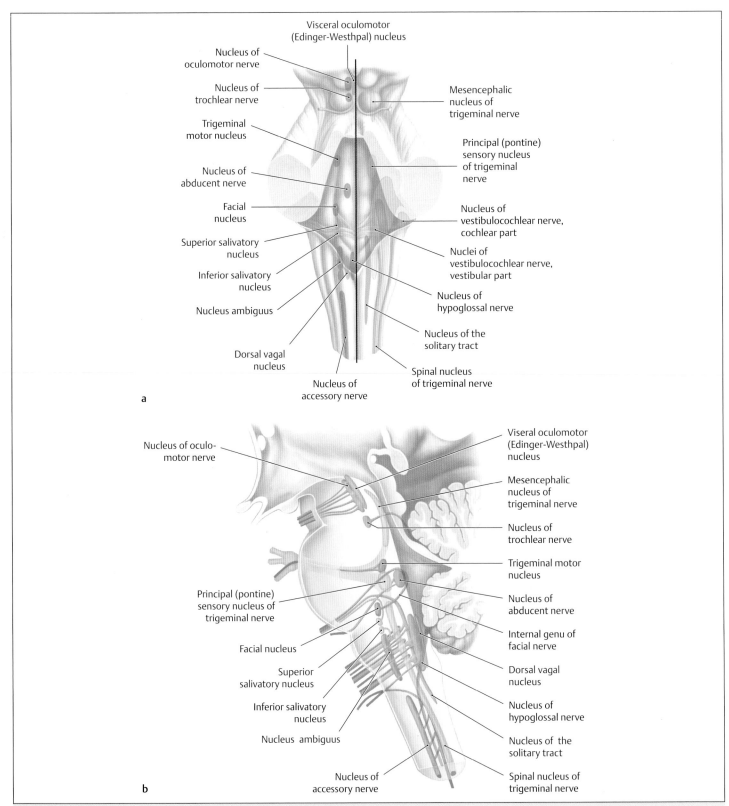

Fig. 4.76 Cranial nerve nuclei in the brainstem. **(a)** Posterior view. **(b)** Midsagittal section.

examination by testing the *brainstem reflexes* (whose relay centers are located in the brainstem). These reflexes are important in the evaluation of comatose patients. Examples are the pupillary reflexes or the gag reflex, which are described more later. In the next section, the cranial nerves and their functions and relationships to speech function will be described in more detail. They are introduced here to clarify their relationship to the brainstem.

4.20.2 Overview of the Nuclei of Cranial Nerves III–XII

See **Table 4.6**.

4.20.3 Location of the Substantia Nigra and Red Nucleus in the Mesencephalon

Both of these nuclei, like the cranial nerve nuclei, are well-defined structures that belong functionally to the *extrapyramidal motor* system (**Fig. 4.77**). Recall that the extrapyramidal motor system is important in refining, fine tuning, and providing feedback on motor or movement activity, including speech motor control. Anatomically, the substantia nigra (important in Parkinson's disease) is part of the cerebral peduncles and therefore is

not located in the tegmentum of the mesencephalon. Owing to their high respective contents of melanin and iron, the substantia nigra and red nucleus appear brown and red, respectively, in sections of fresh brain tissue. Both nuclei extend into the diencephalon and are connected to its nuclei by fiber tracts (see Chapter 4.20.5).

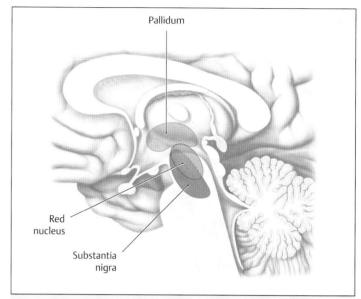

Fig. 4.77 Location of the substantia nigra and red nucleus in the mesencephalon.

Table 4.6 Cranial nerve nuclei in brainstem

Motor nuclei: give rise to efferent (motor) fibers, left in Fig. 4.76a	Sensory nuclei: where afferent (sensory) fibers terminate, right in Fig. 4.76b
Somatic efferent or somatic motor nuclei (red): • Nucleus of oculomotor nerve (CN III) • Nucleus of trochlear nerve (CN IV) • Nucleus of abducent nerve (CN VI) • Nucleus of accessory nerve (CN XI) • Nucleus of hypoglossal nerve (CN XII)	**Somatic afferent (somatic sensory) and vestibulocochlear nuclei (yellow):** *Sensory nuclei associated with the trigeminal nerve (CN V):* • Mesencephalic nucleus of trigeminal nerve (special feature: pseudounipolar ganglion cells ("displaced sensory ganglion") provide direct sensory innervation for muscles of mastication) • Principal (pontine) sensory nucleus of trigeminal nerve • Spinal nucleus of trigeminal nerve
Visceral efferent (visceral motor) nuclei: *Nuclei associated with the parasympathetic nervous system (light blue):* • Visceral oculomotor (Edinger–Westphal) nucleus (CN III) • Superior salivatory nucleus (facial nerve, CN VII) • Inferior salivatory nucleus (glossopharyngeal nerve, CN IX) • Dorsal vagal nucleus (CN X)	*Nuclei of the vestibulocochlear nerve (CN VIII):* • Vestibular part: ◦ Medial vestibular nucleus ◦ Lateral vestibular nucleus ◦ Superior vestibular nucleus ◦ Inferior vestibular nucleus • Cochlear part: ◦ Anterior cochlear nucleus ◦ Posterior cochlear nucleus

Nuclei of the branchial arch nerves (dark blue):
• Trigeminal motor nucleus (CN V)
• Facial nucleus (CN VII)
• Nucleus ambiguus (glossopharyngeal nerve, CN IX; vagus nerve, CN X; accessory nerve, CN XI, cranial root)
	Visceral afferent (visceral sensory) nuclei (green):
	
	• Nucleus of the solitary tract (nuclear complex):
	 ◦ Superior part:
	  – Special visceral afferents (taste) from facial (CN VII), glossopharyngeal (CN IX), and vagus (CN X) nerves
	 ◦ Inferior part:
	  – General visceral afferents from glossopharyngeal (CN IX) and vagus (CN X) nerves

4.20.4 Cross-Sectional Structure of the Brainstem at Different Levels

Transverse sections through the mesencephalon (**Fig. 4.78a**), pons (Fig. **4.78b**), and medulla oblongata (**Fig. 4.78c**), viewed from above.

A feature common to all three sections is the dorsally situated tegmentum ("hood," medium gray), the phylogenetically old part of the brainstem. The tegmentum of the adult brain contains the brainstem nuclei. Anterior to the tegmentum are the large ascending and descending tracts that run to and from the telencephalon. This region is called the cerebral peduncle (crus cerebri) in the mesencephalon, the basilar part (foot) of the pons at the pontine level, and the pyramids in the medulla oblongata. The tegmentum is covered dorsally by the tectum (= "roof") only in the region of the mesencephalon. In the mature brain pictured here, this structure forms the quadrigeminal plate containing the superior and inferior colliculi ("little hills"), shown faintly in **Fig. 4.78a**. The brainstem is covered by the cerebellum at the level of the medulla oblongata and pons and therefore lacks a tectal covering at those levels.

4.20.5 Afferent (Blue) and Efferent (Red) Connections of the Red Nucleus and Substantia Nigra

These two nuclei are important relay stations in the motor system. The *red nucleus* consists of a larger *neorubrum* and a smaller *paleorubrum* (**Fig. 4.79**). It receives afferent axons from the dentate nucleus (dentatorubral tract), superior colliculi (tectorubral tract), inner pallidum (pallidorubral tract), and cerebral cortex (corticorubral tract). The red nucleus sends its axons to the olive (rubro-olivary fibers and reticulo-olivary fibers, part of the central tegmental tract) and to the spinal cord (rubrospinal tract). It coordinates muscle tone, body position, and gait. A lesion of the red nucleus produces resting tremor, abnormal muscle tone (tested as involuntary muscular resistance of the joints in the relaxed patient), and choreoathetosis (involuntary writhing movements, usually involving the distal parts of the limbs). The **substantia nigra** consists of a *compact part* (dark, contains melanin) and a *reticular part* (reddish, contains iron; for simplicity, the entire substantia nigra appears dark in the drawing). Most of its axons project diffusely to other brain areas and are not collected into tracts. Axons from the caudate nucleus (striatonigral fibers), anterior cerebral cortex (corticonigral fibers), putamen, and precentral cortex terminate in the substantia nigra. As mentioned previously, the substantia nigra is implicated in Parkinson's disease, and when disease reduces the number of functioning neurons in the substantia nigra about 70%, the clinical manifestations of Parkinson's disease become apparent (tremor, muscular rigidity, bradykinesia or slow movements, shuffling gait, and imprecise articulation coupled with inadequate loudness and inadequate pitch variation).

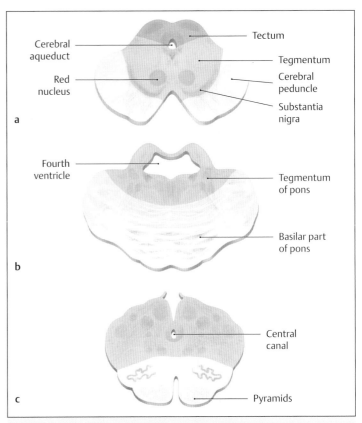

Fig. 4.78 Cross-sectional structure of the brainstem at different levels. (a) Mesencephalon. (b) Pons. (c) Medulla oblongata.

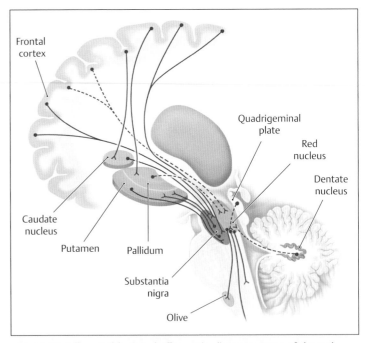

Fig. 4.79 Afferent (blue) and efferent (red) connections of the red nucleus and substantia nigra.

4.21 Brainstem: Descending (Motor) and Ascending (Sensory) Tracts

4.21.1 Descending Tracts in the Brainstem

See **Fig. 4.80**. The descending tracts shown here begin in the telencephalon and terminate partly in the brainstem but mostly in

the spinal cord. The most prominent tract that descends through the brainstem, the *corticospinal tract*, terminates in the spinal cord. Its axons arise from large pyramidal neurons of the primary motor cortex and terminate on or near alpha motor neurons in the anterior horn of the spinal cord. Most of the axons cross to the opposite side (decussate) at the level of the pyramids. The fibers in this part of the pyramidal tract that descend through the brainstem are called *corticospinal fibers*. Those fibers in the pyramidal tract that terminate in the brainstem are called *corticonuclear or corticobulbar fibers*. Corticonuclear axons connect the motor

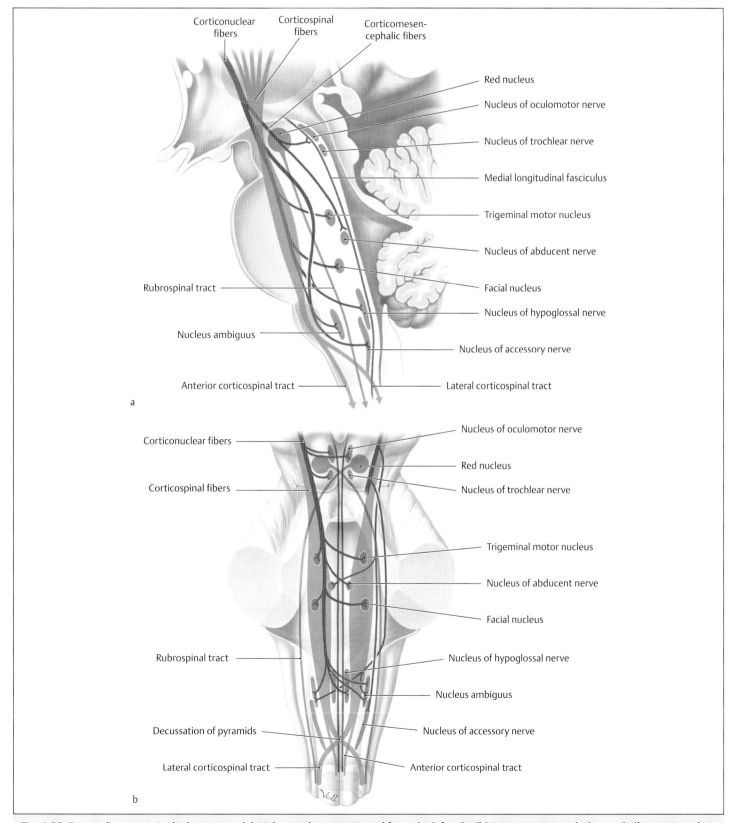

Fig. 4.80 Descending tracts in the brainstem. **(a)** Midsagittal section viewed from the left side. **(b)** Posterior view with the cerebellum removed.

cortex to the brainstem motor nuclei of the cranial nerves. The corticobulbar fibers are very important for the motoric or movement functions necessary for speech and swallowing, as will be seen in detail in the section on the cranial nerves. The corticobulbar tract serves the head and neck; the corticospinal tract serves the trunk, limbs, and rest of the body.

Note: Direct cortical projections to the brainstem nuclei are predominantly

- *Bilateral* for
  - The trigeminal motor nucleus (CN V)
  - Neurons in the facial nucleus (CN VII) that innervate muscles in the forehead
  - Nucleus ambiguus (CN X)
- *Contralateral (crossed)* for
  - The nucleus of the abducent nerve (CN VI)
  - Neurons in the facial nucleus (CN VII) that innervate muscles in the lower face
  - The nucleus of the hypoglossal nerve (CN XII)
- *Ipsilateral* for
  - Neurons in the nucleus of the accessory nerve (CN XI) that innervate the sternocleidomastoid muscle

The pattern of corticonuclear innervation is important in the diagnosis of different lesions, particularly involving the facial nerve (CN VII). Most cortical projections to the brainstem motor nuclei, however, are indirect, involving intermediate neurons, many of which are located in the surrounding reticular formation. Direct cortical control of brainstem motor neurons, specifically for the tongue and face, seems to be a recent evolutionary development, present in primates but not in other mammals. The nuclei of the

oculomotor (CN III) and trochlear (CN IV) nerves, which do not receive direct cortical projections, are synaptically connected with the abducent nucleus through the *medial longitudinal fasciculus*, a brainstem tract that contains both ascending and descending fibers.

4.21.2 Ascending Tracts in the Brainstem

See **Fig. 4.81**.

Two major ascending fiber bundles, the **posterior funiculus** (violet) and the **lateral spinothalamic tract** (dark blue), carry sensory information from the spinal cord to the brainstem. The posterior funiculus consists of the *medial fasciculus gracilis*, from the lower limb and trunk, and the *lateral fasciculus cuneatus*, from thoracic and cervical levels. Many of the fibers in these tracts are the central processes of dorsal root ganglion cells whose peripheral processes are in muscle spindles and tendon stretch receptors (proprioception) and cutaneous touch receptors. The first synapse in this ascending pathway is in the *nucleus gracilis or nucleus cuneatus*; the neurons from these nuclei send their axons in the *medial lemniscus* (lemniskos = "ribbon," Gr.) across the midline to the thalamus. The lateral spinothalamic tract bears pain and temperature information from secondary neurons in the contralateral spinal cord, passing without an additional synaptic relay directly to the thalamus. The other ribbon-like sensory tract in the brainstem—the *lateral lemniscus*—contains axons from the cochlear nuclei, some of which cross the midline in the trapezoid body, to synapse in the inferior colliculus of the quadrigeminal plate.

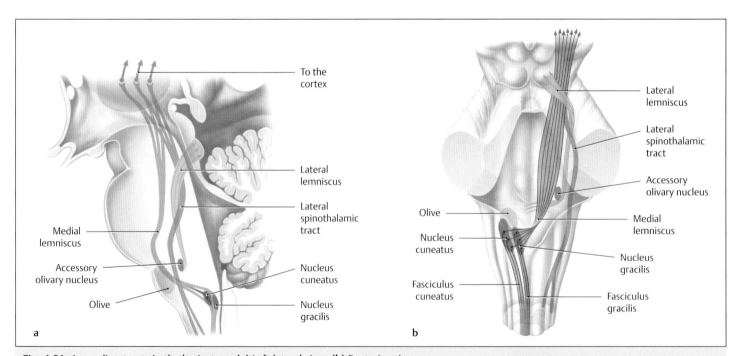

Fig. 4.81 Ascending tracts in the brainstem. **(a)** Left lateral view. **(b)** Posterior view.

4.21.3 Courses of the Major Cerebellar Tracts through the Brainstem

The cerebellum is involved in the coordination of movement, including speech movement, and balance. Descending tracts (red) and ascending tracts (blue) enter the cerebellum through the superior, middle, and inferior cerebellar peduncles (**Fig. 4.82**).

- **Superior cerebellar peduncle:** Contains most of the *efferent* axons from the cerebellum. The only major *afferent* axon tract entering the cerebellum through the superior peduncle is the anterior spinocerebellar pathway.
- **Middle cerebellar peduncle:** Largest of the three peduncles, occupied mostly by *afferent* fibers from contralateral basal pontine nuclei. These afferent fibers are the second step of a massive descending corticopontine to pontocerebellar projection.
- **Inferior cerebellar peduncle:** Contains the *afferent* posterior spinocerebellar and olivocerebellar tracts. The posterior spinocerebellar tract enters ipsilaterally, the olivocerebellar tract from the contralateral (inferior) olivary nuclei.

4.22 Brainstem: Reticular Formation

4.22.1 Definition, Demarcation, and Organization

The *reticular formation (RF)* is a phylogenetically old, morphologically ill-defined collection of numerous small nuclei in the *tegmentum* of the brainstem. These nuclei serve entirely different functions. The morphological term *"reticular formation"* incorrectly implies a homogeneity when in fact it represents different centers. Thus, it would be better to refer to them as *reticular nuclei*, which morphologically are difficult to distinguish from one another. The reticular nuclei use different neurotransmitters to serve their different functions. Considering these facts, the reticular formation can be classified as follows:

- Cytoarchitectonics (morphological classification) takes into account the shape and architecture of the reticular nuclei.
- Transmitter architectonics (chemical classification) takes into account the type of neurotransmitters used by the cells.

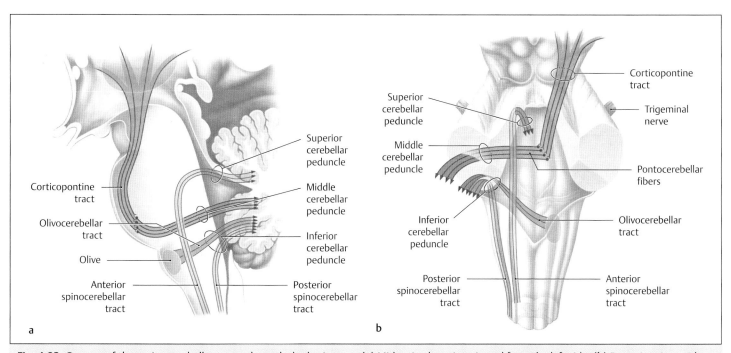

Fig. 4.82 Courses of the major cerebellar tracts through the brainstem. (**a**) Midsagittal section viewed from the left side. (**b**) Posterior view with the cerebellum removed.

- The classification based on functional centers (physiological classification) covers the functions associated with the nuclei.

Note: Cranial nerve nuclei, which are mainly located in the tegmentum of the brainstem (but are usually very well defined morphologically) are not part of the RF but are functionally closely linked with it. Neither the nuclear regions of the "red nucleus" or "substantia nigra" located in the tegmentum of the mesencephalon nor the pontine nuclei are part of the RF.

4.22.2 Functional Centers

Left lateral view of the brainstem bisected (**Fig. 4.83**). Displayed is the position of functional centers as well as the position of functionally relevant cranial nerve nuclei. For further details of the functional centers, see Chapter 4.22.4.

4.22.3 Cyto- and Transmitter Architectonics

Dorsal view of the brainstem after the cerebellum has been removed; left hemisphere: cytoarchitectonics; right hemisphere: transmitter architectonics (**Fig. 4.84**). With the help of

cytoarchitectonics, the reticular nuclei can be divided already in the RF on both sides into three longitudinal zones each:

- *Lateral zone* with small-cell nuclei (parvocellular zone)
- *Medial zone* with large-cell nuclei (magnocellular zone)
- *Median zone* (it lies on both sides of the midline = raphe of the brainstem; the large-cell nuclei located in this zone are thus also referred to as "raphe nuclei").

The axons of the medial and median zone, after a long course, reach other nuclei of the CNS either in cranial direction up to the telencephalon or in caudal direction up to the sacral spinal region. These two zones are mostly responsible for connecting the RF with other regions of the CNS. They are thus called "effectory." However, the axons of the lateral zone largely remain inside the brainstem, connecting individual portions of the RF with one another or interconnecting with cranial nerve nuclei in the brainstem. They are thus also referred to as "association areas." Some nuclei have been labeled as examples.

Note: The division into three longitudinal zones is not equally visible in all portions of the brainstem. It is best visible in the medulla oblongata. As a reference point, the cranial nerve nuclei (they are not part of the RF, see introduction), which are closely interconnected with the RF, have also been marked. Transmitter architectonics can help identify areas in which neurons with a

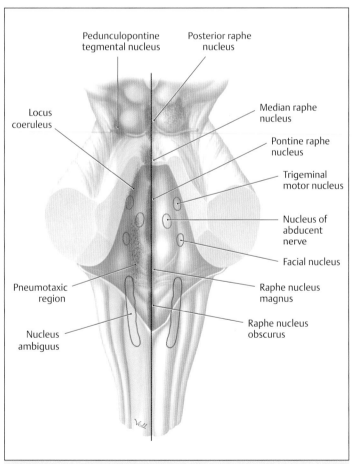

Fig. 4.83 Left lateral view of the brainstem bisected.

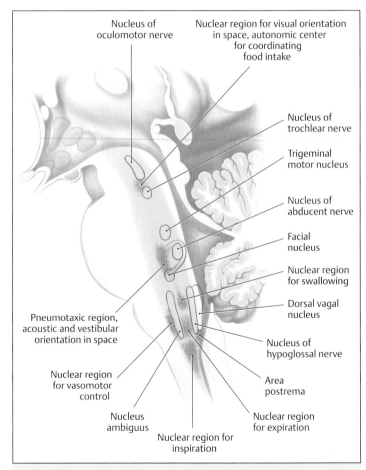

Fig. 4.84 Dorsal view of the brainstem after the cerebellum has been removed.

specific transmitter predominate. Catecholamines (adrenaline, noradrenaline, dopamine) as well as serotonin and acetylcholine are examples shown here.

Note: Raphe nuclei (median zone), which send their axons to the limbic system (modulation of moods and feelings) use serotonin as a transmitter.

Pharmacologically, influencing the effect of serotonin is said to effectively modulate emotions.

4.22.4 Overview of the Functions of the Reticular Formation

See **Fig. 4.85**.

A distinction is drawn between the following functional relationships of the reticular formation with other centers in the CNS:

- **Afferents to the** reticular formation: These originate from nuclei of almost all sensory organs, the telencephalon, diencephalon as well as the cerebellum and spinal cord. They carry auditory, visual, and tactile impulses and to a special degree, pain sensation, but also carry information regarding muscle relaxation, equilibrium, blood pressure, oxygen saturation, and parameters of ingestion.

- **Efferents of the** reticular formation: These extend to the telencephalon and diencephalon but also to the motor nuclei of the cranial nerves and the spinal cord. These efferents have very different effects:
  - Regulating sleep–wake transitions and level of alertness of the telencephalon (so-called *"ARAS"*: **A**scending **R**eticular **A**ctivating **S**ystem)
  - Regulating eye movement
  - "Vital" functions such as regulating blood pressure and respiration
  - Functions of ingestion such as licking, sucking, and chewing
  - Protective reflexes such as gagging and vomiting
  - Control of micturition
  - Regulating muscle tone in the spinal cord
  - Pain inhibition in the spinal cord

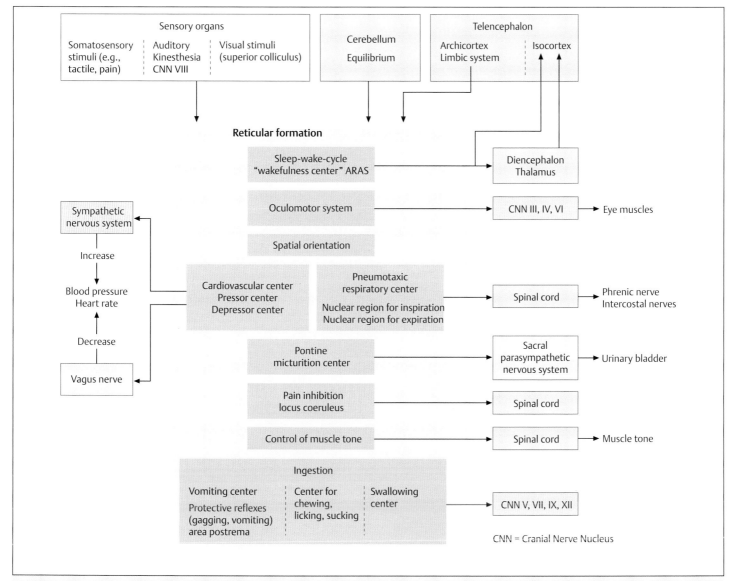

Fig. 4.85 Functions of the reticular formation.

4.23 Mesencephalon and Pons, Transverse Section

4.23.1 Transverse Section through the Mesencephalon (Midbrain)

Superior view (**Fig. 4.86**).

Nuclei: The most rostral cranial nerve nucleus is the relatively small *nucleus of the oculomotor nerve.* In the same transverse plane is the *mesencephalic nucleus of the trigeminal nerve*; other trigeminal nuclei can be identified in sections at lower levels (see Chapter 4.23.3). Unique in the CNS, the mesencephalic nucleus of the trigeminal nerve contains displaced pseudounipolar sensory neurons, closely related to the PNS neurons of the trigeminal ganglion. The peripheral processes of these mesencephalic neurons are proprioceptors in the muscles of mastication. The *superior collicular nucleus* is part of the visual system. The *red nucleus* and *substantia nigra* are involved in coordination of motor activity. The red nucleus and all of the cranial nerve nuclei are located in the tegmentum of the mesencephalon, the superior colliculus is in the tectum (roof) of the mesencephalon, and the substantia nigra is in the cerebral peduncle. Different parts of the reticular formation, a diffuse aggregation of nuclear groups (related to arousal, wakefulness, and levels of consciousness), are visible here and in sections below.

Tracts: The tracts at this level run anterior to the nuclear regions. Prominent descending tracts seen at this level include the pyramidal tract and the corticonuclear fibers that branch from it. Ascending tracts visible at this level include the lateral

spinothalamic tract and the medial lemniscus, both of which terminate in the thalamus.

4.23.2 Transverse Section through the Upper Pons

See **Fig. 4.87.**

Nuclei: The only cranial nerve nucleus appearing in this plane of section is the mesencephalic trigeminal nucleus. It can be seen that the fibers from the nucleus of the trochlear nerve (CN IV) cross to the opposite side (decussate) while still within the brainstem.

Tracts: The ascending and descending tract systems are the same as in Chapters 4.23.1 and 4.23.3. The pyramidal tract appears less compact at this level compared with the previous section due to the presence of intermingled pontine nuclei. This section cuts the tracts (mostly efferent) that exit the cerebellum through the superior cerebellar peduncle. The lateral lemniscus at the dorsal surface of the section is part of the auditory pathway. The relatively large *medial* longitudinal fasciculus ("highway of the brainstem nuclei") extends from the mesencephalon (see Chapter 4.23.1) into the spinal cord. It interconnects the brainstem nuclei and contains a variety of fibers that enter and emerge at various levels. The smaller *dorsal* longitudinal fasciculus connects hypothalamic nuclei with the parasympathetic cranial nerve nuclei. The size and location of the nuclei of the reticular formation, which here are shown graphically within a compact area, vary with the plane of the section. This diagram indicates only the approximate location

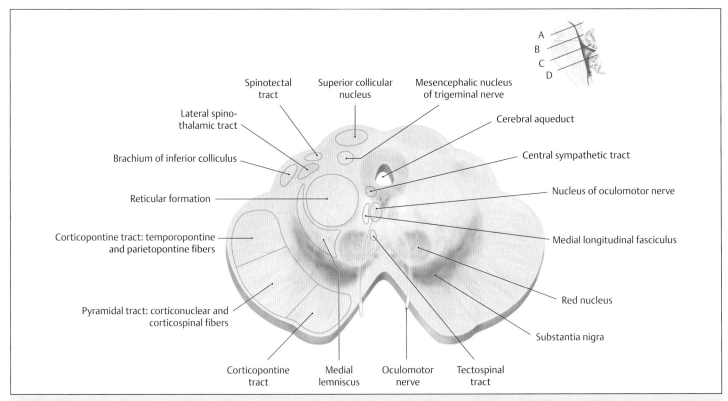

Fig. 4.86 Transverse section through the mesencephalon (midbrain). **A,** mesencephalon; **B,** upper pons; **C,** midportion of the pons; **D,** lower pons.

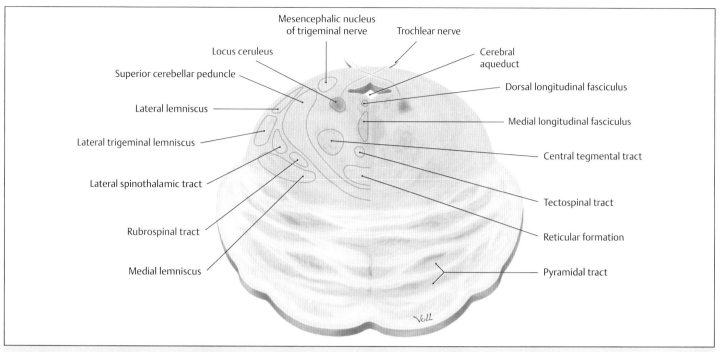

Fig. 4.87 Transverse section through the upper pons.

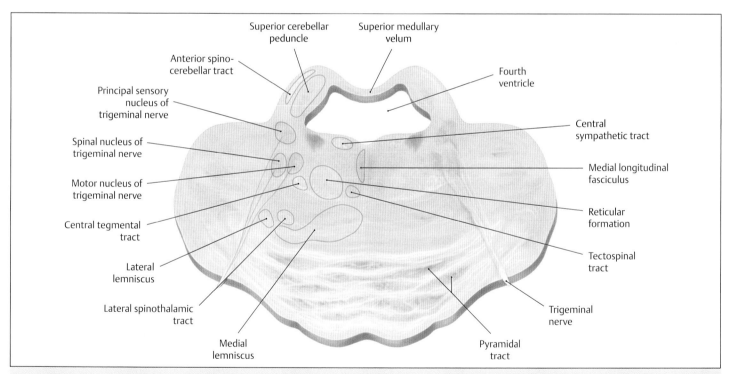

Fig. 4.88 Transverse section through the midportion of the pons nuclei.

of the reticular formation, and other smaller nuclei and fibers may be found within these regions.

4.23.3 Transverse Section through the Midportion of the Pons

Nuclei: The trigeminal nerve leaves the brainstem at the midlevel of the pons, its various nuclei dominating the pontine tegmentum (**Fig. 4.88**). The *principal sensory nucleus* of the trigeminal

nerve relays afferents for touch and discrimination, while its *spinal nucleus* relays pain and temperature fibers. The trigeminal motor nucleus contains the motor neurons for the muscles of mastication. This nucleus, cranial nerve, and its tracts are important for jaw movement, swallowing, and speech.

Tracts: This section cuts the anterior spinocerebellar tract, which passes to the cerebellum, immediately dorsal to the pons.

CSF space: At this level, the cerebral aqueduct has given way to the fourth ventricle, which appears in cross section. It is covered dorsally by the medullary velum.

4.23.4 Transverse Section through the Lower Pons

Nuclei: The lower pons contains a number of cranial nerve nuclei including the nuclei of the vestibulocochlear and abducent nerves, and the facial (motor) nucleus. The rhomboid fossa is covered dorsally by the cerebellum, whose nuclei also appear in this section—the fastigial nucleus, emboliform nucleus, globose nucleus, and dentate nucleus (**Fig. 4.89**).

    Tracts: The trapezoid body with its subnuclei is an important relay station and crossing point in the auditory pathway. The central tegmental tract is an important pathway in the motor system.

4.24 Medulla Oblongata, Transverse Section

4.24.1 Transverse Section through the Upper Medulla Oblongata

Nuclei: The nuclei of the hypoglossal nerve, vagus nerve, vestibulocochlear nerve, and the spinal nucleus of the trigeminal nerve appear in the *dorsal* part of the medulla oblongata. The inferior olivary nucleus, which belongs to the motor system, is located in the *ventral* part of the medulla oblongata. The reticular formation

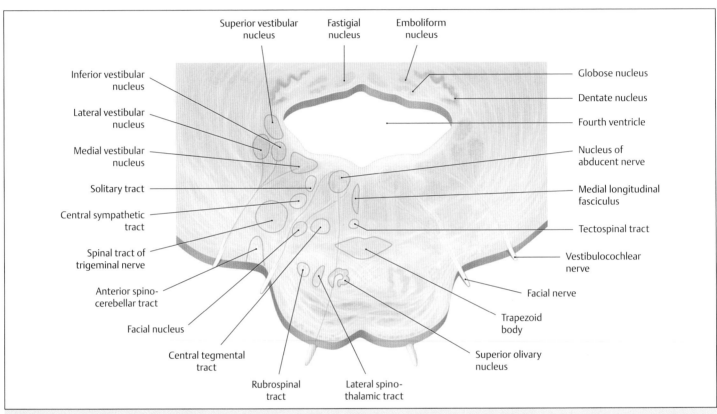

Fig. 4.89 Transverse section through the lower pons.

is interposed between the cranial nerve nuclei and the inferior olivary nucleus (**Fig. 4.90**). It appears in all the transverse sections of this unit.

Tracts: Most of the ascending and descending tracts are the same as in the previous unit. A new structure appearing at this level is the *inferior cerebellar peduncle*, through which afferent tracts pass to the cerebellum.

CSF space: The floor of the fourth ventricle is the rhomboid fossa, which marks the dorsal boundary of this section.

4.24.2 Transverse Section Just above the Middle of the Medulla Oblongata

Nuclei: The only cranial nerve nuclei visible at this level are those of the hypoglossal nerve, vagus nerve, and trigeminal nerve, appearing in the dorsal medulla. The lower portion of the inferior olivary nucleus appears in the ventral medulla (**Fig. 4.91**).

Tracts: The ascending and descending tracts are the same as in the previous unit. Ascending sensory tracts (from nuclei

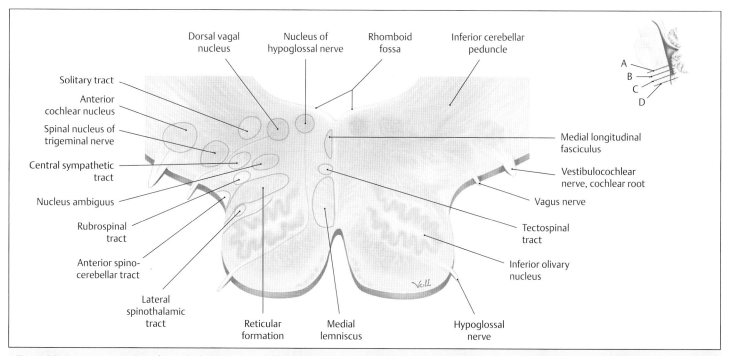

Fig. 4.90 Transverse section through the upper medulla oblongata. **A**, upper; **B**, middle; **C**, just below the middle; **D**, lower medulla oblongata.

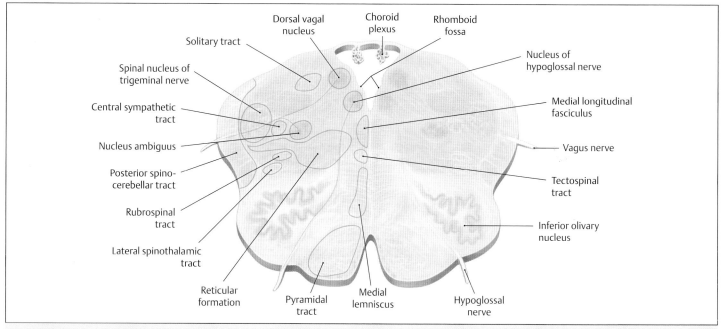

Fig. 4.91 Transverse section just above the middle of the medulla oblongata.

gracilis and cuneatus) decussate in the *medial lemniscus*. The solitary tract carries the gustatory fibers of cranial nerves V, VII, and X. Dorsolateral to it is the *nucleus of the solitary tract* (not shown). The *pyramidal tract* again appears as a compact structure at this level due to the absence of interspersed nuclei and decussating fibers.

4.24.3 Transverse Section Just below the Middle of the Medulla Oblongata

Nuclei: The nuclei of the hypoglossal, vagus, and trigeminal nerves appear at this level. The irregular outline of the inferior olivary nucleus is still just visible in the ventral medulla (**Fig. 4.92**). The nuclei that relay signals from the posterior

funiculus—the nucleus cuneatus and nucleus gracilis—appear prominently in the dorsal part of the section. The tracts that arise from these nuclei decussate in the medial lemniscus (see above).

Tracts: The ascending and descending tracts correspond to those in the previous diagrams. The rhomboid fossa, which is the floor of the fourth ventricle, has narrowed substantially at this level to become the central canal.

4.24.4 Transverse Section through the Lower Medulla Oblongata

The medulla oblongata is continuous with the spinal cord at this level, showing no distinct transition (**Fig. 4.93**).

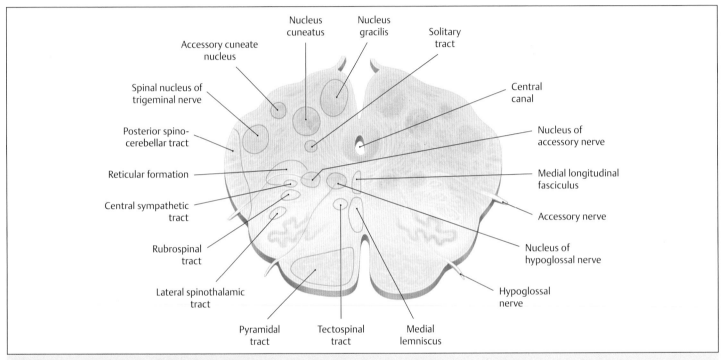

Fig. 4.92 Transverse section just below the middle of the medulla oblongata.

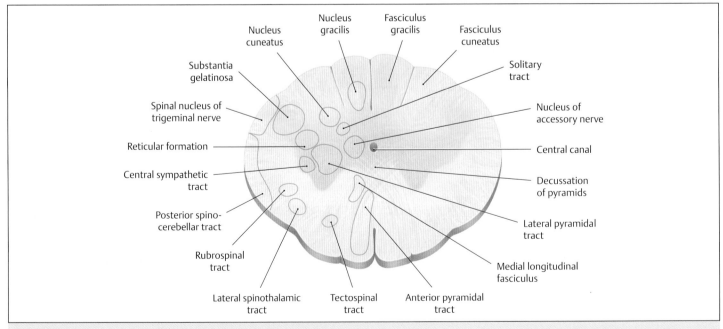

Fig. 4.93 Transverse section through the lower medulla oblongata.

Nuclei: The cranial nerve nuclei visible at this level are the spinal part of the trigeminal nerve and the nucleus of the accessory nerve. This section passes through the caudal ends of the nuclei in the relay station of the posterior funiculus—the nucleus cuneatus and nucleus gracilis.

Tracts: The ascending and descending tracts correspond to those in the previous diagrams of this unit. The section passes through the decussation of the pyramids, and we can now distinguish the anterior pyramidal tract (uncrossed) from the lateral pyramidal tract.

CSF space: This section passes through a portion of the central canal, which is markedly smaller at this level than in Chapter 4.24.3. It may even be obliterated at some sites, but this has no clinical significance.

4.25 Cerebellum, Internal Structure

4.25.1 The Cerebellum, Brainstem, and Diencephalon

Midsagittal section viewed from the left side, displaying the internal structure of the cerebellum (**Fig. 4.94**). The interior of the cerebellum is composed of *white matter* and its exterior of *gray matter (cerebellar cortex,* whose layers are shown in Chapter 4.25.4). This section again shows how the cerebellum abuts the fourth ventricle, in which the choroid plexus can be seen. The superior medullary velum forms the *upper* portion of the roof of

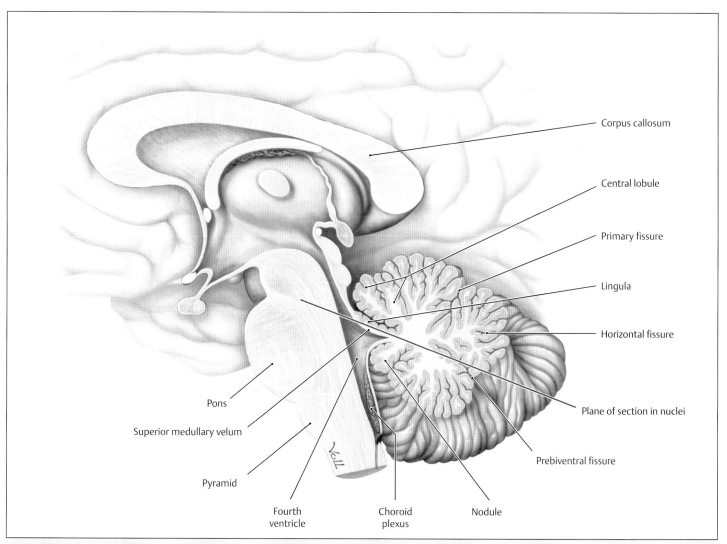

Corpus callosum

Central lobule

Primary fissure

Lingula

Horizontal fissure

Plane of section in nuclei

Prebiventral fissure

Pons

Superior medullary velum

Pyramid

Fourth ventricle

Choroid plexus

Nodule

Fig. 4.94 Midsagittal section viewed from the left side of the cerebellum.

the fourth ventricle; the lingula is closely apposed to its dorsal surface. The *lower* portion of the roof of the fourth ventricle is in contact with the cerebellar nodule. This section demonstrates how the cerebellar cortex is deeply folded into *folia* (gyri, not individually labeled), producing a treelike outline of the white matter called the *arbor vitae* ("tree of life").

4.25.2 Nuclei of the Cerebellum

Section through the superior cerebellar peduncles (plane of section shown in **Fig. 4.95**), viewed from behind. Deep within the cerebellar white matter are four pairs of nuclei that contain most of the *efferent* neurons of the cerebellum (**Fig. 4.95**):

- Fastigial nucleus (green)
- Emboliform nucleus (blue)
- Globose nuclei (blue)
- Dentate nucleus (pink)

The cortical regions have been color-coded to match their target nuclei. The dentate nucleus is the largest of the cerebellar nuclei and extends into the cerebellar hemispheres. The cerebellar nuclei receive projections from Purkinje cells in the cerebellar cortex (see Chapter 4.25.4). While the *efferent fibers* of the cerebellum can be assigned rather easily to anatomical structures, this is not true of the afferent fibers.

4.25.3 Cerebellar Nuclei and the Regions of the Cortex from Which They Receive Projections

See **Table 4.7.**

Table 4.7 Cerebellar nuclei

Cerebellar nucleus	Synonyms	Region of the cerebellar cortex that send axons to the nucleus
Dentate nucleus	Lateral cerebellar nucleus	Lateral part (lateral portions of the cerebellar hemispheres)
Emboliform nucleus	Anterior interpositus nucleus	Intermediate part (medial portions of the cerebellar hemispheres)
Globose nuclei	Posterior interpositus nucleus	Intermediate part (medial portions of the cerebellar hemispheres)
Fastigial nucleus	Medial cerebellar nucleus	Median part (cerebellar vermis)

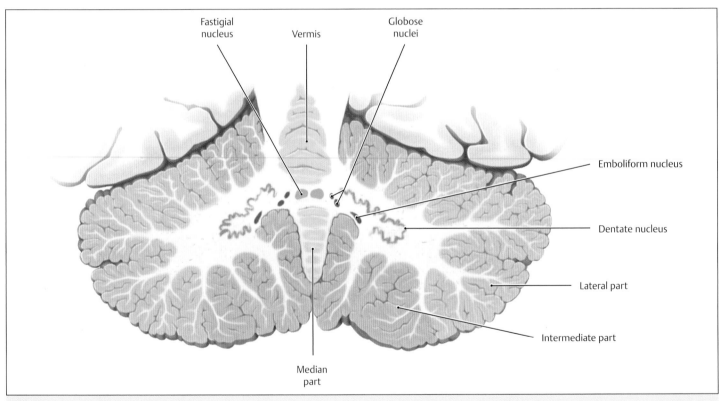

Fig. 4.95 Nuclei of the cerebellum.

4.25.4 Cerebellar Cortex

The cerebellar cortex (**Fig. 4.96**) consists of three layers:

- Molecular layer: outer layer; contains *parallel fibers*, which are the axons of granule cells (blue) from the granular layer. They run parallel to the cerebellar folia and terminate in the molecular layer, where they synapse into the dendrites of the Purkinje cells. This layer also contains axons from the inferior olive and its accessory nuclei *(climbing fibers)* and a small number of inhibitory interneurons *(basket and stellate neurons)*.
- Purkinje layer: Contains the cell bodies of *Purkinje cells* (purple).
- Granular layer: Contains mostly *granule cells* (blue), as well as *mossy* and *climbing fibers* (green and pink, respectively), and *Golgi cells* (not shown; the cell types are viewed in Chapter 4.25.6).

The white matter of the cerebellum is located under the granular layer.

Note: The Purkinje cells are the only efferent cells of the cerebellar cortex. They project to the cerebellar nuclei.

4.25.5 Synaptic Circuitry of the Cerebellum

The cerebellum comprises 10% of the mass of the brain, but contains up to 50% of its neurons. This enormous population (cerebellar granule cells alone may number in excess of 100 billion) is composed of a few cell types arranged in a repetitive, highly ordered array. This repetition of simple elements has led to the description of the cerebellum as an intricate synaptic computer for motor coordination (**Fig. 4.97**).

The basic cerebellar circuitry involves **afferents** including climbing and mossy fibers. *Climbing fibers* originate from the inferior olivary complex and form multiple excitatory synapses on the cell bodies and proximal dendritic tree of Purkinje cells (see Chapter 4.25.4); collateral branches synapse in the (deep) cerebellar nuclei. *Mossy fibers* originate in the vestibular and pontine nuclei and the spinal cord to form excitatory contacts with granule cells in synaptic complexes called cerebellar glomeruli (see Chapter 4.25.4); some branches excite local inhibitory neurons, and collaterals also enter the cerebellar nuclei. The axons of

granule cells form parallel fibers that form excitatory synapses on the dendritic trees of Purkinje cells. The Purkinje cells in turn send their axons mostly to the cerebellar nuclei (see Chapter 4.25.2, above; also to vestibular nuclei), where they make inhibitory synapses. The identities of some neurotransmitters in this pathway have been established: local inhibitory neurons, and Purkinje cells themselves, use γ-aminobutyric acid (GABA), while granule cells employ glutamate. Glutamate is probably also involved at mossy and climbing fiber synapses. The principal cerebellar **efferent** axons arise from the cerebellar nuclei. This circuitry combines direct activation (afferents to granule cells to Purkinje cells) and indirect inhibition (afferents to inhibitory interneurons to Purkinje cells), which may be integrated in a complex spatial pattern and temporal sequence in the cerebellar cortex and deep nuclei to provide indirect feedback control for motor coordination.

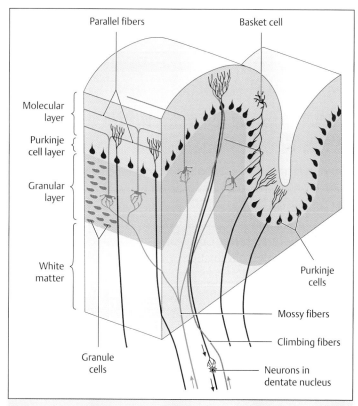

Fig. 4.96 Cerebellar cortex.

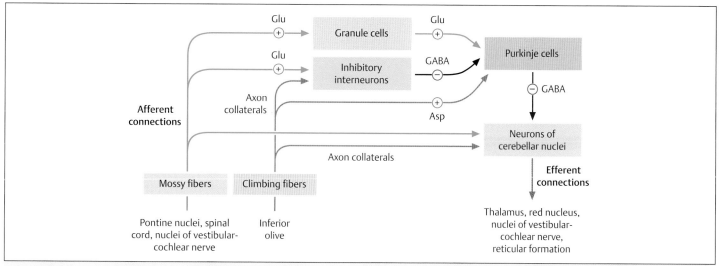

Fig. 4.97 Synaptic circuitry of the cerebellum.

4.25.6 Principal Neurons and Fiber Types in the Cerebellar Cortex

See **Table 4.8**.

Table 4.8 Types of cell bodies and axons in cerebellum

Name	Definition
Climbing fibers	Axons of neurons of the inferior olive and its associated nuclei
Mossy fibers	Axons of neurons of the pontine nuclei, the spinal cord, and vestibular nuclei (pontocerebellar, spinocerebellar, and vestibular tracts)
Parallel fibers (see Chapter 4.25.4)	Axons of granule cells
Granule cells	Interneurons of the cerebellar cortex
Purkinje cells	The only efferent cells of the cerebellar cortex; exert an inhibitory effect

4.26 Cerebellum, Simplified Functional Anatomy and Lesions

4.26.1 Simplified Functional Anatomy of the Cerebellum

Two-dimensional representation of the cerebellum. Left: afferent inputs to the cerebellar cortex; right: paths of cerebellar (efferent) output (**Fig. 4.98**).

The coordination of motor activity by the cerebellum can be divided into three broad categories corresponding to the areas responsible for the coordination:

- Maintenance of posture and balance ("vestibulocerebellum")
- Dynamic control of muscle tone under various loads ("spinocerebellum")
- Integration of activity of various muscle groups during complex tasks ("pontocerebellum")

These categories of cerebellar function require different types of afferent information, and have different output (efferent) paths. Although afferent inputs and their corresponding tracts are not segregated by obvious anatomical boundaries in the cerebellum, there is a functional division that correlates with the evolution of the cerebellar structures (see Chapter 4.26.2). The phylogenetically ancient part of the cerebellum (archicerebellum) receives vestibular input, projects to the fastigial nucleus and lateral vestibular nucleus, and controls trunk musculature through a "medial motor system." Dynamic control of muscle tone requires feedback from muscle and tendon proprioceptors entering the cerebellum through spinocerebellar tracts. This "spinocerebellar" function utilizes more recently evolved paleocerebellar structures, the emboliform and globose cerebellar nuclei, and modulates muscle activity through a "lateral motor system" that involves muscles in the extremities. The most recent evolutionary developments in the cerebellum include the significant expansion of cerebral cortical projections via a relay in the pons, and a reciprocal massive cerebellar projection, through the dentate nucleus, back to the cerebral cortex via the thalamus. The neocerebellum thus sends information back to the cerebral cortex, which controls some musculature directly through corticobulbar (corticonuclear) projections to lower motor neurons controlling the tongue and face, and corticospinal projections to spinal motor neurons controlling the hands. This "pontocerebellar" pathway and function involve complex anticipatory activation of muscle groups to accept a load or limit a motion, and so can be characterized in part as a "planning" or "programming" function.

Note: This simplified outline of cerebellar function does not take into account the complexity of cerebellar contributions to a variety of other tasks. Visual inputs and oculomotor functions, specifically, have not been considered here.

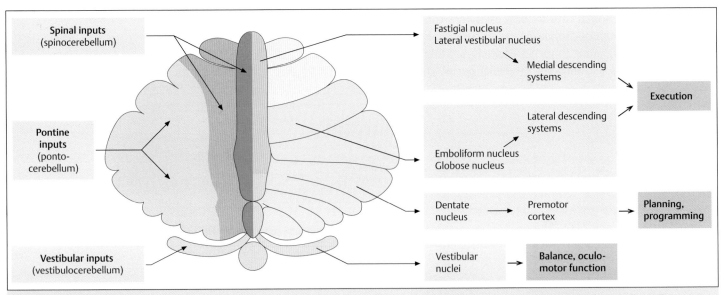

Fig. 4.98 Two-dimensional representation of the cerebellum. (left) Afferent inputs to the cerebellar cortex. (right) Paths of cerebellar (efferent) output.

4.26.2 Synopsis of Cerebellar Classifications and Their Relationships to Motor Deficits

Some cerebellar lesions cause subtle cognitive deficits that cannot be explained simply as a loss of muscle coordination (**Table 4.9**).

4.26.3 Cerebellar Lesions

Cerebellar lesions may remain clinically silent for some time because other brain regions can functionally compensate for them with reasonable effectiveness. Exceptions are direct lesions of the efferent cerebellar nuclei, which cannot be clinically compensated (**Table 4.10**).

Table 4.9 Signs and symptoms of cerebellar damage

Functional classification	Phylogenetic classification	Anatomical classification	Deficit symptoms

Vestibulocerebellum	Archicerebellum	Flocculonodular lobe	• Truncal, stance, and gait ataxia
			  ◦ Vertigo
			  ◦ Nystagmus
			• Vomiting

Spinocerebellum	Paleocerebellum	Anterior lobe, parts of vermis; Posterior lobe, medial parts	• Ataxia, chiefly affecting the lower limb ◦ Oculomotor dysfunction • Speech disorder (asynergy of speech muscles of speech production)

Pontocerebellum (= cerebrocerebellum)	Neocerebellum	Posterior lobe, hemispheres	• Dysmetria and hypermetria (positive rebound)
			  ◦ Intention tremor
			  ◦ Nystagmus
			• Decreased muscle tone[a]

[a]*Speech note:* Lesions to the cerebellum are related to a type of motor speech disorder known as ataxic dysarthria. Ataxic dysarthria is related to the general motor impairment associated with the coordination and fine-tuning of motor output associated with the cerebellum. Ataxic dysarthric speech is evident by irregularity and incoordination of the fine and fast motor movements needed for connected speech. The disorder is characterized by a primary disruption of articulation and prosody. Irregular alternating movements can be heard and seen during tasks such as the AMR production of /pa-ta-ka/ as well as in connected speech. Some suggest the underlying causal links to ataxic dysarthria may be problems of speech motor programming as well as speech execution deficits. The cerebellum is relatively unstudied in such motor speech disorders as apraxia of speech, but the motor planning and programming functions of this "little cabbage" (cerebellum) would seem to suggest that perhaps the motor planning and programming problems apparent in apraxia of speech might make this structure an attractive candidate for future research. Moreover, neuroimaging research is helping to clarify models of cerebellar contributions to speech processing and production, and suggests possible regions of speech localization within the cerebellum.

Table 4.10 Cerebellar symptoms

Asynergy	Lack of coordination among different muscle groups, especially in the performance of fine movements.
Ataxia	Uncoordinated sequence of movements. Truncal ataxia (patient cannot sit quietly upright) is distinguished from stance and gait ataxia (impaired limb movements, such as an unsteady gait in inebriation). The patient stands with the legs spread apart and places his or hand on the wall for stability (**Fig. 4.99a**).
Decreased muscle tone	Ipsilateral muscle weakness and rapid fatigability (asthenia).
Intention tremor	Involuntary, rhythmical wavering movement of the hand when a purposeful movement is attempted, as in the finger–nose test: normal test (**Fig. 4.99b**), test indicating a cerebellar lesion (**Fig. 4.99c**).
Rebound phenomenon	The patient, with eyes closed, is told to move the arm against a resistance from the examiner (**Fig. 4.99d**). When the examiner suddenly releases the arm, it forcefully "rebounds" toward the patient (hypermetria).

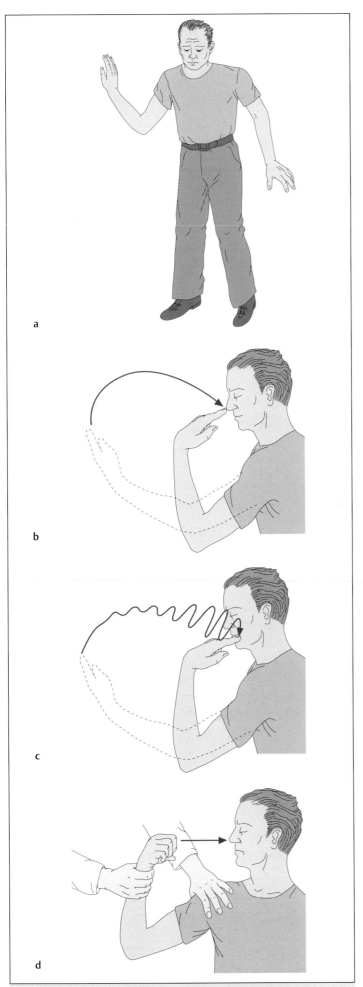

a

b

c

d

Fig. 4.99 Cerebellar symptoms. **(a)** Ataxia. **(b)** Finger-nose test. **(c)** Test indicating a cerebellar lesion. **(d)** Rebound phenomenon.

4.27 Vertebral Column and Vertebrae

Left lateral view (**Fig. 4.100**). The spinal (vertebral) column is divided into four regions: the cervical, thoracic, lumbar, and sacral spines. In the neonate, all regions demonstrate an anteriorly concave curvature. This single concave curvature in the neonate is referred to as the primary curvature of the vertebral column.

During development, the cervical and lumbar regions of the vertebral column develop anteriorly convex curvatures. These changes are referred to as secondary curvatures. The cervical secondary curvature develops as infants begin to hold up their heads. The lumbar secondary curvatures are the result of upright bipedal locomotion.

Kyphosis is a pathological condition where the thoracic primary curvature is abnormally exaggerated (hunchback, rounded back). Lordosis is a pathological condition where the secondary curvatures are exaggerated. Lordosis may occur in either the cervical or lumbar regions (swayback) of the vertebral column. Differing from the abnormal development of primary and secondary curvatures, scoliosis is an abnormal lateral deviation of the vertebral column.

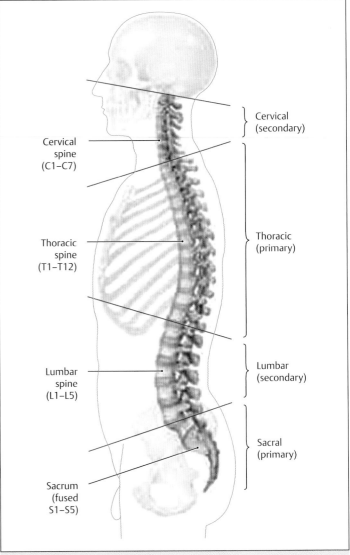

Cervical (secondary)

Cervical spine (C1–C7)

Thoracic (primary)

Thoracic spine (T1–T12)

Lumbar spine (L1–L5)

Lumbar (secondary)

Sacral (primary)

Sacrum (fused S1–S5)

Fig. 4.100 Spinal curvature.

Left lateral view (**Fig. 4.101a**). Posterior view (**Fig. 4.101b**). The vertebral column is divided into four regions: cervical, thoracic, lumbar, and sacral. Each vertebra consists of a vertebral body and vertebral (neural) arch. The vertebral bodies (with intervening intervertebral disks) form the load-bearing component of the vertebral column. The vertebral (neural) arches enclose the vertebral canal, protecting the spinal cord.

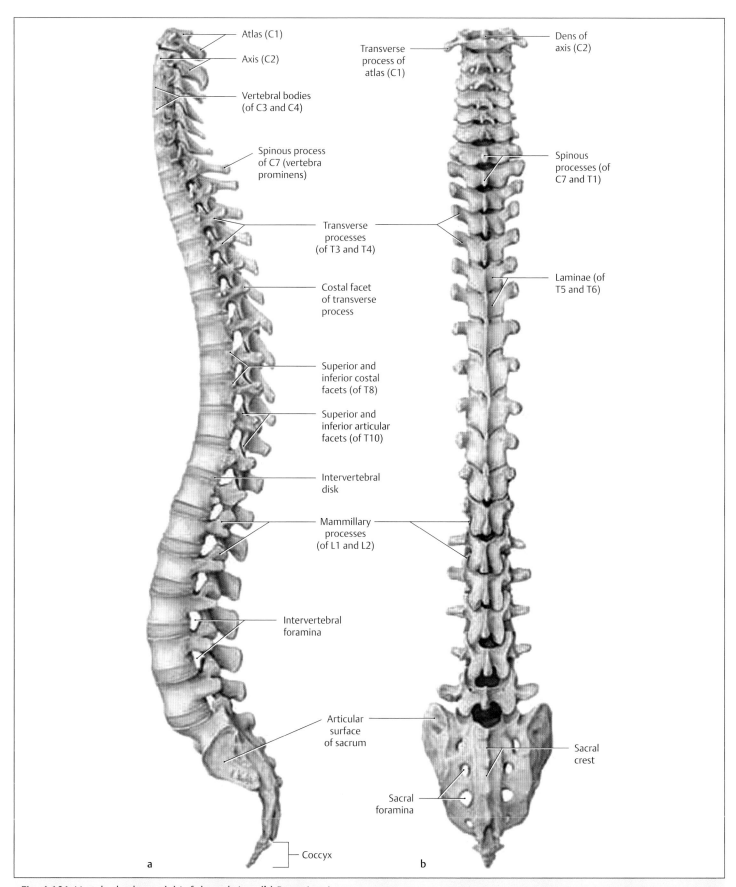

Atlas (C1)

Axis (C2)

Vertebral bodies (of C3 and C4)

Spinous process of C7 (vertebra prominens)

Transverse processes (of T3 and T4)

Costal facet of transverse process

Superior and inferior costal facets (of T8)

Superior and inferior articular facets (of T10)

Intervertebral disk

Mammillary processes (of L1 and L2)

Intervertebral foramina

Articular surface of sacrum

Coccyx

a

Transverse process of atlas (C1)

Dens of axis (C2)

Spinous processes (of C7 and T1)

Laminae (of T5 and T6)

Sacral crest

Sacral foramina

b

Fig. 4.101 Vertebral column. (a) Left lateral view. (b) Posterior view.

Schematic, left oblique posterosuperior view (**Fig. 4.102**). Each vertebra consists of a load-bearing body and an arch that encloses the vertebral foramen. The arch is divided into the pedicle and lamina. Vertebrae have transverse and spinous processes that provide sites of attachment for muscles. Vertebrae articulate at facets on the superior and inferior articular processes. Thoracic vertebrae articulate with ribs at costal facets.

Superior view (**Fig. 4.103**). (a) Cervical vertebra (C4). (b) Thoracic vertebra (T6). (c) Lumbar vertebra (L4). (d) Sacrum. The vertebral bodies increase in size cranially to caudally.

Each vertebra consists of a body and an arch that enclose the vertebral foramen. The types of vertebrae can be distinguished particularly easily by examining their transverse processes. The sacrum has structures that are analogous to the other vertebrae (**Table 4.11**).

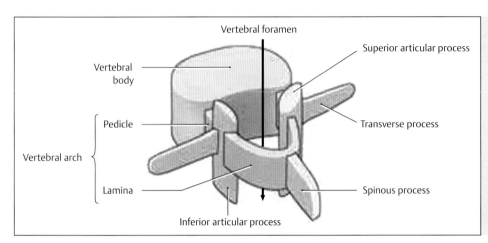

Fig. 4.102 Structure of vertebrae.

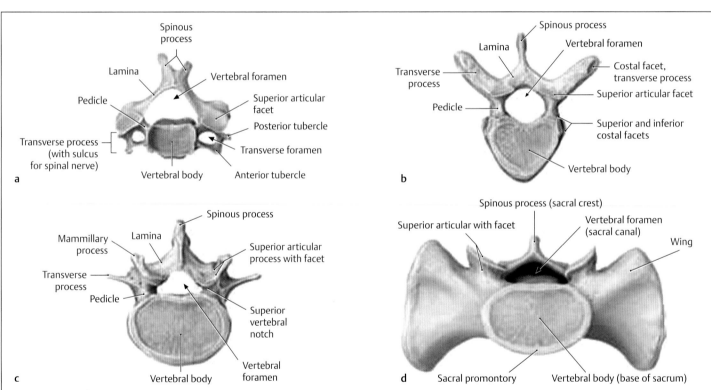

Fig. 4.103 Typical vertebrae. **(a)** Cervical vertebra (C4). **(b)** Thoracic vertebra (T6). **(c)** Lumbar vertebra (L4). **(d)** Sacrum.

Table 4.11 Structural elements of vertebrae

Vertebrae	Body	Foramen	Transverse process	Spinous process
Cervical vertebrae C3–C7	Small (kidney-shaped)	Large (triangular)	Transverse foramina	C3–C5: short C7: long C3–C6: bifid
Thoracic vertebrae T1–T12	Medium (heart-shaped) with costal facets	Small (circular)	Costal facets	Long
Lumbar vertebrae L1–L5	Large (kidney-shaped)	Medium (triangular)	Mammillary processes	Short and broad
Sacrum (fused S1–S5)	Large to small (decreases from base to apex)	Sacral canal (triangular)	Fused (forms wing of sacrum)	Short (median sacral crest)

4.28 Spinal Cord, Segmental Organization

4.28.1 Development of the Spinal Cord

Transverse section, superior view (**Fig. 4.104**).

(a) Early neural tube, (b) intermediate stage, (c) adult spinal cord. The spinal cord develops from the neural tube.

- **Posterior horn:** Develops from the posterior part of the neural tube (the *alar plate*). It contains the afferent (sensory) neurons.
- **Anterior horn:** Develops from the anterior part of the neural tube (the *basal plate*). It contains the efferent (motor) neurons.
- **Lateral column:** Develops from the intervening zone. Present only in the thoracic, lumbar, and sacral regions of the cord, it contains the autonomic (sympathetic and parasympathetic) neurons.

Neurons do not develop from the roof or floor plates. Viewing the spinal cord in transverse section, we see that it consists of gray matter that is arranged about the central canal and is surrounded by white matter. The **gray matter** contains the cell bodies of neurons while the **white matter** consists of nerve fibers (axons).

Note: Axons that have the same function are collected into bundles called *tracts*. Tracts that terminate in the brain are called *ascending*, *afferent*, or *sensory* tracts, while tracts that pass from the brain into the spinal cord are called *descending*, *efferent*, or *motor* tracts.

4.28.2 Structure of a Spinal Cord Segment

See **Fig. 4.105**.

Two main organizational principles are observed in the spinal cord:

1. **Functional organization within a segment** (viewed in a transverse section of the spinal cord). In each spinal cord segment, the *afferent* dorsal rootlets enter the back of the cord while the *efferent* ventral rootlets emerge from the front of the cord. The rootlets in each set combine to form the dorsal (posterior) and ventral (anterior) roots. Each dorsal and ventral root fuse to form a mixed *spinal nerve*, which carries both sensory and motor fibers. Shortly after the fusion of its two roots, the spinal nerve divides into various branches.
2. **Topographical organization of the segments** (viewed in a longitudinal section of the spinal cord). The spinal cord consists of a vertical series of 31 segments (see Chapter 4.28.3), each of which innervates a specific area in the trunk and limbs.

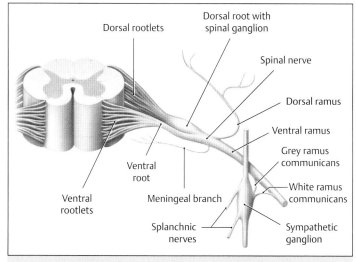

Fig. 4.105 Structure of a spinal cord segment.

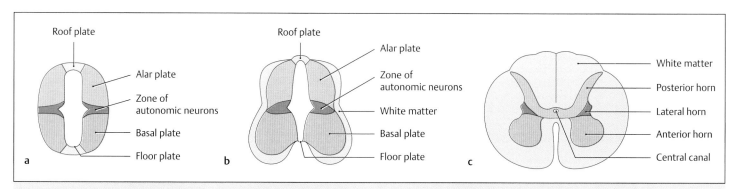

Fig. 4.104 Development of the spinal cord. **(a)** Early neural tube. **(b)** Intermediate stage. **(c)** Adult spinal cord.

4.28.3 Spinal Cord and Spinal Ganglia In Situ

Posterior view with the laminar arches of the vertebral bodies removed (**Fig. 4.106**). The longitudinal growth of the spinal cord lags behind that of the bony vertebral column. As a result, the lower end of the spinal cord in the adult lies at approximately the level of the first lumbar vertebral body (L1, see Chapter 4.28.4). Below L1, the spinal nerve roots descend from the end of the cord to the intervertebral foramina, where they join to form the spinal nerves. The collection of these spinal roots is called the *cauda equina* ("horse's tail").

4.28.4 Spinal Cord Segments and Vertebral Bodies in the Adult

- Midsagittal section, viewed from the right side (**Fig. 4.107**). The spinal cord can be divided into four major regions: cervical cord (C, pink); thoracic cord (T, blue); lumbar cord (L, green); and sacral cord (S, yellow). The spinal cord segments are numbered according to the exit point of their associated nerves and do not necessarily correlate numerically with the nearest skeletal element (see **Table 4.12**). The spinal cord generally terminates at the level of the L1 vertebral body and the region below this is known as the *cauda equina*. The cauda equina consists of dorsal (sensory) and ventral

(motor) spinal nerve roots, and provides safe access for introducing a spinal needle to sample CSF (lumbar puncture).

- Differential growth of the spinal cord and vertebral column may separate spinal cord segments from their associated skeletal elements, with progressively greater "mismatch" occurring at more caudal levels (**Table 4.12**). It is important to know the relationship of the spinal cord segments to the

Table 4.12 Relationship of spinal cord segments to vertebral bodies

Spinal cord segment	Vertebral body	Spinous process
C8	Inferior margin of C6, superior margin of C7	C6
T6	T5	T4
T12	T10	T9
L3	T11	T11
S1	T12	T12

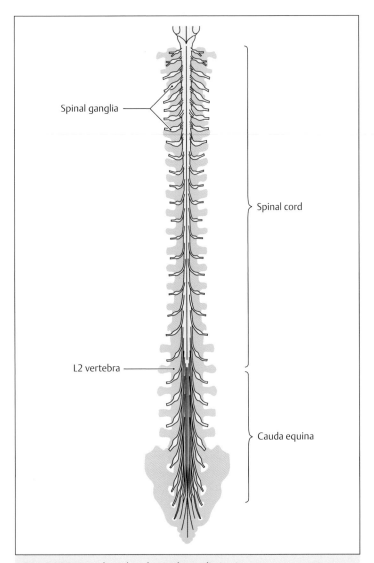

Fig. 4.106 Spinal cord and spinal ganglia in situ.

Spinal ganglia

Spinal cord

L2 vertebra

Cauda equina

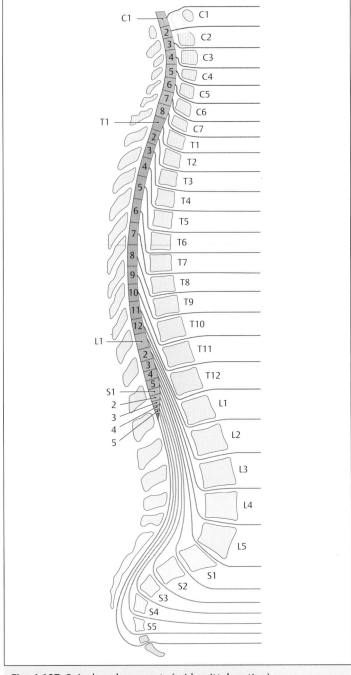

Fig. 4.107 Spinal cord segments (midsagittal section).

associated vertebral bodies when assessing injuries to the vertebral column (e.g., spinal fracture and cord lesions). The parts in the table are only approximations and may differ slightly in individual cases.

Note: There are only seven cervical vertebrae (C1–C7), but eight pairs of cervical nerves (C1–C8).

4.28.5 Simplified Schematic Representation of the Segmental Innervation of the Skin

Distribution of the dermatomes on the body. Sensory innervation of the skin correlates with the sensory roots of the spinal nerves in **Fig. 4.108**. Every spinal cord segment (except for C1, see below) innervates a particular skin area (= dermatome). From a clinical standpoint, it is important to know the precise correlation of dermatomes with spinal cord segments so that the level of a spinal cord lesion can be determined based on the location of the affected dermatome. For example, a lesion of the C8 spinal nerve root is characterized by a loss of sensation on the ulnar (small finger) side of the hand.

   Note: There is no C1 dermatome because the first spinal nerve is purely motor.

4.29 Tracts of the Spinal Cord, Overview

4.29.1 Ascending Tracts in the Spinal Cord

Ascending tracts are afferent (= sensory) pathways that carry information from the trunk and limbs to the brain (**Fig. 4.109**). The most important ascending tracts and their functions are listed below.

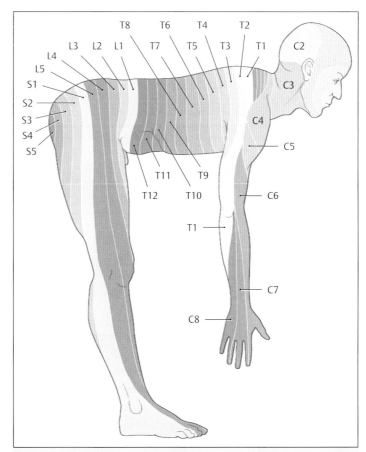

Fig. 4.108 Simplified schematic representation of the segmental innervation of the skin.

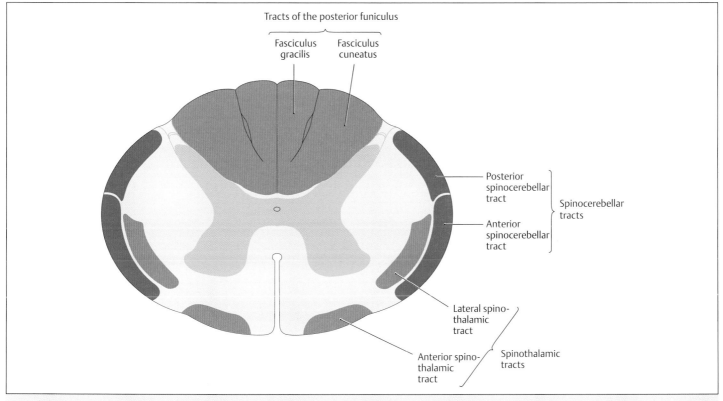

Fig. 4.109 Transverse section through the spinal cord (ascending tracts).

Spinothalamic Tracts

- Anterior spinothalamic tract (coarse touch sensation)
- Lateral spinothalamic tract (pain and temperature sensation)

Tracts of the Posterior Funiculus

- Fasciculus gracilis (fine touch sensation, conscious proprioception of the *lower* limb)
- Fasciculus cuneatus (fine touch sensation, conscious proprioception of the upper limb).

Spinocerebellar Tracts

- Anterior spinocerebellar tract (unconscious proprioception to the cerebellum)
- Posterior spinocerebellar tract (unconscious proprioception to the cerebellum)

Proprioception involves the perception of limb position in space ("position sense"). It lets us know, for example, that our arm is in front of or behind our chest even when our eyes are closed. The information involved in proprioception is complex. Thus, our position sense tells us where our joints are in relation to one another while our motion sense (kinesthesia) tells us the speed and direction of joint movements. Proprioception and kinesthesia are seen as interrelated, and there is considerable disagreement regarding the definition of these terms. Some of this difficulty stems from the British neurologist Sherrington's original description of joint position sense (or the ability to determine exactly where a particular body part is in space) and kinesthesia (or the sensation that the body part has moved) under a more general heading of proprioception. People that have a limb amputated may still have a confused sense of that limb existence on their body, known as phantom limb syndrome. Phantom sensations can occur as passive proprioceptive sensations of the limb's presence, or more active sensations such as perceived movement, pressure, pain, itching, or temperature. Phantom sensations and phantom pain also may be experienced after removal of body parts other than the limbs, such as after amputation of the breast, extraction of a tooth (phantom tooth pain), or removal of an eye (phantom eye syndrome). We also have a "force sense" by which we can perceive the muscular force that is associated with joint movements. Moreover, proprioception takes place on both a conscious (I know that my hand is making a fist in my pants pocket without seeing it) and an unconscious level, enabling us to ride a bicycle and climb stairs without thinking about it.

4.29.2 Descending Tracts in the Spinal Cord

The descending tracts of the spinal cord are concerned with motor function (body movement). They convey information from higher motor centers to the motor neurons in the spinal cord (**Fig. 4.110**).

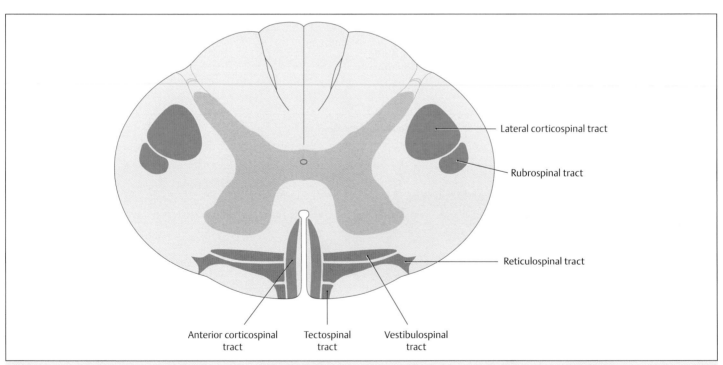

Fig. 4.110 Transverse section through the spinal cord (descending tracts).

Lateral corticospinal tract

Rubrospinal tract

Reticulospinal tract

Anterior corticospinal tract

Tectospinal tract

Vestibulospinal tract

According to a relatively recent classification (not yet fully accepted in clinical medicine), the descending tracts of the spinal cord can be divided into two motor systems:

- **Lateral motor system** (concerned with fine, precise motor skills in the hands):
  - Pyramidal tract (anterior and lateral corticospinal tract)
  - Rubrospinal tract
- **Medial motor system** (innervates medially situated motor neurons controlling trunk movement and stance):
  - Reticulospinal tract
  - Tectospinal tract
  - Vestibulospinal tract

Except for the pyramidal tract, which may be represented as a monosynaptic pathway in a simplified scheme, it is difficult to offer a simple and direct classification of the motor system because sequences of movements are programmed and coordinated in multiple feedback mechanisms called "motor loops." There is no point, then, in listing the various tracts in a simplified table. While the tracts can be distinguished rather clearly from one another at the level of the spinal cord, their fibers are so intermixed at the higher cortical levels that isolated motor disturbances (unlike sensory disturbances) essentially do not occur at the level of the spinal cord.

4.30 Spinal Cord, Topography

4.30.1 Spinal Cord and Spinal Nerve in the Vertebral Canal at the Level of the C4 Vertebra

Transverse section viewed from above (**Fig. 4.111**). The spinal cord occupies the center of the vertebral foramen and is anchored within the subarachnoid space to the spinal dura mater by the denticulate ligament. The root sleeve, an outpouching of the dura

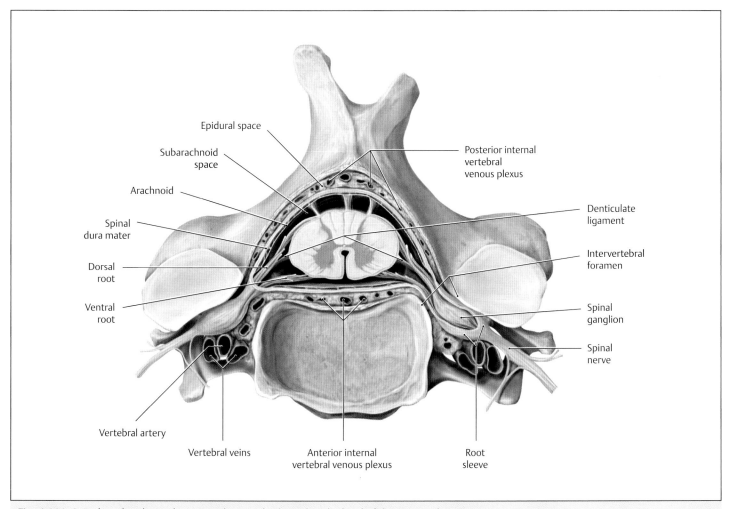

Fig. 4.111 Spinal cord and spinal nerve in the vertebral canal at the level of the C4 vertebra.

mater in the intravertebral foramen, contains the spinal ganglion and the dorsal and ventral roots of the spinal nerve. The spinal dura mater is bounded externally by the epidural space, which contains venous plexuses, fat, and connective tissue. The epidural space extends upward as far as the foramen magnum, where the dura becomes fused to the cranial periosteum.

4.30.2 Cauda Equina at the Level of the L2 Vertebra

Transverse section viewed from below (**Fig. 4.112**). The spinal cord usually ends at the level of the first lumbar vertebra (L1). The space below the lower end of the spinal cord is occupied by the cauda equina and filum terminale in the dural sac, which ends at the level of the S2 vertebra (see Chapter 4.30.3). The epidural space expands at that level and contains extensive venous plexuses and fatty tissue.

4.30.3 Cauda Equina in the Vertebral Canal

Posterior view (**Fig. 4.113**). The laminae and the dorsal surface of the sacrum have been partially removed. The spinal cord in the

adult terminates at approximately level of the first lumbar vertebra (L1). The dorsal and ventral spinal nerve roots extending from the lower end of the spinal cord (conus medullaris) are known collectively as the cauda equina. During lumbar puncture at this level, a needle introduced into the subarachnoid space (lumbar cistern) normally slips past the spinal nerve roots without injuring them.

4.30.4 The Spinal Cord, Dural Sac, and Vertebral Column at Different Ages

Anterior view (**Fig. 4.114**). As an individual grows, the longitudinal growth of the spinal cord increasingly lags behind that of the vertebral column. At birth, the distal end of the spinal cord, the conus medullaris, is at the level of the L3 vertebral body (where lumbar puncture is contraindicated). The spinal cord of a tall adult ends at the T12/L1 level, while that of a short adult extends to the L2/L3 level. The dural sac always extends into the upper sacrum. It is important to consider these anatomical relationships during lumbar puncture. For lumbar puncture (spinal tap) the needle is inserted at the L3/L4 interspace (see Chapter 4.30.5).

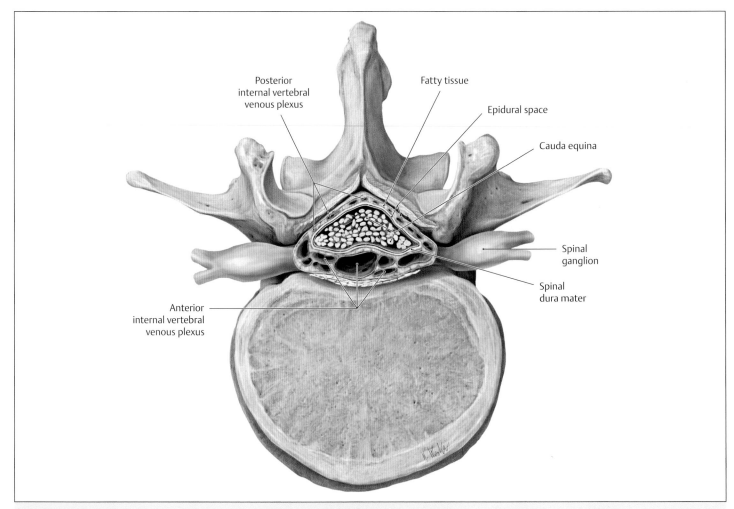

Fig. 4.112 Cauda equina at the level of the L2 vertebra.

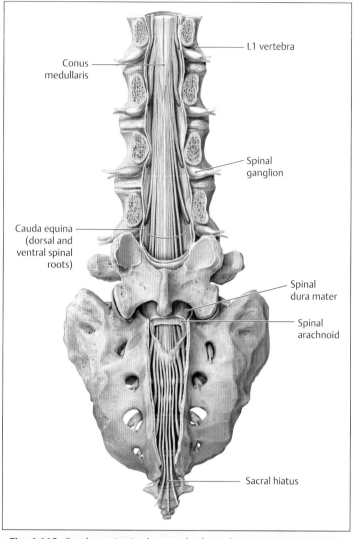

Fig. 4.113 Cauda equina in the vertebral canal.

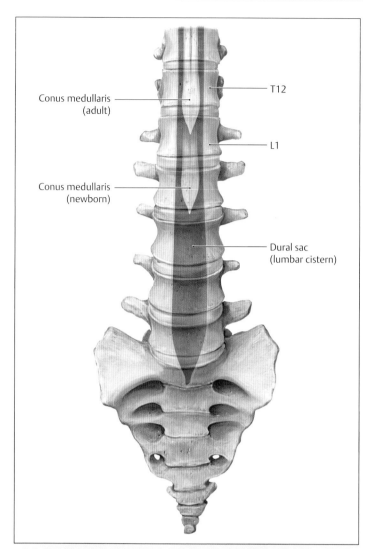

Fig. 4.114 The spinal cord, dural sac, and vertebral column at different ages.

4.30.5 Lumbar Puncture, Epidural Anesthesia, and Lumbar Anesthesia

In preparation for a **lumbar puncture**, the patient bends far forward to separate the spinous processes of the lumbar spine (**Fig. 4.115**). The spinal needle is usually introduced between the spinous processes of the L3 and L4 vertebrae. It is advanced through the skin and into the dural sac (lumbar cistern, see Chapter 4.30.4) to obtain a CSF sample. This procedure has numerous applications, including the diagnosis of meningitis. Lumbar puncture (also known as a spinal tap) is important in the diagnosis of infections and certain inflammatory diseases (e.g., multiple sclerosis, Guillain–Barre syndrome, and vasculitis). Lumbar puncture with CSF analysis is also an important diagnostic tool in sudden-onset headache primarily to test for a type of bleeding around the brain (subarachnoid hemorrhage) and certain malignant conditions. For **epidural anesthesia**, a catheter is placed in the epidural space without penetrating the dural sac (1). **Lumbar anesthesia** is induced by injecting a local anesthetic solution into the dural sac (2). Another option is to pass the needle into the epidural space through the sacral hiatus (3).

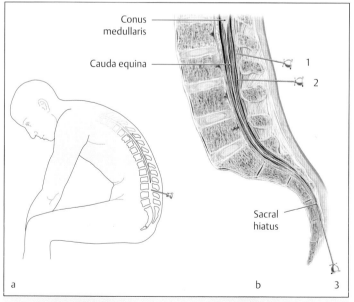

Fig. 4.115 (**a, b**) Lumbar puncture.

5 Cranial Nerves

5.1 Overview of the Cranial Nerves

5.1.1 Functional Components of the Cranial Nerves

The twelve pairs of cranial nerves are designated by Roman numerals according to the order of their emergence from the brainstem (see topographical organization in Chapter 5.1.3).

Note: The first two cranial nerves, the olfactory nerve (CN I) and optic nerve (CN II), are not peripheral nerves in the true sense rather extensions of the brain, that is, they are central nervous system (CNS) pathways that are covered by meninges and contain cell types occurring exclusively in the CNS (oligodendrocytes and microglial cells).

Like the spinal nerves, the cranial nerves may contain both *afferent* and *efferent* axons. These axons belong either to the somatic nervous system, which enables the organism to interact with its environment *(somatic fibers)*, or to the autonomic nervous system, which regulates the activity of the internal organs *(visceral fibers)*. The combinations of these different *general* fiber types in spinal nerves result in four possible compositions that are found chiefly in spinal nerves but also occur in cranial nerves (see functional organization in Chapter 5.1.3).

5.1.2 Color Coding Used in Subsequent Units to Indicate Different Fiber Types

See **Fig. 5.1**.

General somatic afferents (somatic sensation):
- Fibers convey impulses from the skin and striated muscle spindles

General visceral afferents (visceral sensation):
- Fibers convey impulses from the viscera and blood vessels

General visceral efferents (visceromotor function):
- Fibers innervate the smooth muscle of the viscera, intraocular muscles, heart, salivary glands, etc.

General somatic efferents (somatomotor function):
- Fibers innervate striated muscles

Additionally, cranial nerves may contain special fiber types that are associated with particular structures in the head:

Special somatic afferents:
- Fibers conduct impulses from the retina and from the auditory and vestibular apparatus

Special visceral afferents:
- Fibers conduct impulses from the taste buds of the tongue and from the olfactory mucosa

Special visceral efferents:
- Fibers innervate striated muscles derived from the branchial arches *(branchiogenic efferents and branchiogenic muscles)*

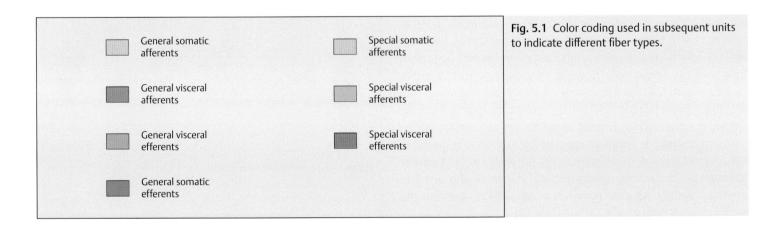

General somatic afferents

General visceral afferents

General visceral efferents

General somatic efferents

Special somatic afferents

Special visceral afferents

Special visceral efferents

Fig. 5.1 Color coding used in subsequent units to indicate different fiber types.

5.1.3 Topographical and Functional Organization of the Cranial Nerves

See **Table 5.1**.

A characteristic feature of the cranial nerves is that their sensory and motor fibers enter and exit the brainstem at the same sites. This differs from the spinal nerves, in which the sensory fibers enter the spinal cord through the dorsal roots while the motor fibers leave the spinal cord through the ventral roots. The cranial nerves are especially important to speech and swallowing in that they innervate the primary head and neck structures responsible for carrying out these acts. On the subsequent pages we will present details on only those cranial nerves that are most associated with speech and swallowing—CN V, VII, VIII, IX, X, XI, and XII.

See **Fig. 5.2** and **Table 5.2**.

Table 5.1 Origin, name, and function of cranial nerves

Topographical origin	Name	Functional fiber type
Telencephalon	• Olfactory nerve (CN I)	• Special visceral afferent
Diencephalon	• Optic nerve (CN II)	• Special somatic afferent
Mesencephalon	• Oculomotor nerve (CN III)[a]	• Somatic efferent
	• Trochlear nerve (CN IV)[a]	• Visceral efferent (parasympathetic)
		• Somatic efferent
Pons	• Trigeminal nerve (CN V)	• Special visceral efferent *(first branchial arch)*
		• Somatic afferent
	• Abducent nerve (CN VI)[a]	• Somatic efferent
	• Facial nerve (CN VII)	• Special visceral efferent *(second branchial arch)*
		• Special visceral afferent
		• Visceral efferent (parasympathetic)
		• Somatic afferent
Medulla oblongata	• Vestibulocochlear nerve (CN VIII)	• Special somatic afferent
	• Glossopharyngeal nerve (CN IX)	• Special visceral efferent *(third branchial arch)*
		• Special visceral afferent
		• Visceral afferent (parasympathetic)
		• Somatic afferent
	• Vagus nerve (CN X)	• Special visceral efferent *(fourth branchial arch)*
		• Special visceral afferent
		• Visceral efferent (parasympathetic)
		• Visceral afferent
		• Somatic afferent
	• Accessory nerve (CN XI)[a]	• Special visceral efferent *(fifth branchial arch)*
		• Somatic efferent
	• Hypoglossal nerve (CN XII)[a]	• Somatic efferent

[a] *Note:* Cranial nerves with somatic efferent fibers innervating the striated muscles also have somatic afferent fibers that conduct proprioceptive impulses from the muscle spindles and other structures (for clarity, not listed above).

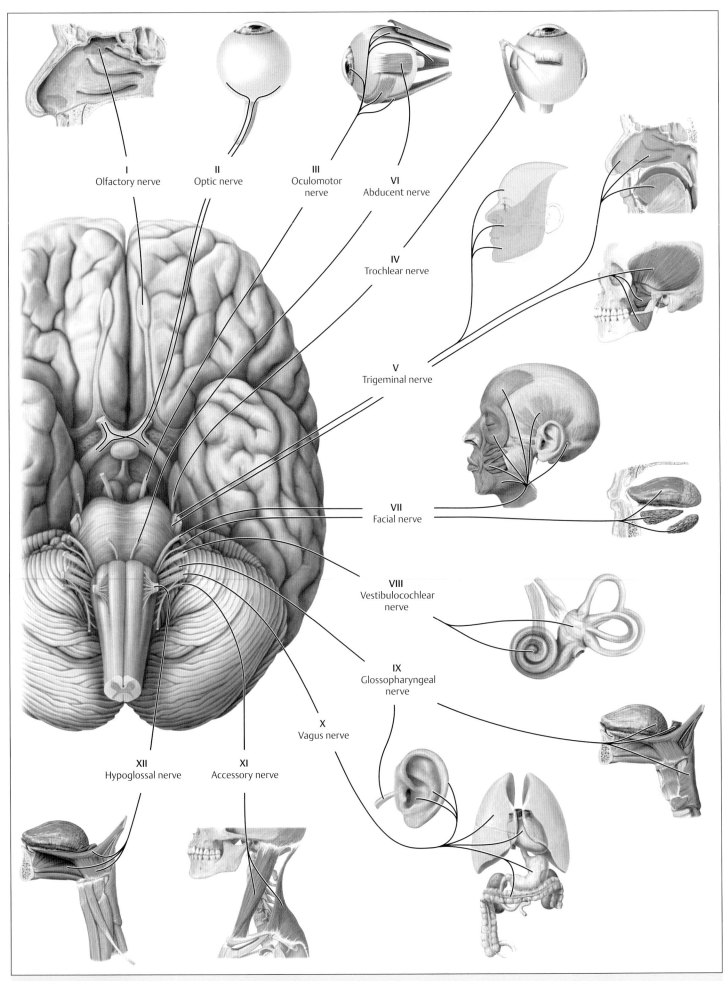

Fig. 5.2 Cranial nerves.

Table 5.2 Cranial nerve function

Cranial nerve		Passage through skull	Fiber A	Fiber E	Sensory territory (afferent) / Target organ (efferent)
CN I: Olfactory n.		Ethmoid bone (cribriform plate)	●		Smell: special viscerosensory fibers from olfactory mucosa of nasal cavity
CN II: Optic n.		Optic canal	●		Sight: special somatosensory fibers from retina
CN III: Oculomotor n.		Superior orbital fissure		●	Somatomotor innervation: to levator palpebrae superioris and four extraocular mm. (superior, medial, and inferior rectus, and inferior oblique)
				●	Parasympathetic innervation: preganglionic fibers to ciliary ganglion; postganglionic fibers to intraocular mm. (ciliary mm. and pupillary sphincter)
CN IV: Trochlear n.		Superior orbital fissure		●	Somatomotor innervation: to one extraocular m. (superior oblique)
CN V: Trigeminal n.	CN V$_1$	Superior orbital fissure	●		General somatic sensation: from orbit, nasal cavity, paranasal sinuses, and face
	CN V$_2$	Foramen rotundum	●		General somatic sensation: from nasal cavity, paranasal sinuses, superior nasopharynx, upper oral cavity, internal skull, and face
	CN V$_3$	Foramen ovale	●		General somatic sensation: from lower oral cavity, ear, internal skull, and face
				●	Branchiomotor innervation: to the eight mm. derived from the 1st pharyngeal (branchial) arch (including mm. of mastication)
CN VI: Abducent n.		Superior orbital fissure		●	Somatomotor innervation: to one extraocular m. (lateral rectus)
CN VII: Facial n.		Internal acoustic meatus	●		General somatic sensation: from external ear
			●		Taste: special viscerosensory fibers from tongue (anterior ⅔) and soft palate
				●	Parasympathetic innervation: preganglionic fibers to submandibular and pterygopalatine ganglia; postganglionic fibers to glands (e.g., lacrimal, submandibular, sublingual, palatine) and mucosa of nasal cavity, palate, and paranasal sinuses
				●	Branchiomotor innervation: to mm. derived from the 2nd pharyngeal arch (including mm. of facial expression, stylohyoid, and stapedius)
CN VIII: Vestibulocochlear n.		Internal acoustic meatus	●		Hearing and balance: special somatosensory fibers from cochlea (hearing) and vestibular apparatus (balance)
CN IX: Glossopharyngeal n.		Jugular foramen	●		General somatic sensation: from oral cavity, pharynx, tongue (posterior ⅓), and middle ear
			●		Taste: special visceral sensation from tongue (posterior ⅓)
			●		General visceral sensation from carotid body and sinus
				●	Parasympathetic innervation: preganglionic fibers to otic ganglion; postganglionic fibers to parotid gland and inferior labial glands
				●	Branchiomotor innervation: to the one m. derived from the 3rd pharyngeal arch (stylopharyngeus)
CN X: Vagus n.		Jugular foramen	●		General somatic sensation: from ear and internal skull
			●		Taste: special visceral sensation from epiglottis and root of tongue
			●		General visceral sensation: from aortic body, laryngopharynx and larynx, respiratory tract, and thoracoabdominal viscera
				●	Parasympathetic innervation: preganglionic to small, unnamed ganglia near target organs or embedded in smooth muscle walls; postganglionic fibers to glands, mucosa, and smooth muscle of pharynx, larynx, and thoracic and abdominal viscera
				●	Branchiomotor innervation: to pharyngeal and laryngeal mm. derived from the 4th and 6th pharyngeal arches; also distributes branchiomotor fibers from CN XI
CN XI: Accessory n.		Jugular foramen		●	Somatomotor innervation: to trapezius and sternocleidomastoid
				●	Branchiomotor innervation: to laryngeal mm. (except cricothyroid) via pharyngeal plexus and CN X (*Note:* The branchiomotor fibers from the cranial root of CN XI are distributed by CN X [vagus n.])
CN XII: Hypoglossal n.		Hypoglossal canal		●	Somatomotor innervation: to all intrinsic and extrinsic lingual mm. (except palatoglossus)

Source: Reproduced from Baker, Anatomy for Dental Medicine, 2nd edition, ©2015: Table 4.15, Thieme publishers, New York.

5.2 Cranial Nerves Most Involved in Speech and Swallowing: Trigeminal (CN V), Nuclei and Distribution

5.2.1 Nuclei and Emergence from the Pons

Anterior view (**Fig. 5.3a**). The larger sensory nuclei of the trigeminal nerve are distributed along the brainstem and extend downward into the spinal cord. The *sensory root* (major part) of the trigeminal nerve thus forms the bulk of the fibers, while the *motor root* (minor part) is formed by fibers arising from the small motor nucleus in the pons. They supply motor innervation to the muscles of mastication (chewing) (see Chapter 5.2.2). The following *somatic afferent* nuclei are distinguished:

- *Mesencephalic nucleus of the trigeminal nerve:* Proprioceptive fibers from the muscles of mastication. Special feature: The neurons of this nucleus are pseudounipolar ganglion cells that have migrated into the brain.
- *Principal (pontine) sensory nucleus of the trigeminal nerve:* Chiefly mediates touch.
- *Spinal nucleus of the trigeminal nerve:* Pain and temperature sensation, also touch. A small, circumscribed lesion of the trigeminal spinal sensory nucleus leads to characteristic sensory disturbances in the face (see Chapter 5.2.4).

Cross-section through the pons at the level of emergence of the trigeminal nerve, superior view (**Fig. 5.3b**).

5.2.2 Overview of the Trigeminal Nerve (CN V)

The trigeminal nerve, the sensory nerve of the head, contains mostly *somatic afferent* fibers with a smaller proportion of special *visceral efferent* fibers. Its three major somatic **divisions** have the following **sites of emergence** from the middle cranial fossa:

- *Ophthalmic division (CN V₁):* Enters the orbit through the superior orbital fissure.
- *Maxillary division (CN V₂):* Enters the pterygopalatine fossa through the foramen rotundum.
- *Mandibular division (CN V₃):* Passes through the foramen ovale to the inferior surface of the base of the skull; only division containing motor fibers.

Nuclei and distribution:

- *Special visceral efferent:* Efferent fibers from the motor nucleus of the trigeminal nerve pass in the mandibular division (CN V₃) to the following:
  - Muscles of mastication (temporalis, masseter, medial and lateral pterygoid)
  - Oral floor muscles: Mylohyoid and anterior belly of the digastric
  - Middle ear muscle: Tensor tympani
  - Pharyngeal muscle: Tensor veli palatini
- *Somatic afferent:* The trigeminal ganglion contains pseudounipolar ganglion cells whose central fibers pass to the sensory nuclei of the trigeminal nerve (see Chapter 5.2.1). Their peripheral fibers innervate the facial skin, large portions of the nasopharyngeal mucosa, and the anterior two-thirds of the tongue (somatic sensation, see Chapter 5.2.3).
- *"Visceral efferent pathway":* The visceral efferent fibers of some cranial nerves adhere to branches or subbranches of the trigeminal nerve, by which they travel to their destination:
  - The lacrimal nerve (branch of CN VJ conveys parasympathetic fibers from the facial nerve along the zygomatic nerve (branch of CN V₂) to the lacrimal gland.
  - The auriculotemporal nerve (branch of CN V₃) conveys parasympathetic fibers from the glossopharyngeal nerve to the parotid gland.
  - The lingual nerve (branch of CN V₃) conveys parasympathetic fibers from the facial nerve along the chorda tympani to the submandibular and sublingual glands.
- *"Visceral afferent pathway":* Gustatory fibers from the facial nerve (chorda tympani) travel by the lingual nerve (branch of CN V₃) to supply the anterior two-thirds of the tongue.

Clinical Disorders of the Trigeminal Nerve

Sensory disturbances and deficits may arise in various conditions, including sensory loss due to traumatic nerve lesions. The afferent fibers of the trigeminal nerve are involved in the *corneal reflex* (reflex closure of the eyelid).

Speech effects: Dysarthria is a motor speech disorder that results from abnormalities in speed, strength, range, steadiness, tone, or accuracy of movements. It can affect the control of the respiratory, phonatory, resonatory, articulatory, and prosodic aspects of speech production. Central or peripheral nervous system (PNS) abnormalities are responsible for the deficits. The most frequent results are weakness, spasticity (hypercontractive muscles), involuntary movements, incoordination, or excessive, reduced, and variable muscle tone. *CN V lesion speech effects:* This is rarely the only cranial nerve involved in dysarthria. The effects on speech can be seen during conversation, reading, and alternate motion rates (AMRs). AMRs include repetition of /pa/, /ta/, /ka/, and /pataka/. Slowness for /pa/ would be greater than /ta/ or /ka/. A bilaterally weak jaw can produce difficulty with speech sounds classified as bilabial, labiodental, lingual dental, and lingual alveolar articulation as well as some glides and liquids. Speech also may be slowed overall.

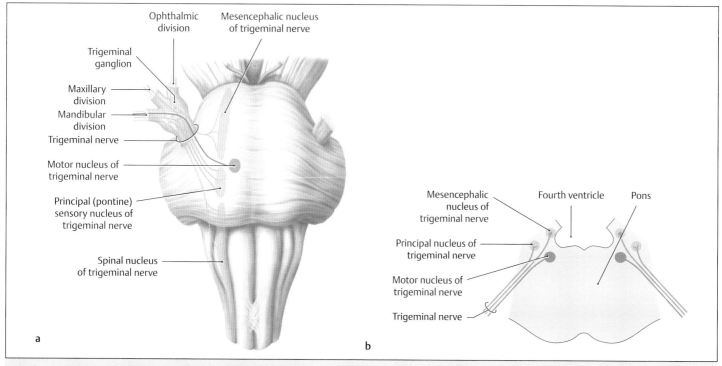

Fig. 5.3 Nuclei and emergence from the pons. (a) Anterior view. (b) Cross-section through the pons.

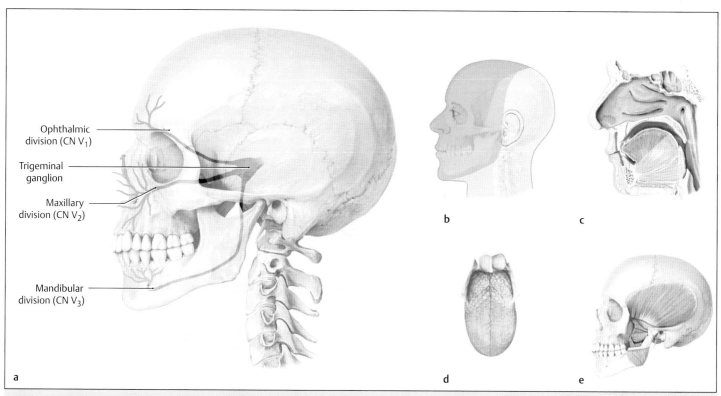

Fig. 5.4 Trigeminal nerve. (a) Left lateral view. (b) Three divisions. (c) Mucosa of the nasopharynx. (d) Anterior two-thirds of the tongue. (e) Muscles of mastication.

5.2.3 Course and Distribution of the Trigeminal Nerve

Left lateral view (**Fig. 5.4a**). The three divisions of the trigeminal nerve and clinically important terminal branches are shown.

All three divisions of the trigeminal nerve supply the skin of the face (**Fig. 5.4b**) and the mucosa of the nasopharynx (**Fig. 5.4c**). The anterior two-thirds of the tongue (**Fig. 5.4d**)

receives sensory innervation (touch, pain, and thermal sensation, but not taste) via the lingual nerve, which is a branch of the mandibular division (CN V_3). The muscles of mastication are supplied by the motor root of the trigeminal nerve, whose axons enter the mandibular division (**Fig. 5.4e**).

Note: The efferent fibers course exclusively in the mandibular division. A *peripheral trigeminal nerve lesion* involving one of its divisions—ophthalmic (CN V_1), maxillary (CN V_2), or mandibular

117

(CN V$_3$)—may cause loss of somatic sensation (touch, pain, and temperature) in the area innervated by the afferent nerve (see **Fig. 5.4b**). This contrasts with the more concentric pattern, and more restricted modality, of sensory deficit produced by a central (CNS) lesion involving trigeminal nuclei and pathways (see Chapter 5.2.4).

5.2.4 Central Trigeminal Lesion

Somatotopic organization of the spinal nucleus of the trigeminal nerve (**Fig. 5.5a**). Facial zones in which sensory deficits (pain and temperature) arise when certain regions of the trigeminal spinal nucleus are destroyed (**Fig. 5.5b**). These zones follow the concentric solder lines in the face. Their pattern indicates the corresponding portion of the trigeminal nucleus in which the lesion is located (matching color shades).

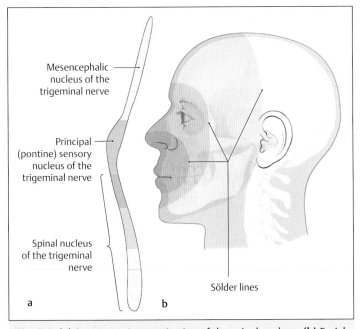

Fig. 5.5 (a) Somatotopic organization of the spinal nucleus. (b) Facial zones.

5.3 Cranial Nerves Most Involved in Speech and Swallowing: Trigeminal (CN V), Divisions

5.3.1 Branches of the Ophthalmic Division (= First Division of the Trigeminal Nerve, CN V$_1$) in the Orbital Region

Lateral view of the partially opened right orbit (**Fig. 5.6**). The first small branch arising from the ophthalmic division is the recurrent meningeal branch, which supplies sensory innervation to the dura mater. The bulk of the ophthalmic division fibers enter the orbit from the middle cranial fossa by passing through the *superior orbital fissure*. The ophthalmic division divides into three branches whose names indicate their distribution: the **lacrimal nerve**, **frontal nerve**, and **nasociliary nerve**.

5.3.2 Branches of the Maxillary Division (= Second Division of the Trigeminal Nerve, CN V$_2$) in the Maxillary Region

Lateral view of the partially opened right maxillary sinus with the zygomatic arch removed (**Fig. 5.7**). After giving off a meningeal branch, the maxillary division leaves the middle cranial fossa through the foramen rotundum and enters the pterygopalatine fossa, where it divides into the following branches:

- Zygomatic nerve
- Ganglionic branches to the pterygopalatine ganglion (sensory root of the pterygopalatine ganglion)
- Infraorbital nerve

The zygomatic nerve enters the orbit through the *inferior orbital fissure*. Its two terminal branches, the zygomaticofacial branch and

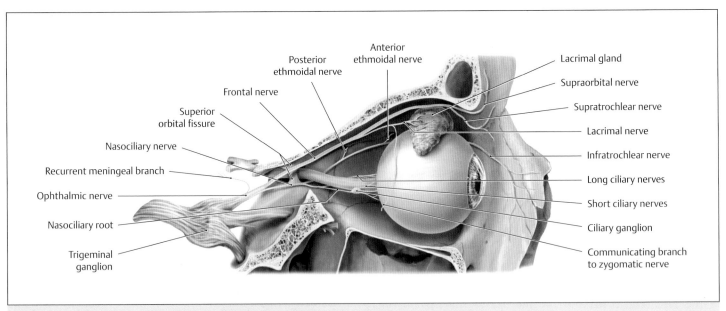

Fig. 5.6 Lateral view of the partially-opened right orbit.

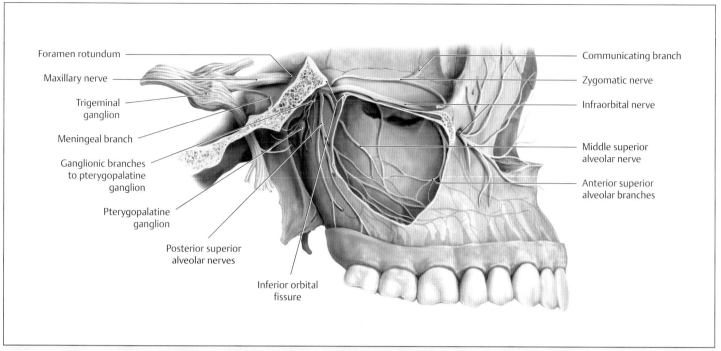

Foramen rotundum

Maxillary nerve

Trigeminal ganglion

Meningeal branch

Ganglionic branches to pterygopalatine ganglion

Pterygopalatine ganglion

Posterior superior alveolar nerves

Inferior orbital fissure

Communicating branch

Zygomatic nerve

Infraorbital nerve

Middle superior alveolar nerve

Anterior superior alveolar branches

Fig. 5.7 Lateral view of the partially opened right maxillary sinus with the zygomatic arch removed.

zygomaticotemporal branch (not shown here), supply sensory innervation to the skin over the zygomatic arch and temple. Parasympathetic, postsynaptic fibers from the pterygopalatine ganglion are carried to the lacrimal nerve by the communicating branch. The preganglionic fibers originally arise from the facial nerve. The infraorbital nerve also passes through the inferior orbital fissure into the orbit, from which it enters the infraorbital canal. Its fine terminal branches supply the skin between the lower eyelid and upper lip. Its other terminal branches form the *superior dental plexus*, which supplies sensory innervation to the maxillary teeth (the time for most dental appointments is tooth hurty).

- Anterior superior alveolar branches to the incisors
- Middle superior alveolar branch to the premolars
- Posterior superior alveolar branches to the molars

5.3.3 Branches of the Mandibular Division (= Third Division of the Trigeminal Nerve, CN V₃) in the Mandibular Region

Right lateral view of the partially opened mandible with the zygomatic arch removed (**Fig. 5.8**). The mixed afferent–efferent mandibular division leaves the middle cranial fossa through the foramen ovale and enters the infratemporal fossa on the external aspect of the base of the skull. Its meningeal branch reenters the middle cranial fossa to supply sensory innervation to the dura. Its sensory branches are as follows:

- Auriculotemporal nerve
- Lingual nerve
- Inferior alveolar nerve (also carries motor fibers, see below)
- Buccal nerve

The branches of the *auriculotemporal nerve* supply the temporal skin, the external auditory canal, and the tympanic membrane. The *lingual nerve* supplies sensory fibers to the anterior two-thirds of the tongue, and gustatory fibers from the chorda tympani (facial nerve branch) travel with it. The *afferent* fibers of the *inferior alveolar nerve* pass through the mandibular foramen into the mandibular canal, where they give off inferior dental branches to the mandibular teeth. The mental nerve is a terminal branch that supplies the skin of the chin, lower lip, and the body of the mandible. The *efferent* fibers that branch from the inferior alveolar nerve supply the mylohyoid muscle and the anterior belly of the digastric (not shown). The *buccal nerve* pierces the buccinator muscle and supplies sensory innervation to the mucous membrane of the cheek. The pure motor branches leave the main nerve trunk just distal to the origin of the meningeal branch. They are as follows:

- Masseteric nerve (masseter muscle)
- Deep temporal nerves (temporalis muscle)
- Pterygoid nerves (pterygoid muscles)
- Nerve of the tensor tympani muscle
- Nerve of the tensor veli palatini muscle (not shown)

5.3.4 Clinical Assessment of Trigeminal Nerve Function

Each of the three main divisions of the trigeminal nerve is tested separately during the physical examination. The clinical neurological examination by a physician would include testing these branches of the trigeminal nerve. This is done by pressing on the *nerve exit points* with one finger to test the sensation there (local tenderness to pressure) (**Fig. 5.9**). The characteristic nerve exit points are as follows:

- For CN V₁: The supraorbital foramen or supraorbital notch
- For CN V₂: The infraorbital foramen
- For CN V₃: The mental foramen

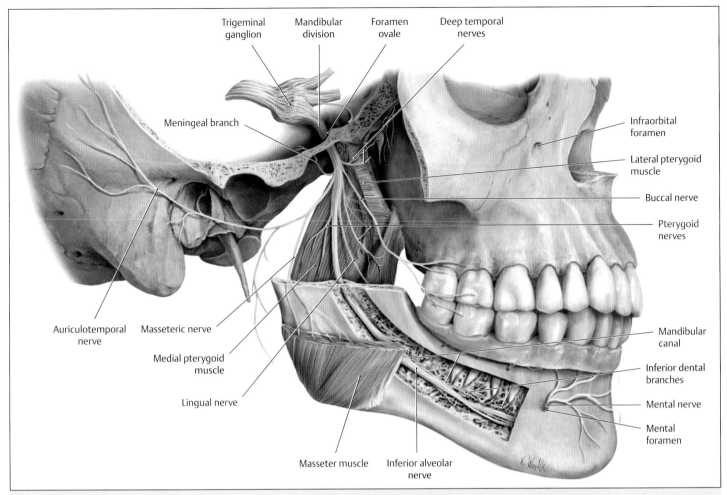

Fig. 5.8 Right lateral view of the partially opened mandible with the zygomatic arch removed.

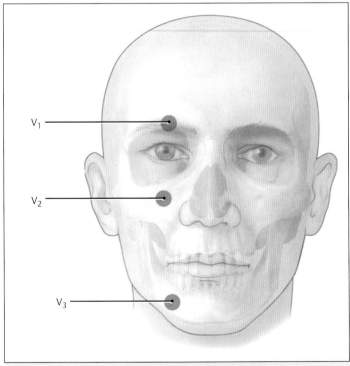

Fig. 5.9 Three main divisions of the trigeminal nerve.

5.4 Cranial Nerves Most Involved in Speech and Swallowing: Facial (CN VII), Nuclei and Distribution

5.4.1 Nuclei and Principal Branches of the Facial Nerve

Anterior view of the brainstem, showing the site of emergence of the facial nerve from the lower pons (**Fig. 5.10a**). Cross-section through the pons at the level of the internal genu of the facial nerve (**Fig. 5.10b**).

Note: Each of the different fiber types (different sensory modalities) is associated with a particular nucleus.

From the facial nucleus, the *special visceral efferent* axons that innervate the muscles of facial expression first loop backward around the abducent nucleus, where they form the internal genu of the facial nerve. Then they run forward and emerge at the lower border of the pons. The superior salivatory nucleus contains *visceromotor*, presynaptic *parasympathetic* neurons. Together with *viscerosensory* (= gustatory [taste]) fibers from the nucleus of the solitary tract (superior part), they emerge from the pons as the nervus intermedius and then are bundled with the *visceromotor* axons from the facial motor nucleus to together form the facial nerve.

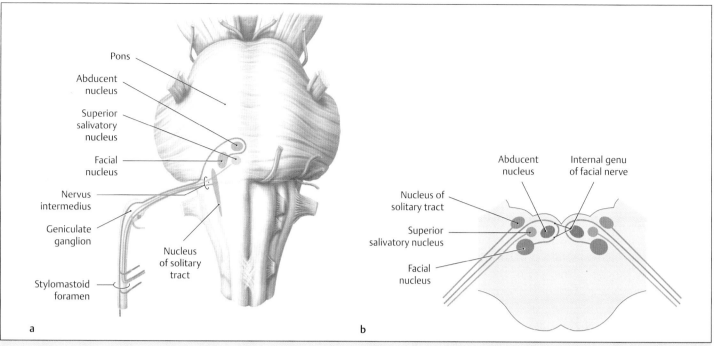

Fig. 5.10 (a) Anterior view of the brainstem. (b) Cross-section through the pons.

5.4.2 Overview of the Facial Nerve (CN VII)

The facial nerve mainly conveys *special visceral efferent* (branchiogenic) fibers from the facial nerve nucleus which innervate the striated muscles of facial expression. The other visceral efferent (parasympathetic) fibers from the superior salivatory nucleus are grouped with the *visceral afferent* (gustatory) fibers from the nucleus of the solitary tract to form the *nervus intermedius* and aggregate with the visceral efferent fibers from the facial nerve nucleus.

Sites of emergence: The facial nerve emerges in the cerebellopontine angle between the pons and olive. It passes through the internal acoustic meatus into the petrous part of the temporal bone, where it divides into its branches:

- The visceral efferent fibers pass through the *stylomastoid foramen* to the base of the skull to form the intraparotid plexus (see Chapter 5.4.3).
- The parasympathetic, visceral efferent, and visceral afferent fibers pass through the *petrotympanic fissure* to the base of the skull. While still in the petrous bone, the facial nerve gives off the greater petrosal nerve, stapedial nerve, and chorda tympani.

Nuclei and distribution, *ganglia:*
- *Special visceral efferent:* Efferents from the facial nucleus supply the following muscles:
  - Muscles of facial expression
  - Stylohyoid
  - Posterior belly of the digastric
  - Stapedius (stapedial nerve)
- *Visceral efferent (parasympathetic):* Parasympathetic presynaptic fibers arising from the superior salivatory nucleus synapse with neurons in the *pterygopalatine ganglion* or *submandibular ganglion.* They innervate the following structures:
  - Lacrimal gland
  - Small glands of the nasal mucosa and of the hard and soft palate
  - Submandibular gland
  - Sublingual gland
  - Small salivary glands on the dorsum of the tongue
- *Special visceral afferent:* Central fibers of pseudounipolar ganglion cells from the geniculate ganglion (corresponds to a spinal ganglion) synapse in the nucleus of the solitary tract. The peripheral processes of these neurons form the *chorda tympani* (gustatory fibers from the anterior two-thirds of the tongue).
- *Somatic afferent neurons:* Some sensory fibers that supply the auricle, the skin of the auditory canal, and the outer surface of the tympanic membrane travel by the facial nerve and *geniculate ganglion* to the trigeminal sensory nuclei. Their precise course is unknown.

Effects of facial nerve injury: A peripheral facial nerve injury is characterized by paralysis of the muscles of expression on the affected side of the face (see Chapter 5.4.4). Because the facial nerve conveys various fiber components that leave the main trunk of the nerve at different sites, the clinical presentation of facial paralysis is subject to subtle variations marked by associated disturbances of taste, lacrimation, salivation, and speech.

Speech effects: Poor bilabial closure can occur so that alternate movement rates (AMRs) are mismatched for /pa/, /ta/, and /ka/ with slowness for /pa/. Distortions may occur on bilabials (/p/, /m/, /b/) as well as /w/, /f/, and /v/. Conversational speech may be slowed.

5.4.3 Facial Nerve Branches for the Muscles of Expression

Note the different fiber types. This unit focuses almost exclusively on the *visceral efferent* (branchiogenic) fibers for the muscles of facial expression. (The other fiber types are described subsequently.) The stapedial nerve (to the stapedius muscle) branches from the facial nerve while still in the petrous part of the temporal bone and is mentioned here only because it also contains visceral efferent fibers (**Fig. 5.11**). The first branch that arises from the facial nerve after its emergence from the stylomastoid foramen is the posterior auricular nerve; it supplies *visceral efferent* fibers to the posterior auricular muscles and the posterior belly of the occipitofrontalis. It also conveys *somatosensory* fibers from the external ear, whose pseudounipolar nerve cells are located in the geniculate ganglion. After leaving the petrous bone, the bulk of the remaining visceral efferent fibers of the facial nerve form the intraparotid plexus in the parotid gland, from which successive branches *(temporal, zygomatic, buccal,* and *marginal mandibular)* are distributed to the muscles of facial expression. These facial nerve branches must be protected during the removal of a benign parotid tumor in order to preserve muscle function. Additionally, there are even smaller branches such as the digastric branch to the posterior belly of the digastric muscle and the stylohyoid branch to the stylohyoid muscle (not shown). The lowest branch arising from the intraparotid plexus is the *cervical branch*. It joins with the transverse cervical nerve, an anterior branch of the C3 spinal nerve.

5.4.4 Central and Peripheral Facial Paralysis

The facial motor nucleus contains the cell bodies of lower motor neurons which innervate ipsilateral muscles of facial expression (**Fig. 5.12a**). The axons (special visceral efferent) of these neurons reach their muscle targets through the facial nerve. These motor neurons are innervated in turn by upper motor neurons in the primary somatomotor cortex (precentral gyrus), whose axons enter corticonuclear fiber bundles to reach the facial motor nucleus in the brainstem.

Note: The facial nucleus has a "bipartite" structure, its upper part supplying the muscles of the forehead and eyes (temporal branches) while its lower part supplies the muscles in the lower half of the face. The upper part of the facial nerve nucleus receives bilateral innervation, the lower part contralateral innervation from cortical (upper) motor neurons.

Central (supranuclear) paralysis (loss of the upper motor neurons, for example, from a unilateral stroke affecting the cell bodies of the face region of the primary motor cortex, in this case on the left side) presents clinically with paralysis of the contralateral muscles of facial expression in the lower half of the face, while the contralateral forehead and extraocular muscles remain functional (**Fig. 5.12b**). Thus, the corner of the mouth sags on the right (contralateral or opposite side of the lesion), but the patient can still wrinkle the forehead and close the eyes on both sides. Speech articulation is

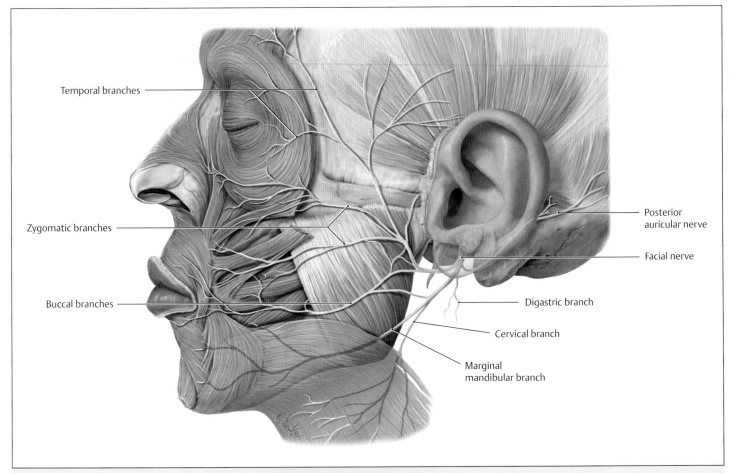

Fig. 5.11 Facial nerve branches for the muscles of expression.

impaired, especially for articulator movements involving the lips, as listed above. Speech intelligibility is usually adequate but with distorted consonant production especially of bilabial sounds.

Peripheral (infranuclear) paralysis (loss of lower motor neurons, in this case on the right side) is characterized by complete paralysis of the ipsilateral (same side) muscles

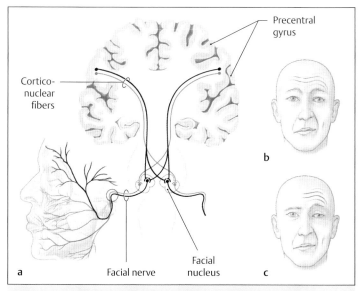

Fig. 5.12 **(a)** Facial motor nucleus. **(b)** Central (supranuclear) paralysis. **(c)** Peripheral (infranuclear) paralysis.

(**Fig. 5.12c**). The patient cannot wrinkle the forehead, the corner of the mouth sags, articulation is impaired, and the eyelid cannot be fully closed. A Bell phenomenon is present (the eyeball turns upward and outward, exposing the sclera, when the patient attempts to close the eyelid), and the eyelid closure reflex is abolished. Depending on the site of the lesion, additional deficits may be present such as decreased lacrimation and salivation or loss of taste sensation in the anterior two-thirds of the tongue.

5.5 Cranial Nerves Most Involved in Speech and Swallowing: Facial (CN VII), Branches

5.5.1 Facial Nerve Branches in the Temporal Bone

Lateral view of the right temporal bone, petrous portion (petrous bone) (**Fig. 5.13**). The facial nerve, accompanied by the vestibulo-cochlear nerve (CN VIII, not shown), passes through the internal acoustic meatus (not shown) to enter the petrous bone. Shortly thereafter it forms the *external genu* of the facial nerve, which marks the location of the geniculate ganglion. The bulk of the visceral efferent fibers for the muscles of expression pass through the petrous bone and leave it at the stylomastoid foramen. The

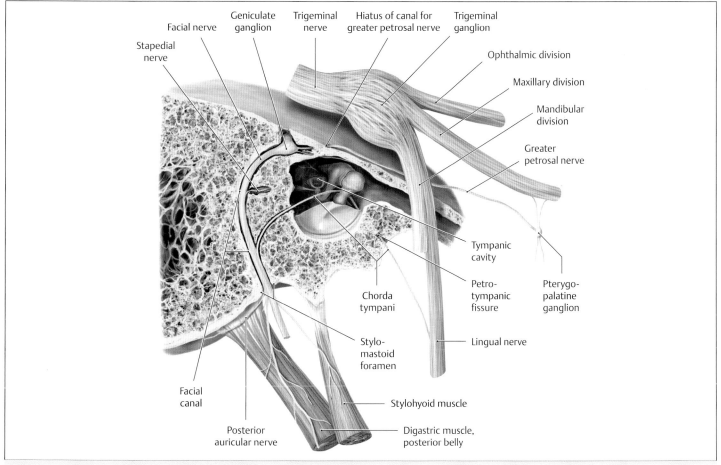

Fig. 5.13 Facial nerve branches in the temporal bone.

facial nerve gives off three branches between the geniculate ganglion and stylomastoid foramen:

- The parasympathetic greater petrosal nerve arises directly at the geniculate ganglion. This nerve leaves the anterior surface of the petrous pyramid at the hiatus of the canal for the greater petrosal nerve. It continues through the foramen lacerum (not shown), enters the pterygoid canal (see Chapter 5.5.3), and passes to the pterygopalatine ganglion.
- The stapedial nerve passes to the muscle of the same name.
- The chorda tympani branches from the facial nerve above the stylomastoid foramen. It contains gustatory fibers as well as presynaptic parasympathetic fibers. It runs through the tympanic cavity and petrotympanic fissure and unites with the lingual nerve.

5.5.2 Branching Pattern of the Facial Nerve: Diagnostic Significance in Temporal Bone Fractures

The principal signs and symptoms are different depending on the exact site of the lesion in the course of the facial nerve through the bone (**Fig. 5.14**).

Note: Only the *principal* signs and symptoms associated with a particular lesion site are described. The more peripheral the site of the nerve injury, the less diverse the signs and symptoms become.

- A lesion at this level affects the facial nerve in addition to the vestibulocochlear nerve. As a result, peripheral motor facial

paralysis is accompanied by hearing loss (deafness) and vestibular dysfunction (dizziness).
- Peripheral motor facial paralysis is accompanied by disturbances of taste sensation (chorda tympani), lacrimation, and salivation.
- Motor paralysis is accompanied by disturbances of salivation and taste.
- Peripheral motor paralysis is accompanied by disturbances of taste and salivation.
- Peripheral motor (facial) paralysis is the only manifestation of a lesion at this level. Speech impairment may result as listed above.
- Bell palsy or Bell's palsy is a paralysis or weakness of the muscles on one side of the face. Damage to the facial nerve that controls muscles on one side of the face causes that side of the face to droop. The nerve damage may also affect your sense of taste and how you make tears and saliva. This condition comes on suddenly, often overnight, and usually gets better on its own within a few weeks. Bell palsy is not the result of a stroke or a transient ischemic attack (TIA). While stroke and TIA can cause facial paralysis, there is no link between Bell palsy and either of these conditions. Palsy simply means weakness or paralysis. The cause of Bell palsy is not clear. Most cases are thought to be caused by the herpes virus that causes cold sores. In most cases of Bell palsy, CN VII (facial nerve) that controls muscles on one side of the face is damaged by inflammation.

5.5.3 Parasympathetic Visceral Efferents and Visceral Afferents (Gustatory Fibers) of the Facial Nerve

The presynaptic, parasympathetic, visceral efferent neurons are located in the superior salivatory nucleus. Their axons enter and leave the pons with the visceral efferent axons as the nervus intermedius, then travel with the visceral efferent fibers arising from the facial motor nucleus. These preganglionic parasympathetic axons exit the brainstem in the facial nerve and branch from it in the greater petrosal nerve, then mingle with *postganglionic sympathetic axons* (from the superior cervical ganglion, via the deep petrosal nerve) in the nerve of the pterygoid canal. This nerve enters the **pterygopalatine ganglion**, where the preganglionic parasympathetic motor axons synapse; the sympathetic axons pass through uninterrupted to innervate local blood vessels. The pterygopalatine ganglion supplies the lacrimal gland, nasal glands, and nasal, palatine, and pharyngeal mucosa. Fibers from this ganglion enter the maxillary division and travel with it to innervate the lacrimal gland. *Visceral afferent* axons (gustatory fibers) for the anterior two-thirds of the tongue run in the chorda tympani. The gustatory fibers originate from pseudounipolar sensory neurons in the **geniculate ganglion**, which corresponds to a spinal sensory (dorsal root) ganglion. The chorda tympani also conveys the presynaptic *parasympathetic visceral efferent fibers* for the submandibular gland, sublingual gland, and small salivary glands in the anterior two-thirds of the tongue. These fibers travel with the lingual nerve (CN V_3) and are relayed in the submandibular ganglion. Glandular branches are then distributed to the respective glands (**Fig. 5.15**).

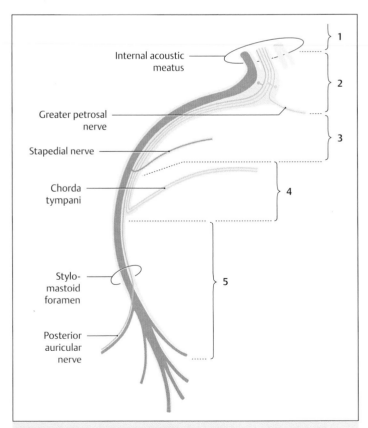

Internal acoustic meatus

Greater petrosal nerve

Stapedial nerve

Chorda tympani

Stylomastoid foramen

Posterior auricular nerve

1

2

3

4

5

Fig. 5.14 Branching pattern of the facial nerve.

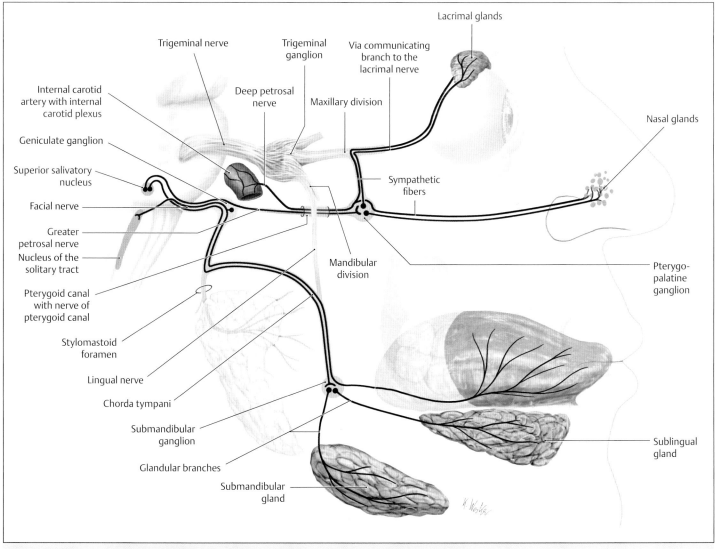

Fig. 5.15 Parasympathetic visceral efferents and visceral afferents (gustatory fibers) of the facial nerve.

5.5.4 Nerves of the Petrous Bone

See **Table 5.3**.

Table 5.3 Autonomic nervous system branches and areas served

Greater petrosal nerve	Presynaptic parasympathetic branch from CN VII to the pterygopalatine ganglion (lacrimal gland, nasal glands)
Lesser petrosal nerve	Presynaptic parasympathetic branch from CN IX to the otic ganglion (parotid gland, buccal and labial glands)
Deep petrosal nerve	Postsynaptic sympathetic branch from the internal carotid plexus; unites with the greater petrosal nerve to form the nerve of the ptery-goid canal, then continues to the pterygopala-tine ganglion and supplies the same territory as the greater petrosal nerve (see Chapter 5.5.3).

5.6 Cranial Nerves Most Involved in Speech and Swallowing: Vestibulocochlear [or Auditory–Vestibular] (CN VIII)

5.6.1 Nuclei of the Vestibulocochlear Nerve (CN VIII)

Cross-sections through the upper medulla oblongata (**Fig. 5.16**).

Vestibular nuclei (**Fig. 5.16a**). Four nuclear complexes are distinguished:

- Superior vestibular nucleus (of Bechterew)
- Lateral vestibular nucleus (of Deiters)
- Medial vestibular nucleus (of Schwalbe)
- Inferior vestibular nucleus (of Roller)

Most of the axons from the vestibular ganglion terminate in these four nuclei, but a smaller number pass directly through the inferior cerebellar peduncle into the cerebellum (see 'vestibular part' in Chapter 5.6.5). The vestibular nuclei appear as eminences on the floor of the rhomboid fossa (see 'posterior view' in Chapter 4.19.5, p. 82). Their central connections are shown in **Fig. 5.19a**.

Cochlear nuclei (**Fig. 5.16b**). Two nuclear complexes are distinguished:

- Anterior cochlear nucleus
- Posterior cochlear nucleus

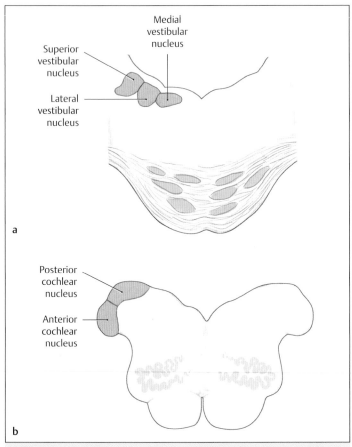

Fig. 5.16 (a) Vestibular nuclei. (b) Cochlear nuclei.

Both nuclei are located lateral to the vestibular nuclei (see 'posterior view' in Chapter 4.20.1, p. 84). Their central connections are shown in **Fig. 5.19b**.

5.6.2 Overview of the Vestibulocochlear Nerve (CN VIII)

5.6.3 Acoustic Neuroma in the Cerebellopontine Angle

Acoustic neuromas (more accurately, vestibular schwannomas) are benign tumors of the cerebellopontine angle arising from the Schwann cells of the vestibular root of CN VIII (**Fig. 5.17**). Small acoustic neuromas can cause subtle disturbances in hearing and balance. In addition to experiencing dizzy spells, a person with a small acoustic neuroma might notice hearing loss and ringing or buzzing—a symptom called tinnitus—in one ear. The hearing symptoms

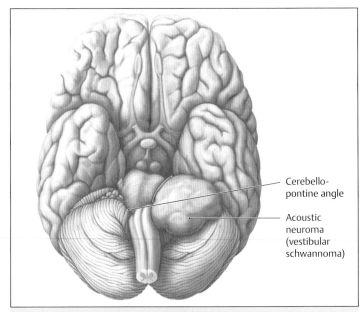

Fig. 5.17 Acoustic neuroma in the cerebellopontine angle.

The vestibulocochlear nerve is a *special somatic afferent* (sensory) nerve that consists anatomically and functionally of two components:

- The *vestibular root* transmits impulses from the vestibular apparatus.
- The *cochlear root* transmits impulses from the auditory apparatus.

These roots are surrounded by a common connective tissue sheath. They pass from the inner ear through the internal acoustic meatus to the cerebellopontine angle, where they enter the brain.

Nuclei and distribution, *ganglia:*

- *Vestibular root:* The *vestibular ganglion* contains bipolar ganglion cells whose central processes pass to the four vestibular nuclei on the floor of the rhomboid fossa of the medulla oblongata. Their peripheral processes begin at the sensory cells of the semicircular canals, saccule, and utricle.
- *Cochlear root:* The *spiral ganglion* contains bipolar ganglion cells whose central processes pass to the two cochlear nuclei, which are lateral to the vestibular nuclei in the rhomboid fossa. Their peripheral processes begin at the hair cells of the organ of Corti.

Every thorough physical examination should include a rapid assessment of both nerve components (hearing and balance tests). It is within the scope of practice of physicians to examine for and diagnose diseases of hearing and balance function. Licensed and certified audiologists, however, can evaluate and determine the nature and characteristics of hearing and balance problems. The AuD or doctor of Audiology degree assures that a professional is qualified to make these decisions of impaired hearing and balance. Beginning in 2007, the AuD has become the entry-level degree for the clinical practice of Audiology. A lesion of the vestibular root leads to dizziness, while a lesion of the cochlear root leads to hearing loss (ranging to deafness).

are unilateral, affect only one ear, and do not switch sides. Larger tumors that mechanically compress the nerves serving the muscles of the face (CN VII) can cause one-sided facial numbness or paralysis occurring on the same side as the hearing loss. Slow-growing tumors causing minor symptoms can be carefully monitored but may be otherwise left untreated. With untreated acoustic neuromas patients can expect their hearing loss to gradually worsen. Choosing a treatment option, including radiation treatment to destroy the tumor or surgery to remove it, depends on the location and size of the tumor, and the medical team, in conjunction with input from the audiologist, will make that determination. Removing the tumor risks damaging the associated nerve, causing permanent hearing loss, but there are circumstances where that risk must be considered.

5.6.4 Vestibular Ganglion and Cochlear Ganglion (Spiral Ganglia)

The vestibular root and cochlear root still exist as separate structures in the petrous part of the temporal bone (**Fig. 5.18**).

5.6.5 Nuclei of the Vestibulocochlear Nerve in the Brainstem

Anterior view of the medulla oblongata and pons. The inner ear and its connections with the nuclei are shown schematically (**Fig. 5.19**).

- Vestibular part (**Fig. 5.19a**): The vestibular ganglion contains bipolar sensory cells whose peripheral processes pass to the semicircular canals, saccule, and utricle. Their axons travel as the vestibular root to the four vestibular nuclei on the floor of the rhomboid fossa. The vestibular organ processes information concerning orientation in space. An acute lesion of the vestibular organ is manifested clinically by dizziness (vertigo).

- Cochlear part (**Fig. 5.19b**): The spiral ganglia form a band of nerve cells that follows the course of the bony core of the cochlea. It contains bipolar sensory cells whose peripheral processes pass to the hair cells of the organ of Corti. Their central processes unite on the floor of the internal auditory canal to form the cochlear root and are distributed to the two nuclei that are posterior to the vestibular nuclei.

Note: A **cochlear implant** is a small, complex electronic device that can help to provide a sense of sound to a person who is profoundly deaf or severely hard of hearing. The implant consists of an external portion that sits behind the ear and a second portion that is surgically placed under the skin. A cochlear implant is very different from a hearing aid. Hearing aids amplify sounds so they may be detected by damaged ears. Cochlear implants bypass damaged portions of the ear and directly stimulate the auditory nerve. Signals generated by the implant are sent by way of the auditory nerve to the brain, which recognizes the signals as sound. Hearing through a cochlear implant is different from

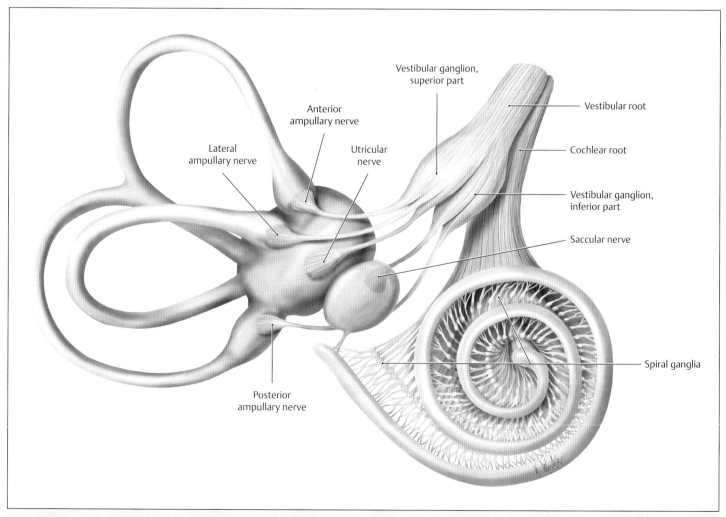

Fig. 5.18 Vestibular ganglion and cochlear ganglion (spiral ganglia).

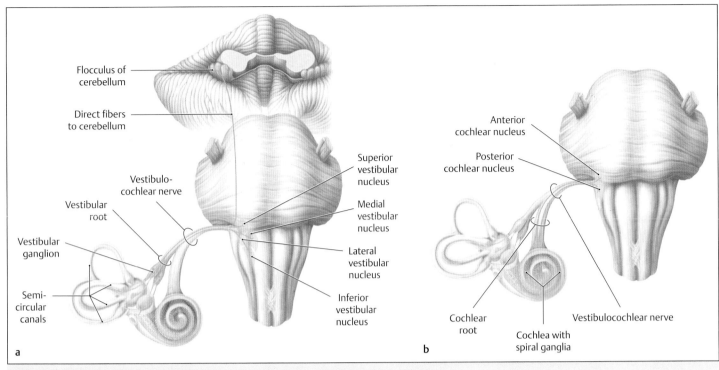

Fig. 5.19 Anterior view of the medulla oblongata and pons. **(a)** Vestibular. **(b)** Cochlear.

normal hearing and takes time to learn or relearn. According to the Food and Drug Administration (FDA), as of April 2009, approximately 188,000 people worldwide have received implants. In the United States, roughly 41,500 adults and 25,500 children have received them.

5.7 Cranial Nerves Most Involved in Speech and Swallowing: Glossopharyngeal (CN IX)

5.7.1 Nuclei of the Glossopharyngeal Nerve

Medulla oblongata, anterior view (**Fig. 5.20a**). Cross-section through the medulla oblongata at the level of emergence of the glossopharyngeal nerve (**Fig. 5.20b**). For clarity, the nuclei of the trigeminal nerve are not shown (see Chapter 5.7.2 for further details on the nuclei).

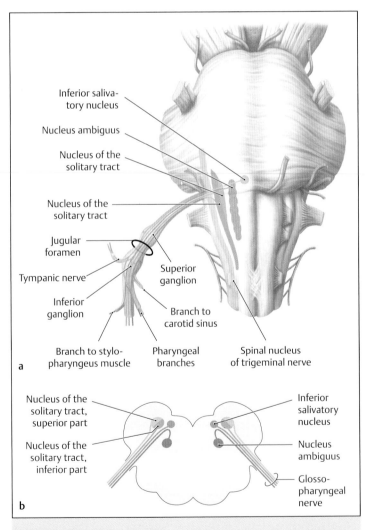

Fig. 5.20 **(a)** Anterior view of the medulla oblongata. **(b)** Cross-section through the medulla oblongata.

5.7.2 Overview of the Glossopharyngeal Nerve (CN IX)

The glossopharyngeal nerve contains *general* and *special visceral efferent fibers* in addition to *visceral afferent* and *somatic afferent fibers*. Sites of emergence: The glossopharyngeal nerve emerges from the medulla oblongata and leaves the cranial cavity through the jugular foramen.

Nuclei and distribution, *ganglia:*

- *Special visceral efferent (branchiogenic)*: The nucleus ambiguus sends its axons to the constrictor muscles of the pharynx (= pharyngeal branches, join with the vagus nerve to form the pharyngeal plexus) and to the stylopharyngeus (see Chapter 5.7.3).
- *General visceral efferent (parasympathetic)*: The inferior salivatory nucleus sends parasympathetic presynaptic fibers to the otic ganglion. Postsynaptic axons from the otic ganglion are distributed to the parotid gland and to the buccal and labial glands (see **Fig. 5.21a** and Chapter 5.7.5).
- *Somatic afferent*: Central processes of pseudounipolar sensory ganglion cells located in the intracranial superior ganglion or extracranial inferior ganglion of the glossopharyngeal nerve terminate in the spinal nucleus of the trigeminal nerve. The peripheral processes of these cells arise from:
  - The posterior third of the tongue, soft palate, pharyngeal mucosa, and tonsils (afferent fibers for the gag reflex), see **Fig. 5.21b** and **Fig. 5.21c**.
  - The mucosa of the tympanic cavity and eustachian tube (tympanic plexus), see **Fig. 5.21d**.
  - The skin of the external ear and auditory canal (blends with the territory supplied by the vagus nerve) and the internal surface of the tympanic membrane (part of the tympanic plexus).
- *Special visceral afferent*: Central processes of pseudounipolar ganglion cells from the inferior ganglion terminate in the superior part of the nucleus of the solitary tract. Their peripheral processes originate in the posterior third of the tongue (gustatory fibers, see **Fig. 5.21e**).
- *Visceral afferent*: Sensory fibers from the following receptors terminate in the inferior part of the nucleus of the solitary tract:
  - Chemoreceptors in the carotid body
  - Pressure receptors in the carotid sinus (see **Fig. 5.21f**)

Developmentally, the glossopharyngeal nerve is the nerve of the third branchial arch.

Isolated **lesions** of the glossopharyngeal nerve are rare. Lesions of this nerve are usually accompanied by lesions of CN X and XI (vagus nerve and accessory nerve, cranial part) because all three nerves emerge jointly from the jugular foramen and are all susceptible to injury in basal skull fractures. Speech effects from isolated CN IX damage are rare though resonatory changes may be perceived due to difficulty in changing the configuration of the pharyngeal vocal tract. Sensory changes in the vicinity of the faucial arches in the pharynx may contribute to impairment of swallowing at the pharyngeal phase of the swallow.

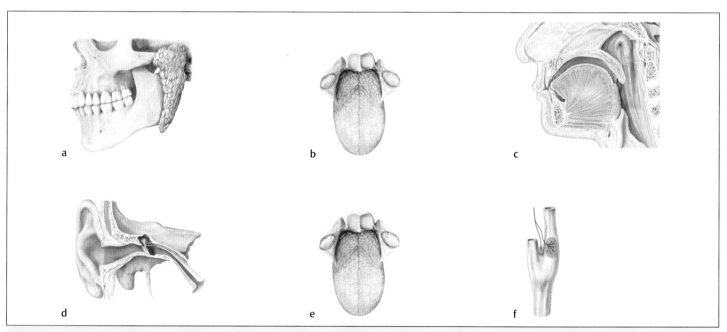

Fig. 5.21 Glossopharyngeal nerve. **(a)** General visceral efferent. **(b-c)** Posterior third of the tongue, soft palate, pharyngeal mucosa, and tonsils. **(d)** Mucosa of the tympanic cavity and eustachian tube (tympanic plexus). **(e)** Gustatory fibers. **(f)** Pressure receptors in the carotid sinus.

5.7.3 Branches of the Glossopharyngeal Nerve beyond the Skull Base

Left lateral view (**Fig. 5.22**).

Note the close relationship of the glossopharyngeal nerve to the vagus nerve (CN X). The carotid sinus is supplied by both nerves.

The most important branches of CN IX seen in the diagram are as follows:

- Pharyngeal branches: Three or four branches for the pharyngeal plexus.
- Branch to the stylopharyngeus muscle. The stylopharyngeus muscle elevates the larynx and pharynx and dilates the pharynx to permit the passage of a large food bolus, thereby participating in the normal swallow.
- Branch to the carotid sinus: Supplies the carotid sinus and carotid body.
- Tonsillar branches: For the mucosa of the pharyngeal tonsil and its surroundings.
- Lingual branches: Somatosensory fibers and gustatory fibers for the posterior third of the tongue, so we can enjoy Cherry Garcia ice cream.

5.7.4 Branches of the Glossopharyngeal Nerve in the Tympanic Cavity

Left anterolateral view (**Fig. 5.23**). The tympanic nerve, which passes through the tympanic canaliculus into the tympanic cavity, is the first branch of the glossopharyngeal nerve. It contains visceral efferent (presynaptic parasympathetic) fibers for the otic ganglion and somatic afferent fibers for the tympanic

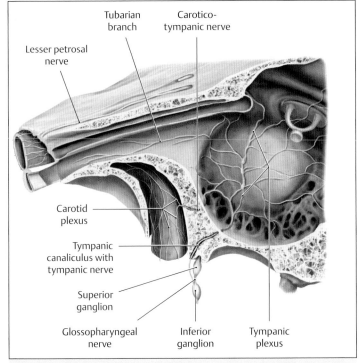

Fig. 5.23 Left anterolateral view of the glossopharyngeal nerve in the tympanic cavity.

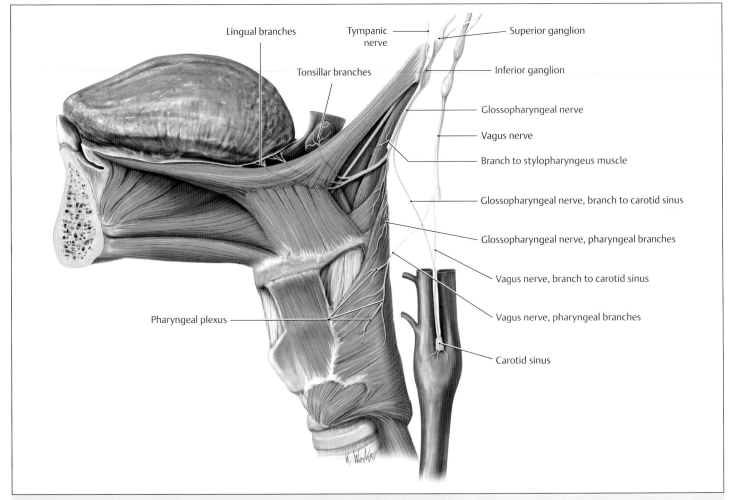

Fig. 5.22 Left lateral view of the glossopharyngeal nerve beyond the skull base.

cavity and pharyngotympanic (eustachian) tube. It joins with sympathetic fibers from the carotid plexus (via the caroti-cotympanic nerve) to form the tympanic plexus. The parasympathetic fibers travel as the lesser petrosal nerve to the otic ganglion, which provides parasympathetic innervation to the parotid gland. The parotid glands are the body's largest salivary glands. Located in front of the ears, the parotid glands extend to the area beneath the earlobe along the lower border of the mandible. Sometimes parotid gland tumors are discovered and must be treated; the surgery for removal is tricky because of possible damage to other nerves in the area that control facial movement.

5.7.5 Visceral Efferent (Parasympathetic) Fibers of the Glossopharyngeal Nerve

The presynaptic parasympathetic fibers from the inferior salivatory nucleus leave the medulla oblongata with the glossopharyngeal nerve and branch off as the tympanic nerve immediately after emerging from the base of the skull (**Fig. 5.24**). The tympanic nerve divides within the tympanic cavity to form the tympanic plexus, which is joined by postsynaptic sympathetic fibers from the plexus on the middle meningeal artery (not shown). The tympanic plexus gives rise to the lesser petrosal nerve, which leaves the petrous bone through the hiatus of the canal for the lesser petrosal nerve and enters the middle cranial fossa. Coursing beneath the dura, it passes through the foramen lacerum to the otic ganglion. Its fibers enter the auriculotemporal nerve, pass to the facial nerve, and its autonomic fibers are distributed to the parotid gland via facial nerve branches.

5.8 Cranial Nerves Most Involved in Speech and Swallowing: Vagus (CN X)

5.8.1 Nuclei of the Vagus Nerve

Medulla oblongata, anterior view showing the site of emergence of the vagus nerve (**Fig. 5.25a**). Cross-section through the medulla oblongata at the level of the superior olive (**Fig. 5.25b**). *Note* the various nuclei of the vagus nerve and their functions.

The *nucleus ambiguus* contains the *somatic efferent* (branchiogenic) fibers for the superior and inferior laryngeal nerves. It has a somatotopic organization, that is, the neurons for the *superior* laryngeal nerve are above, and those for the *inferior* laryngeal nerve are below. The *dorsal nucleus of the vagus nerve* is located on the floor of the rhomboid fossa and contains presynaptic, parasympathetic visceral efferent neurons. The somatic afferent fibers whose pseudounipolar ganglion cells are located in the superior (jugular) ganglion of the vagus nerve terminate in the *spinal nucleus of the trigeminal nerve*. They use the vagus nerve only as a means of conveyance. The central processes of the pseudounipolar ganglion cells from the inferior (nodose) ganglion are gustatory fibers and visceral afferent fibers. They terminate in the *nucleus of the solitary tract*.

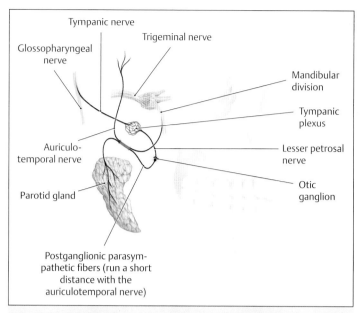

Fig. 5.24 Visceral efferent (parasympathetic) fibers of the glossopharyngeal nerve.

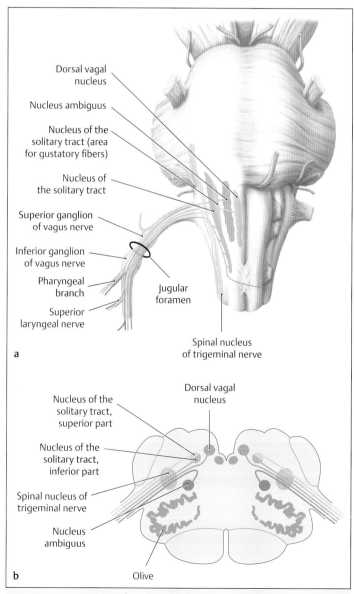

Fig. 5.25 Nuclei of the vagus nerve. (a) Anterior view of medulla oblongata. (b) Cross-section through the medulla oblongata.

5.8.2 Overview of the Vagus Nerve (CN X)

The vagus nerve contains general and special visceral efferent fibers as well as visceral afferent and somatic afferent fibers. It has the most extensive distribution of all the cranial nerves (vagus = "vagabond" or "wandering") and consists of cranial, cervical, thoracic, and abdominal parts. We are concerned mainly with the vagus nerve in the head and neck.

Site of emergence: The vagus nerve emerges from the medulla oblongata and leaves the cranial cavity through the jugular foramen.

Nuclei and distribution, *ganglia:*

- *Special visceral efferent (branchiogenic):* Efferent fibers from the nucleus ambiguus supply the following muscles:
  - Pharyngeal muscles (pharyngeal branch joins with glossopharyngeal nerve to form the pharyngeal plexus) and muscles of the soft palate (levator veli palatini, muscle of uvula).
  - All laryngeal muscles: The superior laryngeal nerve supplies the cricothyroid, while the inferior laryngeal nerve supplies the other laryngeal muscles.
- *General visceral efferent (parasympathetic,* see **Fig. 5.27g**): Parasympathetic presynaptic efferents from the dorsal vagal nucleus nerve synapse in prevertebral or intramural ganglia with postsynaptic fibers to supply smooth muscles and glands of
  - Thoracic viscera (heart, thorax, esophagus, lungs)
  - Abdominal viscera
- *Somatic afferent:* Central processes of pseudounipolar ganglion cells located in the *superior (jugular) ganglion* of the vagus nerve terminate in the spinal nucleus of the trigeminal nerve. The peripheral fibers originate from
  - The dura in the posterior cranial fossa (meningeal branch, see **Fig. 5.27f**),
  - A small area of the skin of the pinna (see **Fig. 5.27b**) and external auditory canal (auricular branch, see **Fig. 5.27c**). The auricular branch is the only cutaneous branch of the vagus nerve.
- *Special visceral afferent:* Central processes of pseudounipolar ganglion cells from the inferior nodose ganglion terminate in the superior part of the nucleus of the solitary tract. Their peripheral processes supply the taste buds on the epiglottis (see **Fig. 5.27d**).
- *General visceral afferent:* These nerves supply the following areas:
  - Mucosa of the lower pharynx at its junction with the esophagus (see **Fig. 5.27a**)
  - Laryngeal mucosa above (superior laryngeal nerve) and below (inferior laryngeal nerve) the glottic aperture (see **Fig. 5.27a**)

Speech notes: Unilateral pharyngeal branch lesion lead to mild to moderate hypernasality and nasal air emission during pressure consonants. Hypernasality can be severe if weakness is bilateral. Speech may be breathy, hoarse, reduced in loudness, have diplophonia ("two tones"), reduced pitch, or pitch breaks if the lesion is below the pharyngeal branch but including the superior and recurrent laryngeal branches. An inability to change pitch might exist if the superior laryngeal nerve is damaged, sparing the pharyngeal and recurrent laryngeal nerves. Unilateral recurrent laryngeal nerve lesions that spare the superior laryngeal nerve and pharyngeal branch cause a breathy-hoarse vocal quality, decreased loudness, and sometimes diplophonia and pitch breaks. Bilateral weakness or paralysis causes stridor or noisy inhalation.

5.8.3 Branches of the Vagus Nerve (CN X) in the Neck

The vagus nerve gives off four sets of branches in the neck: pharyngeal branches, the superior laryngeal nerve, the recurrent laryngeal nerve, and the cervical cardiac branches (**Fig. 5.26a**).

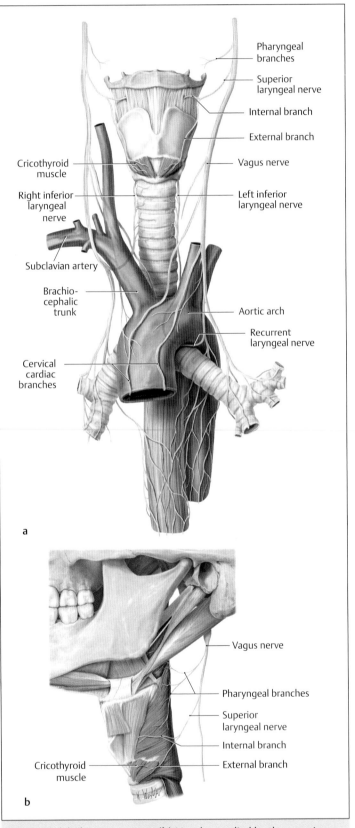

Fig. 5.26 **(a)** The vagus nerve. **(b)** Muscle supplied by the superior laryngeal nerve.

The inferior laryngeal nerve is the terminal branch of the recurrent laryngeal nerve. It winds around the subclavian artery on the right side and around the aortic arch on the left side. On that side it is in close relationship to the left main bronchus. A lesion of the inferior laryngeal nerve (e.g., due to pressure from a bronchial carcinoma or from an aortic aneurysm) may lead to hoarseness (intrinsic laryngeal muscles). The inferior laryngeal nerve passes close to the posterolateral aspect of the thyroid gland, making it susceptible to injury during thyroid operations. For this reason, an otolaryngologist should assess the function of the laryngeal muscles prior to thyroid surgery, and a speech–language pathologist with experience and expertise in phonatory disorders is frequently consulted as well.

Muscle supplied by the superior laryngeal nerve (**Fig. 5.26b**).

5.8.4 Visceral and Sensory Distribution of the Vagus Nerve (CN X)

See **Fig. 5.27**.

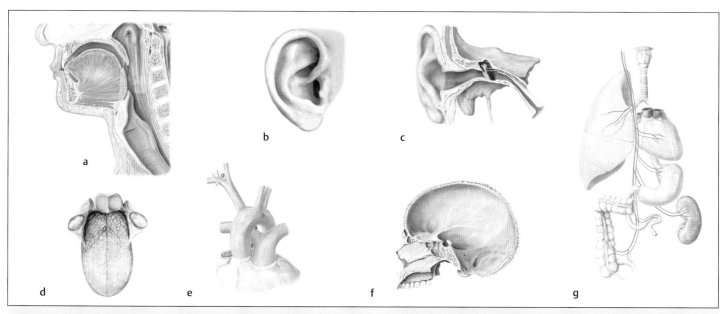

Fig. 5.27 Visceral and sensory distribution of the vagus nerve (CN X). **(a)** Laryngeal mucosa above and below the glottic aperture. **(b)** Pinna. **(c)** External auditory canal. **(d)** Epiglottis. **(e)** Laryngeal nerve and the cervical cardiac branches. **(f)** Meningeal branch. **(g)** Parasympathetic presynaptic efferents.

5.9 Larynx: Topography

5.9.1 Topography of the Larynx

Left lateral view. Superficial dissection (**Fig. 5.28a**).

Deep dissection (cricothyroid and left thyroid lamina removed with pharyngeal mucosa retracted) (**Fig. 5.28b**).

Neurovascular structures enter the larynx posteriorly. The larynx receives sensory and motor innervation from branches of the vagus nerve (CN X).

Sensory innervation: The upper larynx (above the vocal folds) receives sensory innervation from the internal laryngeal nerve, and the infraglottic cavity receives sensory innervation from the recurrent laryngeal nerve.

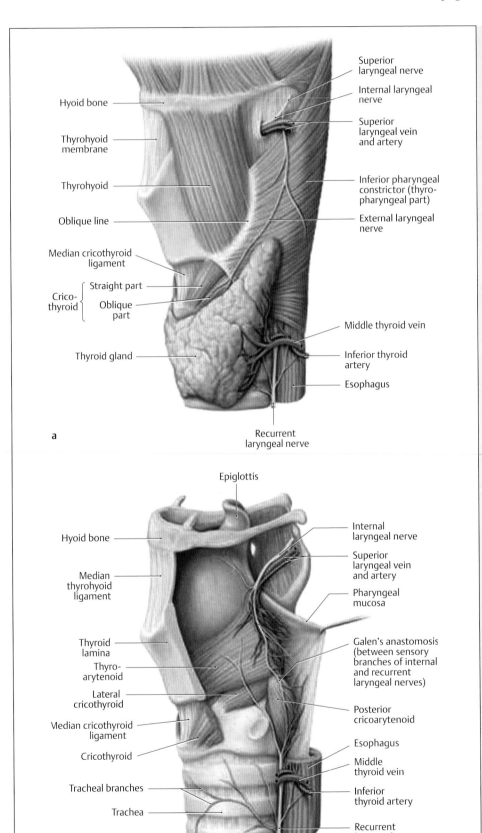

a

b

Fig. 5.28 Topography of the larynx.
(a) Superficial dissection. **(b)** Deep dissection. (Reproduced from Baker, Anatomy for Dental Medicine, 2nd edition, ©2015, Thieme publishers, New York. Illustration by Karl Wesker/Markus Voll.)

Motor innervation: The cricothyroid receives motor innervation from the external laryngeal nerve, and the rest of the intrinsic muscles of the larynx receive motor innervation from the recurrent laryngeal nerve.

5.9.2 Approaches to the Larynx and Trachea

Midsagittal section, left lateral view (**Fig. 5.29**). When an acute edematous obstruction of the larynx (e. g., due to an allergic reaction) poses an acute risk of asphyxiation, the following surgical approaches are available for creating an emergency airway:

- Division of the median cricothyroid ligament (cricothyrotomy)
- Incision of the trachea (tracheotomy) at a level just below the cricoid cartilage (high tracheotomy) or just superior to the jugular notch (low tracheotomy)

5.9.3 Vagus Nerve Lesions

The vagus nerve (CN X) provides branchiomotor innervation to the pharyngeal and laryngeal muscles and somatic sensory innervation to the larynx (**Fig. 5.30**).

Note: The vagus nerve also conveys parasympathetic motor fibers and visceral sensory fibers to and from the thoracic and abdominal viscera.

Branchiomotor innervation: The nucleus ambiguus contains the cell bodies of lower motor neurons whose branchiomotor fibers travel in CN IX, X, and XI. The nuclei of the vagus nerve are located in the middle region of the nucleus ambiguus in the brainstem (the cranial portions of the nucleus send axons via the glossopharyngeal nerve, and the caudal portions send axons via the accessory nerve). Fibers emerge from the middle portion of

the nucleus ambiguus as roots and combine into CN X, which passes through the jugular foramen. Branchiomotor fibers are distributed to the pharyngeal plexus via the pharyngeal branch and the cricothyroid muscle via the external laryngeal nerve (a branch of the superior laryngeal nerve). The remaining branchiomotor fibers leave the vagus nerve as the recurrent laryngeal nerves, which ascend along the trachea to reach the larynx.

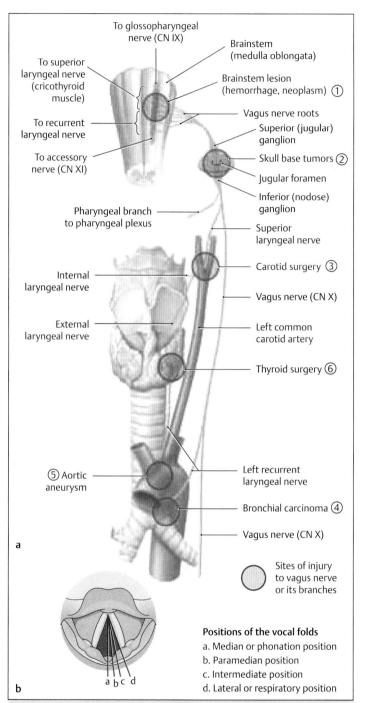

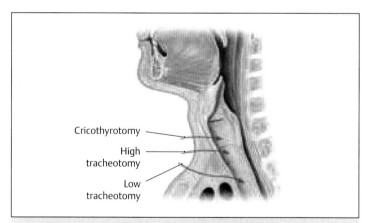

Fig. 5.29 The larynx and trachea. Midsagittal section, left lateral view. (Reproduced from Baker, Anatomy for Dental Medicine, 2nd edition, ©2015, Thieme publishers, New York. Illustration by Karl Wesker/Markus Voll.)

Fig. 5.30 Vagus nerve lesions. **(a)** Lesions of the laryngeal nerves. **(b)** Position of the vocal folds. (Reproduced from Baker, Anatomy for Dental Medicine, 2nd edition, ©2015, Thieme publishers, New York. Illustration by Karl Wesker/Markus Voll.)

Sensory innervation: General somatic sensory fibers travel from the laryngeal mucosa to the spinal nucleus of the trigeminal nerve via the vagus nerve. The cell bodies of these primary sensory neurons are located in the inferior (nodose) ganglion.

Note: The superior (jugular) ganglion contains the cell bodies of viscerosensory neurons.

See **Table 5.4**.

5.9.4 Vocal Folds

The vocal fold, which is exposed to severe mechanical stresses, is covered by nonkeratinized squamous epithelium, unlike the adjacent subglottic space, which is covered by ciliated respiratory epithelium (**Fig. 5.31**). The mucosa of the vocal folds and subglottic space overlies loose connective tissue. Chronic irritation of the subglottic mucosa (e.g., from cigarette smoke) may cause chronic edema in the subglottic space, resulting in a harsh voice. Degenerative changes in the vocal fold mucosa may lead to thickening, loss of elasticity, and squamous cell carcinoma.

Table 5.4 Vagus nerve lesions

Lesions of the laryngeal nerves (**Fig. 5.30a**) may cause sensory loss or motor paralysis, which disrupts the position of the vocal folds (**Fig. 5.30b**).

Level of nerve lesion and effects on vocal fold position		Sensory loss
① Central lesion (brainstem or higher)		
E.g., due to tumor or hemorrhage. Spastic paralysis (if nucleus ambiguus is disrupted), flaccid paralysis, and muscle atrophy (if motor neurons or axons are destroyed).	b, c	None
② Skull base lesion[a]		
E.g., due to nasopharyngeal tumors. Flaccid paralysis of all intrinsic and extrinsic laryngeal muscles on affected side. Glottis cannot be closed, causing severe hoarseness.	b, c	Entire affected (ipsilateral) side
③ Superior laryngeal nerve lesions[a]		
E.g., due to carotid surgery. Hypotonicity of the cricothyroid, resulting in mild hoarseness with a weak voice, especially at high frequencies.	d	Above vocal fold
④, ⑤, ⑥, Recurrent laryngeal nerve lesions[b]		
E.g., due to bronchial carcinoma ④, aortic aneurysm ⑤, or thyroid surgery ⑥. Paralysis of all intrinsic laryngeal muscles on affected side. This results in mild hoarseness, poor tonal control, rapid voice fatigue, but not dyspnea.	a, b	Below vocal fold

Source: Reproduced from Baker, Anatomy for Dental Medicine, 2nd edition, ©2015: Table 13.3, Thieme publishers, New York.

[a] Other motor deficits include drooping of the soft palate and deviation of the uvula toward the cough reflexes, difficulty swallowing (dysphagia), and hypernasal speech due to deficient closure of the pharyngeal isthmus. Sensory defects include the sensation of a foreign body in the throat.

[b] Transection of both recurrent laryngeal nerves can cause significant dyspnea and inspiratory stridor (high-pitched noise indicating obstruction), necessitating tracheotomy in acute cases.

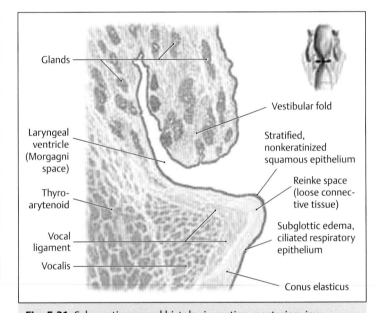

Glands — Vestibular fold — Laryngeal ventricle (Morgagni space) — Stratified, nonkeratinized squamous epithelium — Reinke space (loose connective tissue) — Thyro-arytenoid — Subglottic edema, ciliated respiratory epithelium — Vocal ligament — Vocalis — Conus elasticus

Fig. 5.31 Schematic coronal histologic section, posterior view. (Reproduced from Baker, Anatomy for Dental Medicine, 2nd edition, ©2015, Thieme publishers, New York. Illustration by Karl Wesker/Markus Voll.)

5.10 Endotracheal Intubation

5.10.1 Equipment and Positioning of the Head for Endotracheal Intubation

Endotracheal (ET) tube with an inflatable cuff (left) and laryngoscope with handle and curved spatula (right) (**Fig. 5.32a**). Unfavorable and optimal positioning of the head for endotracheal intubation (**Fig. 5.32b** and **Fig. 5.32c**).

Endotracheal intubation, inserting a tube into the trachea of a patient, is the safest way to keep the airways clear to allow for effective ventilation. Depending on access there are four ways to achieve endotracheal intubation:

- Orotracheal = via the mouth (gold standard)
- Nasotracheal = via the nose (performed if orotracheal intubation is not possible)
- Pertracheal = intubation through tracheostomy (used for long-term ventilation)
- Cricothyrotomy (used only in emergencies when there is the threat of impending suffocation)

Endotracheal intubation requires the use of a laryngoscope and an ET tube (**Fig. 5.32a**). The tubes are available in different sizes (10–22 cm) and diameters (2.5–8 mm). They have a circular cross piece that has a proximal connector for a ventilation hose and a beveled distal end. An inflatable cuff on the ET ensures that the trachea is hermetically sealed (see **Fig. 5.34**). With orotracheal intubation, the oral, pharyngeal, and tracheal axes should lie on a straight line (the so-called "sniffing position", see **Fig. 5.32c**). This facilitates direct visualization of the laryngeal inlet (see **Fig. 5.33**) and shortens the distance between the teeth and glottis in young adults (13–16 cm).

Note: In patients with suspected cervical spine injury, manipulation of the head position without maintaining the stability of the cervical spine is contraindicated.

5.10.2 Placement of the Laryngoscope and the Endotracheal Tube (ET)

Handling and placement of the laryngoscope from the perspective of the physician (**Fig. 5.33a**). Placement of the ET tube (**Fig. 5.33b**). To place the ET tube, the physician stands at the head of the patient and introduces the spatula of the laryngoscope into the patient's mouth. The spatula is then used to push the patient's tongue to the left to get a clear view of the larynx. Under direct visualization, the spatula tip is then advanced until it lies in the vallecula. *Note:* If the spatula is introduced too deep, its tip reaches behind the epiglottis, and orientation is difficult. The physician then pulls the spatula in the direction of floor of mouth without using the upper teeth as a fulcrum. This elevates the

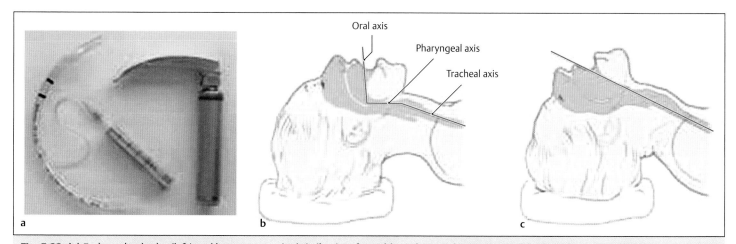

Fig. 5.32 **(a)** Endotracheal tube (left) and laryngoscope (right). **(b, c)** Unfavorable and optimal positioning of the head for endotracheal intubation. (Reproduced from Baker, Anatomy for Dental Medicine, 2nd edition, ©2015, Thieme publishers, New York. Illustration by Karl Wesker/Markus Voll.)

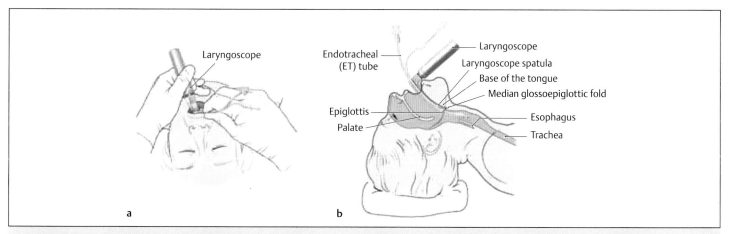

Fig. 5.33 **(a)** Handling and placement of the laryngoscope from the perspective of the physician. **(b)** Placement of the endotracheal tube. (Reproduced from Baker, Anatomy for Dental Medicine, 2nd edition, ©2015, Thieme publishers, New York. Illustration by Karl Wesker/Markus Voll.)

epiglottis and the base of the tongue such that the physician now has an unobstructed view of the laryngeal inlet (see **Fig. 5.34a**). The physician then pushes the ET tube through the rima glottidis into the trachea (see **Fig. 5.34b**). Placement under laryngoscopic control ensures that the ET tube is placed in the trachea and does not accidentally enter the esophagus.

Note: The ET tube has markings in centimeter increments that serve as an orientation aid to the physician. The distance from the upper teeth to the center of the trachea in the adult is about 22 cm and in newborns is about 11 cm. Distances greater than these might indicate that the tube is inserted too deeply and is in the right main bronchus.

5.10.3 View of the Laryngeal Inlet and Location of the Endotracheal Tube after Intubation

Laryngoscopic view of larynx, epiglottis, and median glossoepiglottic fold (**Fig. 5.34a**).

Median sagittal section viewed from the right of an ET tube in situ with its cuff inflated (**Fig. 5.34b**). The inflatable cuff seals the trachea in all directions and eliminates leakage during ventilation and prevents aspiration of foreign bodies, mucus, or gastric juice.

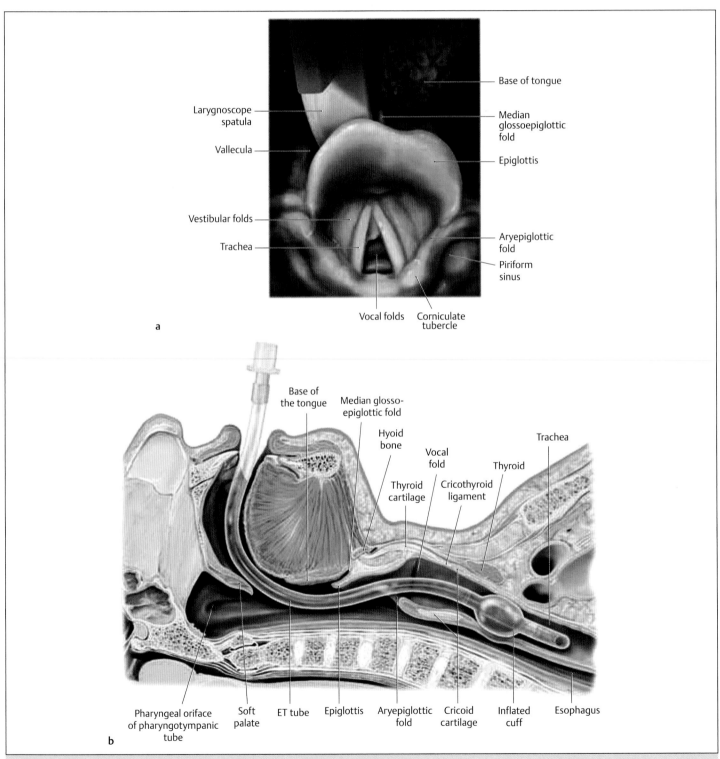

Fig. 5.34 (a) Laryngoscopic view of larynx, epiglottis, and median glossoepiglottic fold. (b) Median sagittal section viewed from the right of an endotracheal tube in situ with its cuff inflated. (Reproduced from Baker, Anatomy for Dental Medicine, 2nd edition, ©2015, Thieme publishers, New York. Illustration by Karl Wesker/Markus Voll.)

To check if the ET tube has been placed correctly, the physician looks at the patient's chest to evaluate if chest movement is symmetrical, he auscultates for equal breath sounds over both lung fields and the absence of breath sounds over the stomach. Further indicators that the ET tube is placed correctly include vapor condensation on the inside of the ET tube with exhalation and measurement of end-tidal carbon dioxide. If there is any doubt as to the positioning of the tube, it should be removed.

5.11 Cranial Nerves Most Involved in Speech and Swallowing: Accessory (CN XI) and Hypoglossal (CN XII)

5.11.1 Nucleus and Course of the Accessory Nerve

Posterior view of the brainstem (with the cerebellum removed) (**Fig. 5.35**). For didactic reasons, the muscles are displayed from the right side (see Chapter 5.11.3 for further details).

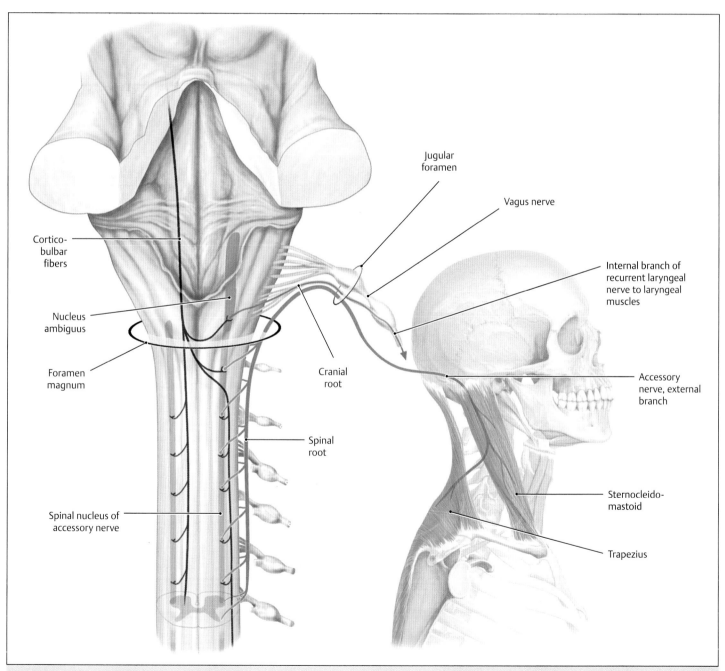

Fig. 5.35 Posterior view of the brainstem (with the cerebellum removed).

5.11.2 Lesion of the Accessory Nerve (on the Right Side)

Posterior view (**Fig. 5.36a**). Paralysis of the trapezius muscle causes drooping of the shoulder on the affected side. Right anterolateral view (**Fig. 5.36b**). With paralysis of the sternocleidomastoid muscle, it is difficult for the patient to turn the head to the opposite side against a resistance.

5.11.3 Overview of the Accessory Nerve (CN XI)

The accessory nerve is considered by some authors to be an *independent* part of the vagus nerve (CN X). It contains both visceral and somatic efferent fibers, and has one cranial and one spinal root.

Sites of emergence: The spinal root emerges from the spinal cord, passes superiorly, and enters the skull through the *foramen magnum,* where it joins with the cranial root from the medulla oblongata. Both roots then leave the skull together through *the jugular foramen.*

Nuclei and distribution:

- *Cranial root:* The special visceral efferent fibers of the accessory nerve that arise from the caudal part of the nucleus ambiguus join the vagus nerve and are distributed with the recurrent laryngeal nerve. The recurrent laryngeal nerve is a branch of the vagus nerve (CN X) and, as mentioned previously, when damaged, may cause paralytic dysphonia including air wastage on phonation along with hoarse, harsh, voice quality. These portions of CN X and CN XI travel adjacently, but the fibers of the recurrent laryngeal nerve (CN X) innervate all of the laryngeal muscles except the cricothyroid.
- *Spinal root:* The spinal nucleus of the accessory nerve forms a narrow column of cells in the anterior horn of the spinal cord at the level of C2 (cervical segment 2)—C5/6. After emerging from the spinal cord, its somatic efferent fibers form the external branch of the accessory nerve, which supplies the trapezius and sternocleidomastoid muscles.

Effects of Accessory Nerve Injury

A unilateral lesion results in the following deficits:

- *Trapezius paralysis,* characterized by drooping of the shoulder and difficulty raising the arm above the horizontal (the trapezius supports the serratus anterior in elevating the arm past 90 degrees). The part of the accessory nerve that supplies the trapezius is vulnerable during operations in the neck (e.g., lymph node biopsies).
- *Sternocleidomastoid paralysis,* characterized by torticollis (wry neck, i.e., difficulty turning the head to the opposite side). Spasmodic torticollis, sometimes referred to as cervical dystonia, also can be caused by many other conditions. See LaPointe et al[6].

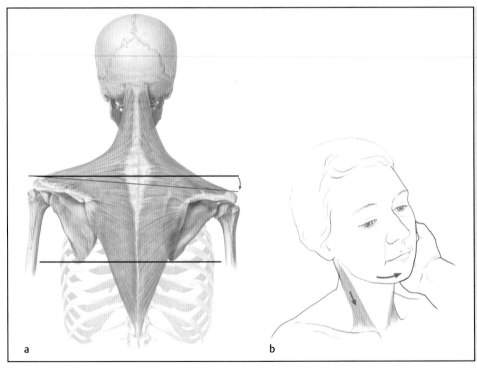

a

b

Fig. 5.36 Lesion of the accessory nerve (on the right side). **(a)** Posterior view. **(b)** Right anterolateral view.

5.11.4 Nuclei of the Hypoglossal Nerve

Cross-section through the medulla oblongata at the level of the olive (**Fig. 5.37a**). This section passes through the nucleus of the hypoglossal nerve. It can be seen that the nucleus lies just beneath the rhomboid fossa and raises the floor of the fossa to form the hypoglossal trigone. Because each nucleus is close to the midline, it is common for more extensive lesions to involve the nuclei on both sides, producing the clinical manifestations of a bilateral nuclear lesion.

Anterior view (**Fig. 5.37b**). The neurons contained in this nuclear column correspond to the alpha motor neurons of the spinal cord.

5.11.5 Overview of the Hypoglossal Nerve (CN XII)

The hypoglossal nerve is a purely somatic efferent nerve that supplies the musculature of the tongue.
Nucleus and site of emergence: The nucleus of the hypoglossal nerve is located in the floor of the rhomboid fossa. Its somatic efferent fibers emerge from the medulla oblongata, leaving the cranial cavity through the hypoglossal canal and descending lateral to the vagus nerve. The hypoglossal nerve enters the root of the tongue above the hyoid bone and distributes its fibers there.
Distribution: The hypoglossal nerve supplies all intrinsic and extrinsic muscles of the tongue (except for the palatoglossus, CNX). The ventral fibers of C1 and C2 travel with the hypoglossal nerve but leave it again after a short distance to form the superior root of the (deep) ansa cervicalis.

Effects of hypoglossal nerve injury:

- Central hypoglossal paralysis (supranuclear): The tongue deviates away from the side of the lesion.
- Nuclear or peripheral paralysis: The tongue deviates toward the affected side due to a preponderance of muscular action on the healthy side.

Speech effects: The most perceivable speech characteristic is imprecise articulation. Difficulty (slowed range or velocity of movement) with the tip or back of the tongue may occur with bilateral lingual weakness. The speech sounds most disrupted are /s/, /sh/, /ch/, /r/, and /l/. Velars (/d/, /t/) also can be distorted. In addition, vowels may be affected. For AMRs /pa/ should be normal, while /ta/ and /ka/ may be imprecise, irregular, and slow. Unilateral paralysis of the tongue usually results in only mild articulatory imprecision, but bilateral hypoglossal nerve impairment can create more severe impairments in lingual movement and speech intelligibility.

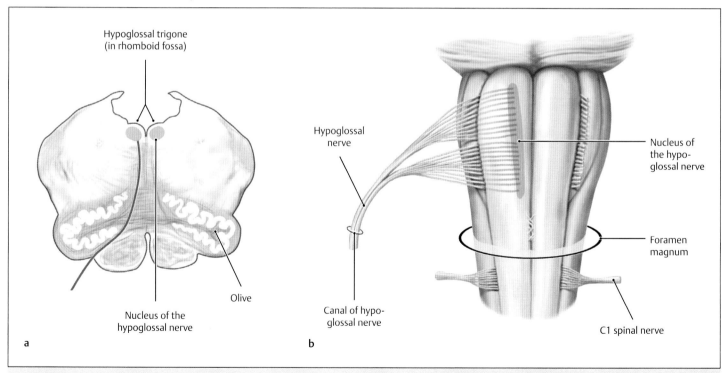

Fig. 5.37 Nuclei of the hypoglossal nerve. (a) Cross-section through the medulla oblongata. (b) Anterior view.

5.11.6 Distribution of the Hypoglossal Nerve

The nucleus of the hypoglossal nerve is innervated (upper motor neurons) by cortical neurons from the contralateral side (**Fig. 5.38**). With a unilateral *nuclear or peripheral* lesion of the hypoglossal nerve, the tongue deviates toward the side of the lesion when protruded because of the relative dominance of the healthy genioglossus muscle (**Fig. 5.38c**). When both nuclei are injured, the tongue cannot be protruded and tongue movements are minimal or greatly reduced in velocity and range of movement (flaccid paralysis).

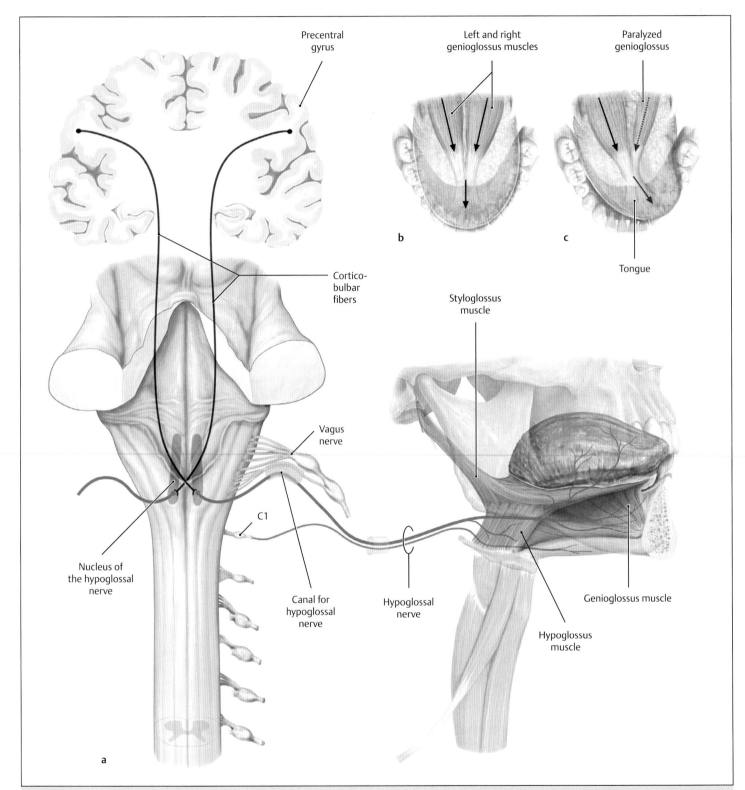

Fig. 5.38 Hypoglossal nerve. **(a)** Central and peripheral course. **(b)** Function of the genioglossus muscle. **(c)** Deviation of the tongue toward the paralyzed side.

6 Blood Vessels, Vascular System

6.1 Overview of the Human Vascular System

6.1.1 Schematic Representation of the Circulatory System

Special circulatory organs are needed to transport and distribute the blood, ensuring that it is made accessible to all the cells in the body, including the human nervous system (**Fig. 6.1**). These organs consist of the heart and vascular system (blood vessels and lymphatics). The **system of blood vessels** consists of arteries, capillaries, and veins. The *arteries* carry the blood from the heart and distribute it throughout the body. The *veins* return the blood to the heart. The exchange of gases, nutrients, and waste products takes place in the *capillary* region. All blood vessels leading away from the heart are called arteries and all vessels leading toward the heart are called veins, regardless of their oxygen content (the umbilical vein, e.g., carries oxygen-rich blood). The blood flow in this closed vascular system is maintained by the **pumping action of the heart**. The **lymphatic system** runs parallel to the venous system. It originates with blind-ended vessels in the capillary region, collects the *extracellular* fluid that is deposited there, and returns it to the venous blood through *lymphatic vessels*. *Lymph nodes* are interposed along these pathways to filter the lymph. Functionally, the circulatory system is divided into two main circuits:

- **The pulmonary circulation:** *Deoxygenated venous blood* from the upper and lower body regions is returned through the superior and inferior vena cava to the *right* atrium. It then enters the *right* ventricle, which pumps it through the pulmonary arteries to the lungs.
- **The systemic circulation:** *Oxygen-enriched blood* from the lungs returns through the pulmonary veins to the *left* atrium. From the left atrium it enters the *left* ventricle, which pumps the blood through the aorta into the systemic circulation. A special part of the systemic circuit is the **portal circulation**, which includes two successive capillary beds. *Before* venous blood returns to the inferior vena cava from the capillary beds of the unpaired abdominal organs (stomach, bowel, pancreas,

and spleen), it is carried by the portal vein to the capillary bed of the liver. This ensures that nutrient-rich blood from the digestive organs undergoes numerous filtering and metabolic processes in the liver before it is returned to the inferior vena cava via the hepatic veins.

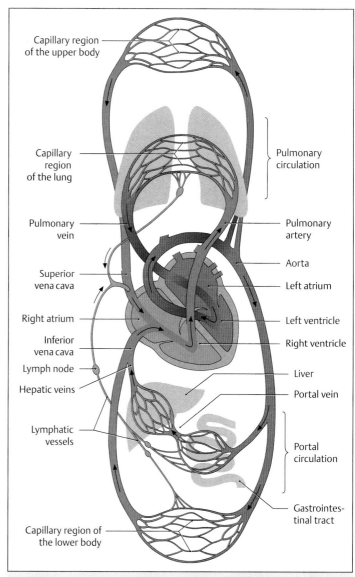

Fig. 6.1 Schematic representation of the circulatory system.

6.1.2 Basic Functional Diagram of the Circulatory System

(No distinction is made between the systemic and pulmonary systems in the diagram; after Klinke, Silbernagl)

Blood is transported through the circulatory system along a *pressure gradient* created by the different pressure levels in the arterial and venous systems (**Fig. 6.2**). While the average blood pressure in the *arterial high-pressure system* is approximately 100 mm Hg (13.3 N), the pressure in the venous *low-pressure system* generally does not exceed 20 mm Hg (2.6 N). The two systems meet in the capillary region of the terminal vascular bed, where metabolic exchange takes place. When the heart expels blood during systole, the *arteries surrounding the heart (elastic-type* arteries) can temporarily expand to accommodate the ejected blood volume. During the diastole that follows, the vessel lumen undergoes an *elastic recoil* that transforms the intermittently ejected blood volumes into continuous flow. *Arteries distant from the heart (muscular-type* arteries) can actively expand *(vasodilation)* and contract *(vasoconstriction)*, providing a very effective means of controlling vascular resistance and regulating local blood flow. The veins are also called *capacitance vessels* because of the high volume of blood contained within the veins. They can accommodate 80% of the total blood volume and thus serve an important reservoir function.

6.1.3 Overview of the Principal Arteries in the Systemic Circulation

Normally, 7 to 8% of human body weight is from blood. In adults, this amounts to 4 to 5 quarts of blood. This essential fluid carries out the critical functions of transporting oxygen and nutrients to our cells and getting rid of carbon dioxide, ammonia, and other waste products. In addition, it plays a vital role in our immune system and in maintaining a relatively constant body temperature (**Fig. 6.3**). Blood is a highly specialized tissue composed of many different kinds of components. Four of the most important ones are red cells, white cells, platelets, and plasma. All humans produce these blood components—there are no populational or regional differences. Without this constant nourishment provided by blood cells we cannot live. Vascular disorders such as stroke are a major cause of brain and nervous system damage. Neuroscientists and speech–language pathologists have a special interest in vascular disorders since they are responsible for so many cases of aphasia and motor speech disorders.

6.1.4 Overview of the Principal Veins in the Systemic Circulation

The venous system is composed of superficial veins, deep veins, and also perforator veins, which interconnect the superficial and deep venous systems (**Fig. 6.4**).

Note: The portal circulation (portal vein), which carries nutrient-rich blood (shown here in purple) from the digestive organs directly to the liver (compare with the left side of **Fig. 6.1**).

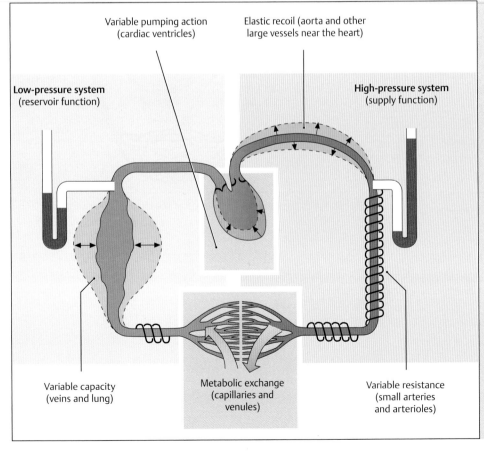

Variable pumping action (cardiac ventricles)

Elastic recoil (aorta and other large vessels near the heart)

Low-pressure system (reservoir function)

High-pressure system (supply function)

Variable capacity (veins and lung)

Metabolic exchange (capillaries and venules)

Variable resistance (small arteries and arterioles)

Fig. 6.2 Basic functional diagram of the circulatory system.

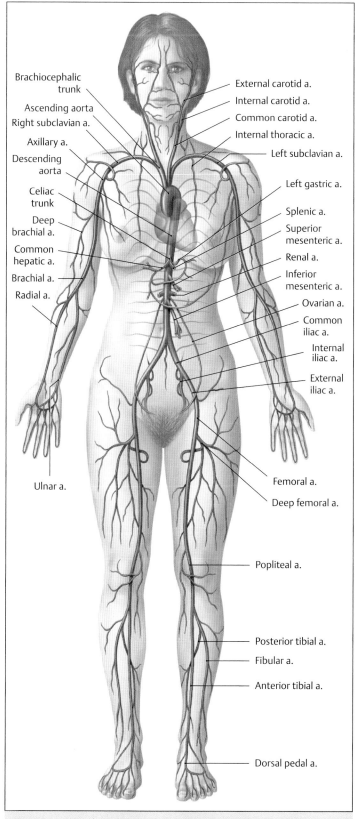

Fig. 6.3 Principal arteries in the systemic circulation.

Brachiocephalic trunk
Ascending aorta
Right subclavian a.
Axillary a.
Descending aorta
Celiac trunk
Deep brachial a.
Common hepatic a.
Brachial a.
Radial a.
Ulnar a.

External carotid a.
Internal carotid a.
Common carotid a.
Internal thoracic a.
Left subclavian a.
Left gastric a.
Splenic a.
Superior mesenteric a.
Renal a.
Inferior mesenteric a.
Ovarian a.
Common iliac a.
Internal iliac a.
External iliac a.
Femoral a.
Deep femoral a.
Popliteal a.
Posterior tibial a.
Fibular a.
Anterior tibial a.
Dorsal pedal a.

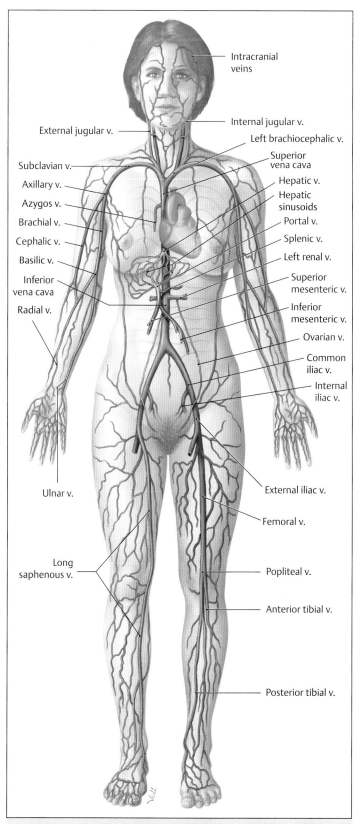

Fig. 6.4 Principal veins in the systemic circulation.

External jugular v.
Subclavian v.
Axillary v.
Azygos v.
Brachial v.
Cephalic v.
Basilic v.
Inferior vena cava
Radial v.
Ulnar v.
Long saphenous v.

Intracranial veins
Internal jugular v.
Left brachiocephalic v.
Superior vena cava
Hepatic v.
Hepatic sinusoids
Portal v.
Splenic v.
Left renal v.
Superior mesenteric v.
Inferior mesenteric v.
Ovarian v.
Common iliac v.
Internal iliac v.
External iliac v.
Femoral v.
Popliteal v.
Anterior tibial v.
Posterior tibial v.

6.2 Arteries of the Head, Overview and External Carotid Artery

6.2.1 Overview of the Arteries of the Head

Left lateral view (**Fig. 6.5**). The common carotid artery divides into the internal carotid artery and external carotid artery at the carotid bifurcation, which is at the approximate level of the fourth cervical vertebra. The carotid body (not shown) is located at the carotid bifurcation. It contains chemoreceptors that respond to oxygen deficiency in the blood (hypoxia) and to changes in pH (both are important in the regulation of breathing). While the external carotid artery divides into eight branches (see Chapter 6.2.4), the internal carotid artery does not branch further before entering the skull, where it mainly supplies blood to the brain. It also gives off branches that supply areas of the facial skeleton.

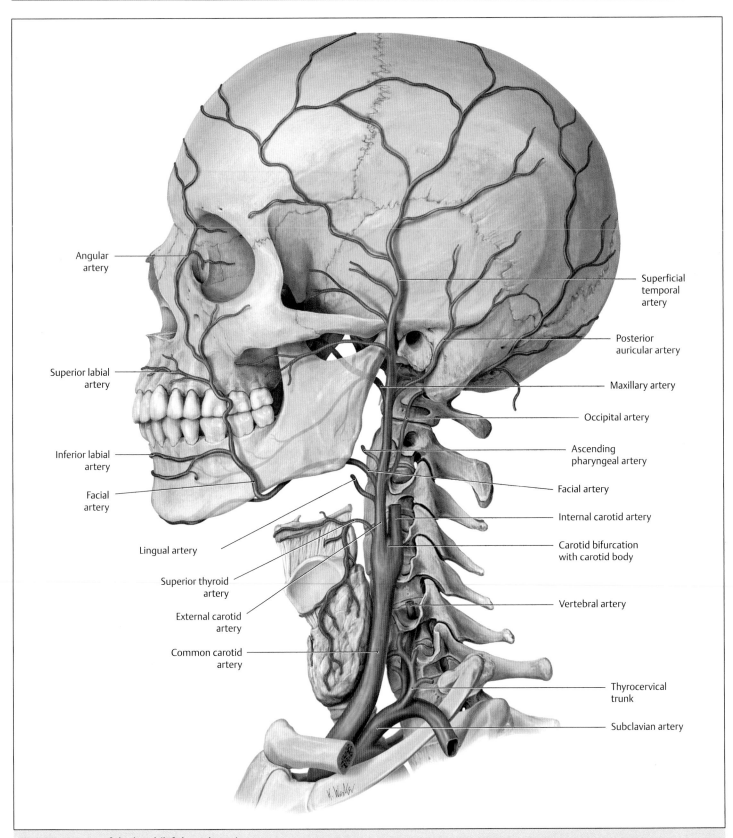

Angular
artery

Superficial
temporal
artery

Posterior
auricular artery

Superior labial
artery

Maxillary artery

Occipital artery

Inferior labial
artery

Ascending
pharyngeal artery

Facial
artery

Facial artery

Internal carotid artery

Lingual artery

Carotid bifurcation
with carotid body

Superior thyroid
artery

Vertebral artery

External carotid
artery

Common carotid
artery

Thyrocervical
trunk

Subclavian artery

Fig. 6.5 Arteries of the head (left lateral view).

6.2.2 Branches of the External Carotid Artery

See **Fig. 6.6**.

The four groups of branches of the external carotid artery are shown in different colors (anterior branches: red, medial branch: blue, posterior branches: green, terminal branches: brown).

Certain branches of the external carotid artery (facial artery, red) communicate with branches of the internal carotid artery (terminal branches of the ophthalmic artery, purple) through anastomoses in the facial region (**Fig. 6.6b**).

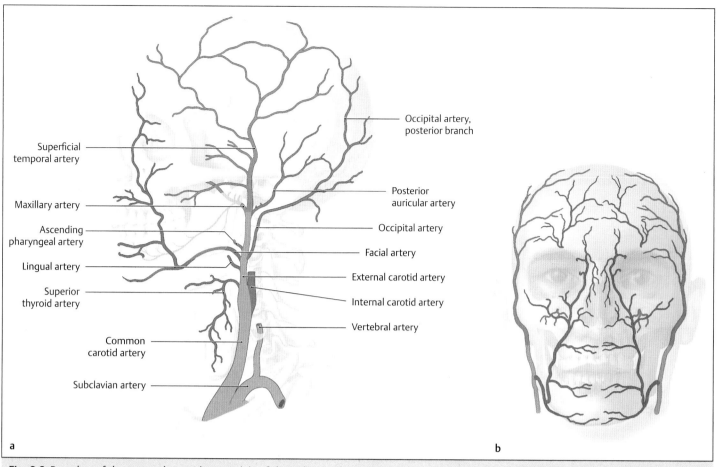

Fig. 6.6 Branches of the external carotid artery. **(a)** Left lateral view. **(b)** Anterior view.

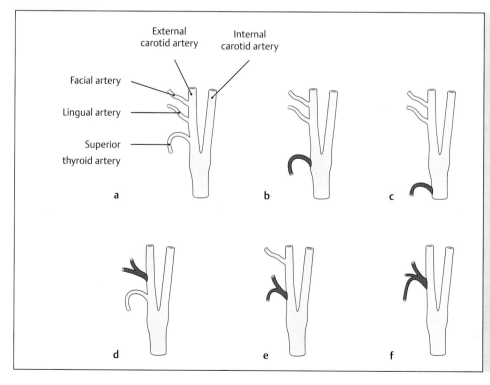

Fig. 6.7 Branches of the external carotid artery **(a)** Facial artery, lingual artery, and superior thyroid artery arise from the external carotid artery. **(b, c)** Superior thyroid artery arises at the level of the carotid bifurcation. **(d–f)** Two or three branches combine to form a common trunk: linguofacial, thyrolingual, or thyrolinguofacial.

6.2.3 Branches of the External Carotid Artery: Typical Anatomy and Variants

- In typical cases (50%), the facial artery, lingual artery, and superior thyroid artery arise from the external carotid artery above the carotid bifurcation (**Fig. 6.7a**).
- Variants (**Fig. 6.7b–f**):

- The superior thyroid artery arises at the level of the carotid bifurcation (20%) or from the common carotid artery (10%) (**Fig. 6.7b,c**).
- Two or three branches combine to form a common trunk: Linguofacial trunk (18%), thyrolingual trunk (2%), or thyrolinguofacial trunk (1%) (**Fig. 6.7d–f**).

147

6.2.4 Overview of the Branches of the External Carotid Artery

(More distal branches are described in the units below.)
Subsequent units deal with the arteries of the head as they are grouped in **Table 6.1**, followed by the branches of the internal carotid artery and the veins.

6.3 External Carotid Artery: Anterior, Medial, and Posterior Branches

6.3.1 Facial Artery, Occipital Artery, and Posterior Auricular Artery and Their Branches

Left lateral view (**Fig. 6.8a**). An important anterior branch of the external carotid artery is the **facial artery**, which gives off branches in the neck and face. The principal *cervical branch* is the ascending palatine artery; the *tonsillar branch* is ligated (tied off) during tonsillectomy. Of the *facial branches*, the superior and inferior labial arteries combine to form an arterial circle around the mouth. The *terminal branch* of the facial artery, the angular artery, anastomoses with the dorsal nasal artery. The latter vessel is the terminal branch of the ophthalmic artery, which arises from the internal carotid artery. Because there are extensive arterial anastomoses, facial injuries have a tendency to not only bleed profusely but also tend to heal quickly and well owing to the copious blood supply. The pulse of the facial artery is palpable at the anterior border of the masseter muscle insertion on the mandibular ramus. The

principal branches of the **posterior auricular artery** include the posterior tympanic artery and the parotid artery (**Fig. 6.8b**).

6.3.2 Superior Thyroid Artery, Ascending Pharyngeal Artery and Their Branches

Left lateral view (**Fig. 6.9**). The superior thyroid artery is typically the first branch to arise from the external carotid artery. One of the anterior branches, it supplies the larynx and thyroid gland. The ascending pharyngeal artery springs from the medial side of the external carotid artery, usually arising above the level of the superior thyroid artery. The level at which a vessel branches from the external carotid artery does not necessarily correlate with the course of the vessel.

Table 6.1 Branches of the external carotid artery

Name of the branches	Distribution
Anterior branches:	
• Superior thyroid artery	• Larynx, thyroid gland
• Lingual artery	• Oral floor, tongue
• Facial artery	• Superficial facial region
Medial branch:	
• Ascending pharyngeal artery	• Plexus to the skull base
Posterior branches:	
• Occipital artery	• Occiput
• Posterior auricular artery	• Ear
Terminal branches:	
• Maxillary artery	• Masticatory muscles, posteromedial part of the facial skeleton, meninges
• Superficial temporal artery	• Temporal region, part of the ear

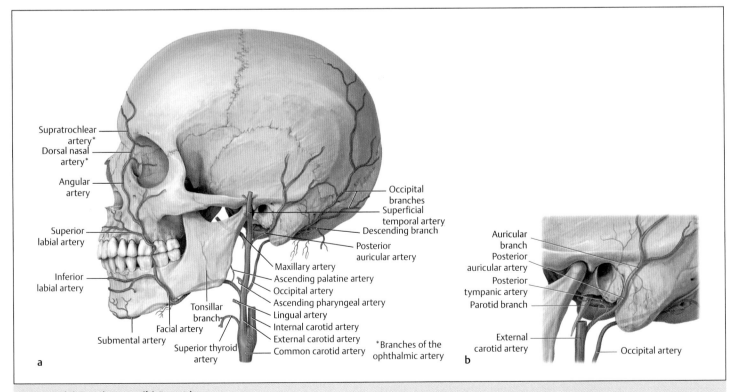

Fig. 6.8 (a) Facial artery. (b) Parotid artery.

6.3.3 Origin of the Ascending Pharyngeal Artery: Typical Case and Variants

- In **typical cases** (70%), the ascending pharyngeal artery arises from the external carotid artery (**Fig. 6.10a**).
- Variants: The ascending pharyngeal artery arises from (**Fig. 6.10b**) the occipital artery (20%), (**Fig. 6.10c**) the internal carotid artery (8%), or (**Fig. 6.10d**) the facial artery (2%).

6.3.4 Lingual Artery and Its Branches

Left lateral view (**Fig. 6.11**). The lingual artery is the second anterior branch of the external carotid artery. It has a relatively large caliber, providing the tongue with its rich blood supply. It also gives off branches to the plexus and tonsils.

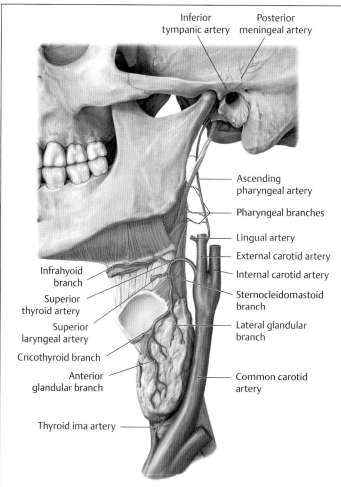

Fig. 6.9 Superior thyroid artery (left lateral view).

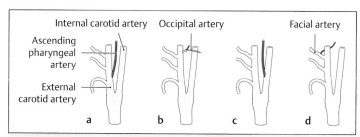

Fig. 6.10 (a) The ascending pharyngeal artery arises from the external carotid artery. (b) Occipital artery. (c) Internal carotid artery. (d) Facial artery.

6.3.5 Branches of the External Carotid Artery and Their Distribution: Anterior, Medial, and Posterior Branches with Their Principal Distal Branches

See **Table 6.2**.

Table 6.2 Branches of the external carotid artery and their distribution

Branch	Distribution
Anterior branches:	
• Superior thyroid artery (see Chapter 6.3.2)	
– Glandular branches	• Thyroid gland
– Superior laryngeal artery	• Larynx
– Sternocleidomastoid branch	• Sternocleidomastoid muscle
• Lingual artery (see Chapter 6.3.4)	
– Dorsal lingual branches	• Base of tongue, epiglottis
– Sublingual artery	• Sublingual gland, tongue, oral floor, oral cavity
– Deep lingual artery	• Tongue
• Facial artery (see Chapter 6.3.1)	
– Ascending palatine artery	• Pharyngeal wall, soft palate, pharyngotympanic tube
– Tonsillar branch	• Palatine tonsil (main branch)
– Submental artery	• Oral floor, submandibular gland
– Labial arteries	• Lips
– Angular artery	• Nasal root
Medial branch:	
• Ascending pharyngeal artery (see Chapter 6.3.2)	
– Pharyngeal branches	• Pharyngeal wall
– Inferior tympanic artery	• Mucosa of middle ear
– Posterior meningeal artery	• Dura, posterior cranial fossa
Posterior branches:	
• Occipital artery (see Chapter 6.3.1)	
– Occipital branches	• Scalp, occipital region
– Descending branch	• Posterior neck muscles
• Posterior auricular branch (see Chapter 6.3.1)	
– Stylomastoid artery	• Facial nerve in the facial canal
– Posterior tympanic artery	• Tympanic cavity
– Auricular branch	• Posterior side of auricle
– Occipital branch	• Occiput
– Parotid branch	• Parotid gland

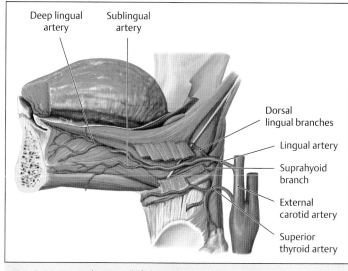

Fig. 6.11 Lingual artery (left lateral view).

6.4 Arteries of the Brain: Blood Supply and the Circle of Willis

6.4.1 Overview of the Arterial Supply to the Brain

Left lateral view (**Fig. 6.12**). The parts of the brain in the anterior and middle cranial fossae receive their blood supply from branches of the internal carotid artery, while parts of the brain in the posterior cranial fossa are supplied by branches of the vertebral and basilar arteries; the latter is formed by the confluence of the two vertebral arteries. The carotid and basilar arteries are connected by a vascular ring called the *circle of Willis (see* Chapter 6.4.3 and Chapter 6.4.4). In many cases the circle of Willis allows for compensation of decreased blood flow in one vessel with increased "collateral" blood flow through another vessel (important in patients with stenotic lesions of the afferent arteries, see Chapter 6.4.5). As a general overview of blood supply and nourishment to the brain, *the two principal arterial systems that supply the brain and keep it healthy and functioning are the vertebral and internal carotid arterial systems*.

6.4.2 The Four Anatomical Divisions of the Internal Carotid Artery

Anterior view of the left internal carotid artery (**Fig. 6.13**). The internal carotid artery consists of four topographically distinct parts between the carotid bifurcation (see Chapter 6.4.1) and the point where it divides into the anterior and middle cerebral arteries (MCAs). The parts (separated in the figure by white disks) are as follows:

(1) Cervical part (red): Located in the lateral pharyngeal space.
(2) Petrous part (yellow): Located in the carotid canal of the petrous bone.
(3) Cavernous part (green): Follows an S-shaped curve in the cavernous sinus.
(4) Cerebral part (purple): Located in the chiasmatic cistern of the subarachnoid space.

Except for the cervical part, which generally does not give off branches, all the other parts of the internal carotid artery give off numerous branches. The *intracranial* parts of the internal carotid artery are subdivided into five segments (C1–C5) based on clinical criteria:

- C1–C2: The supraclinoid segments, located within the cerebral part. C1 and C2 lie above the anterior clinoid process of the lesser wing of the sphenoid bone.
- C3–C5: The infraclinoid segments, located within the cavernous sinus.

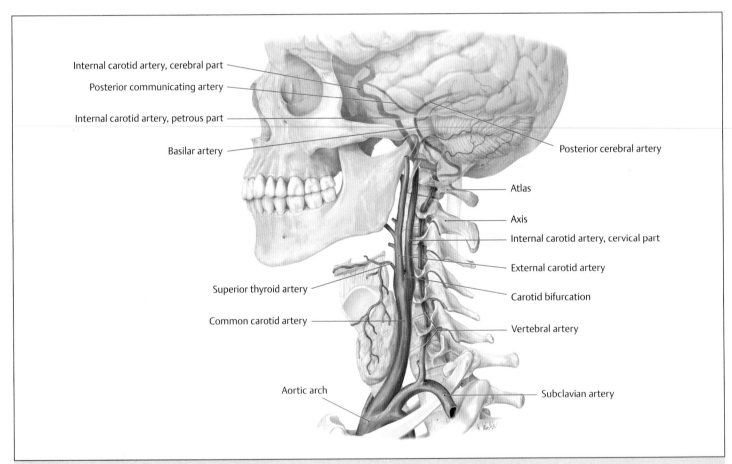

Internal carotid artery, cerebral part
Posterior communicating artery
Internal carotid artery, petrous part
Basilar artery
Superior thyroid artery
Common carotid artery
Aortic arch

Posterior cerebral artery
Atlas
Axis
Internal carotid artery, cervical part
External carotid artery
Carotid bifurcation
Vertebral artery
Subclavian artery

Fig. 6.12 Arterial supply to the brain (left lateral view).

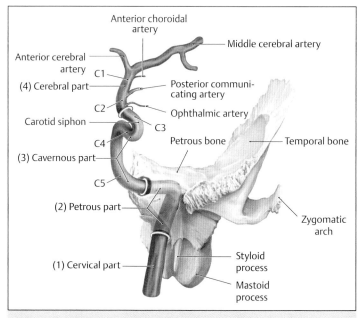

Fig. 6.13 Anterior view of the left internal carotid artery.

Anterior choroidal artery

Middle cerebral artery

Anterior cerebral artery C1

(4) Cerebral part

Posterior communicating artery

C2

Ophthalmic artery

Carotid siphon

C3

C4

Petrous bone

Temporal bone

(3) Cavernous part

C5

(2) Petrous part

Zygomatic arch

(1) Cervical part

Styloid process

Mastoid process

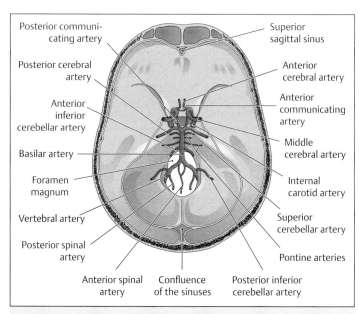

Fig. 6.14 Projection of the circle of Willis onto the base of the skull.

Posterior communicating artery

Superior sagittal sinus

Posterior cerebral artery

Anterior cerebral artery

Anterior inferior cerebellar artery

Anterior communicating artery

Basilar artery

Middle cerebral artery

Foramen magnum

Internal carotid artery

Vertebral artery

Superior cerebellar artery

Posterior spinal artery

Pontine arteries

Anterior spinal artery

Confluence of the sinuses

Posterior inferior cerebellar artery

6.4.3 Projection of the Circle of Willis onto the Base of the Skull

Superior view (**Fig. 6.14**). The two vertebral arteries enter the skull through the foramen magnum and unite behind the clivus to form the unpaired basilar artery. This vessel then divides into the two posterior cerebral arteries (additional vessels that normally contribute to the circle of Willis are shown in **Fig. 6.15**).

Note: Each MCA is the direct continuation of the internal carotid artery on that side. Clots ejected by the left heart will frequently embolize to the MCA territory. Because the left cerebral hemisphere is usually dominant for language (upward of 95% of right handers and 60% of left handers), the MCA is the part of the carotid system usually associated with aphasia. It is common to see the hospital chart note of a person with aphasia as suffering an "LMCA CVA" (left, middle cerebral artery, cerebrovascular accident).

6.4.4 Variants of the Circle of Willis (after Lippert and Pabst)

The vascular connections within the circle of Willis are subject to considerable variation. As a rule, the segmental hypoplasias shown here do not significantly alter the normal functions of the arterial ring.

- In most cases, the circle of Willis is formed by the following arteries: the anterior, middle, and posterior cerebral arteries; the anterior and posterior communicating arteries; the internal carotid arteries; and the basilar artery (**Fig. 6.15a**).
- Occasionally, the anterior communicating artery is absent (**Fig. 6.15b**).
- Both anterior cerebral arteries may arise from one internal carotid artery (10% of cases) (**Fig. 6.15c**).
- The posterior communicating artery may be absent or hypoplastic on one side (10% of cases) (**Fig. 6.15d**).
- Both posterior communicating arteries may be absent or hypoplastic (10% of cases) (**Fig. 6.15e**).
- The posterior cerebral artery may be absent or hypoplastic on one side (**Fig. 6.15f**).
- Both posterior cerebral arteries may be absent or hypoplastic. In addition, the anterior cerebral arteries may arise from a common trunk (**Fig. 6.15g**).

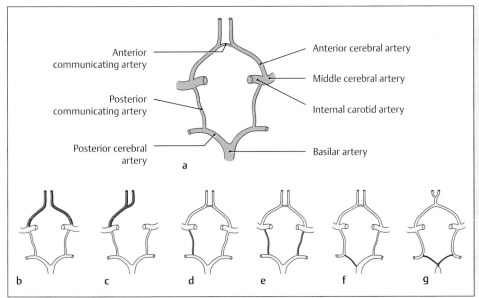

Fig. 6.15 Variants of the circle of Willis. **(a)** The anterior, middle and posterior cerebral arteries; the anterior and posterior communicating arteries; the internal carotid arteries; and the basilar artery. **(b)** The anterior communicating artery is absent. **(c)** Both anterior cerebral arteries may arise from one internal carotid artery. **(d)** The posterior communicating artery may be absent or hypoplastic on one side. **(e)** Both posterior communicating arteries may be absent or hypoplastic. **(f)** The posterior cerebral artery may be absent or hypoplastic on one side. **(g)** Both posterior cerebral arteries may be absent or hypoplastic.

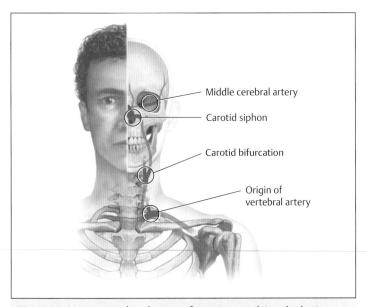

Fig. 6.16 Stenoses and occlusions of arteries supplying the brain.

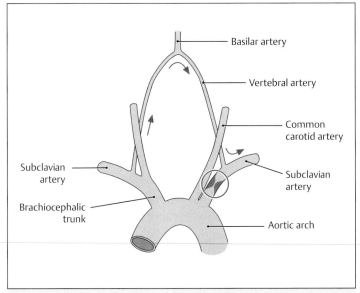

Fig. 6.17 Anatomical basis of subclavian steal syndrome.

6.4.5 Stenoses and Occlusions of Arteries Supplying the Brain

Atherosclerotic lesions in older patients may cause the narrowing (stenosis) or complete obstruction (occlusion) of arteries that supply the brain (**Fig. 6.16**). Stenoses most commonly occur at arterial bifurcations, and the sites of predilection are shown. Isolated stenoses that develop gradually may be compensated for by collateral vessels. When stenoses occur simultaneously at multiple sites, the circle of Willis cannot compensate for the diminished blood supply, and cerebral blood flow becomes impaired (varying degrees of cerebral ischemia, see p. 165).

Note: The damage is manifested clinically in the brain, but the cause is located in the vessels that supply the brain. Because stenoses are treatable, their diagnosis has major therapeutic implications. Unplug a clog or fix a stenosis and blood flows again.

6.4.6 Anatomical Basis of Subclavian Steal Syndrome

"Subclavian steal" usually results from stenosis of the left subclavian artery (red circle) located proximal to the origin of the vertebral artery. This syndrome involves a stealing of blood from the *vertebral artery* by the subclavian artery. When the left arm is exercised, as during yard work, insufficient blood may be supplied to the arm to accommodate the increased muscular effort (the patient complains of muscle weakness). Dr. Harold Klawans has written an interesting collection about people with neurological syndromes. His book Toscanini's Fumble tells of the famous conductor's difficulty with the orchestral baton because of subclavian steal syndrome.[7] As a result, blood is "stolen" from the vertebral artery circulation and there is a reversal of blood flow in the vertebral artery on the *affected* side (*arrows*) (**Fig. 6.17**). This leads to deficient blood flow in the basilar artery and may deprive the brain of blood, producing a feeling of light-headedness.

6.5 Arteries of the Cerebrum

6.5.1 Arteries at the Base of the Brain

The cerebellum and temporal lobe have been removed on the left side to display the course of the posterior cerebral artery. This view was selected because most of the arteries that supply the brain enter the cerebrum from its basal aspect (**Fig. 6.18**).

Note: The three principal arteries of the cerebrum, the anterior, middle, and posterior cerebral arteries, arise from different sources. The anterior and middle cerebral arteries are branches of the internal carotid artery, while the posterior cerebral arteries are terminal branches of the basilar artery. The vertebral arteries, which fuse to form the basilar artery, distribute branches to the spinal cord, brainstem, and cerebellum (anterior spinal artery, posterior spinal arteries, superior cerebellar artery, and anterior and posterior inferior cerebellar arteries).

6.5.2 Segments of the Anterior, Middle, and Posterior Cerebral Arteries

See **Table 6.3**.

Table 6.3 Arterial segments

Artery	Parts 5	Segments
Anterior cerebral artery	• Precommunicating part • Postcommunicating part	• A1 = segment proximal to the anterior communicating artery • A2 = segment distal to the anterior communicating artery
Middle cerebral artery (MCA)	• Sphenoidal part • Insular part	• M1 = first horizontal segment of the artery (horizontal part) • M2 = segment on the insula
Posterior cerebral artery	• Precommunicating part • Postcommunicating part	• P1 = segment between the basilar artery bifurcation and posterior communicating artery • P2 = segment between the posterior communicating artery and anterior temporal branches • P3 = lateral occipital artery • P4 = medial occipital artery

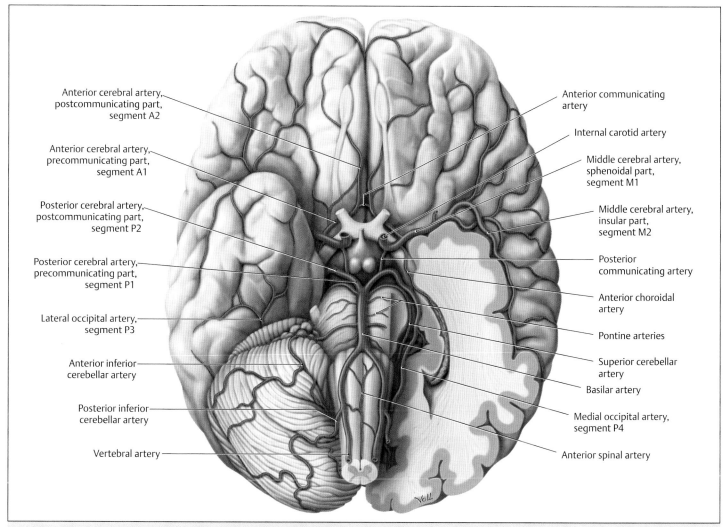

Anterior cerebral artery, postcommunicating part, segment A2

Anterior cerebral artery, precommunicating part, segment A1

Posterior cerebral artery, postcommunicating part, segment P2

Posterior cerebral artery, precommunicating part, segment P1

Lateral occipital artery, segment P3

Anterior inferior cerebellar artery

Posterior inferior cerebellar artery

Vertebral artery

Anterior communicating artery

Internal carotid artery

Middle cerebral artery, sphenoidal part, segment M1

Middle cerebral artery, insular part, segment M2

Posterior communicating artery

Anterior choroidal artery

Pontine arteries

Superior cerebellar artery

Basilar artery

Medial occipital artery, segment P4

Anterior spinal artery

Fig. 6.18 Arteries at the base of the brain.

6.5.3 Terminal Branches of the Middle Cerebral Artery on the Lateral Cerebral Hemisphere

Left lateral view (**Fig. 6.19**). Most of the blood vessels on the lateral surface of the brain are terminal branches of the MCA. They can be subdivided into two main groups:

• Inferior terminal (cortical) branches: Supply the temporal lobe cortex
• Superior terminal (cortical) branches: Supply the frontal and parietal lobe cortex

Deeper structures supplied by these branches are not shown in the diagram.

6.5.4 Course of the Middle Cerebral Artery in the Interior of the Lateral Sulcus

Left lateral view (**Fig. 6.20**). On its way to the lateral surface of the cerebral hemisphere, the MCA first courses on the base of the brain; this is the sphenoidal part of the MCA. It then continues through the lateral sulcus along the insula, which is the sunken portion of the cerebral cortex. When the temporal and parietal lobes are spread apart with a retractor, as shown here, we can see the arteries of the insula (which receive their blood from the insular part of the middle cerebral artery; see Chapter 6.5.1). When viewed in an angiogram, the branches of the insular part of the MCA resemble the arms of a candelabrum, giving rise to

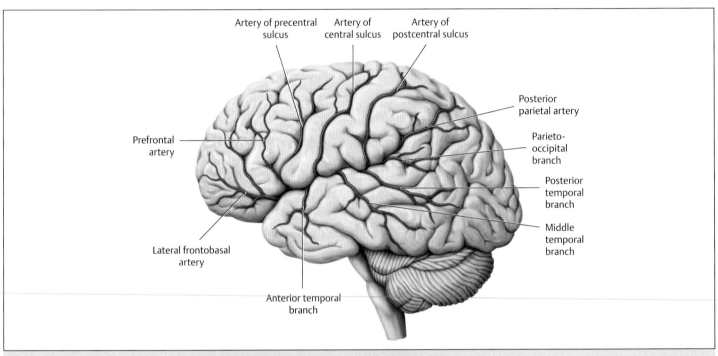

Fig. 6.19 Terminal branches of the middle cerebral artery on the lateral cerebral hemisphere.

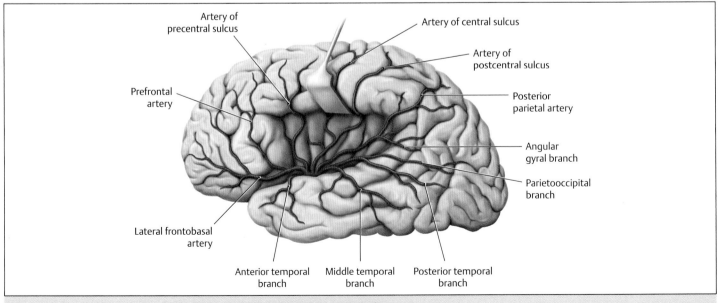

Fig. 6.20 Course of the middle cerebral artery in the interior of the lateral sulcus.

the term "candelabrum artery" for that arterial segment. Recall that the left MCA is most associated with the cortical language areas and damage or CVAs (strokes) here are most likely to result in aphasia.

6.5.5 Branches of the Anterior and Posterior Cerebral Arteries on the Medial Surface of the Cerebrum

Right cerebral hemisphere viewed from the medial side, with the left cerebral hemisphere and brainstem removed (**Fig. 6.21**). The medial surface of the brain is supplied by branches of the anterior and posterior cerebral arteries. While the *anterior cerebral artery* arises from the internal carotid artery, the *posterior cerebral artery* arises from the basilar artery (which is formed by the junction of the left and right vertebral arteries).

6.6 Arteries of the Cerebrum, Distribution

6.6.1 Distribution Areas of the Main Cerebral Arteries

Lateral view of the left cerebral hemisphere (**Fig. 6.22a**), medial view of the right cerebral hemisphere (**Fig. 6.22b**). Most of the lateral surface of the brain is supplied by the *middle* cerebral artery (green), whose branches ascend to the cortex from the depths of the insula. The branches of the *anterior* cerebral artery supply the frontal pole of the brain and the cortical areas near the cortical margin (red and pink). The *posterior* cerebral artery supplies the occipital pole and lower portions of the temporal lobe (blue). The central gray and white matter have a complex blood supply (yellow) that includes the anterior choroidal artery. The anterior and posterior cerebral arteries supply most of the medial surface of the brain.

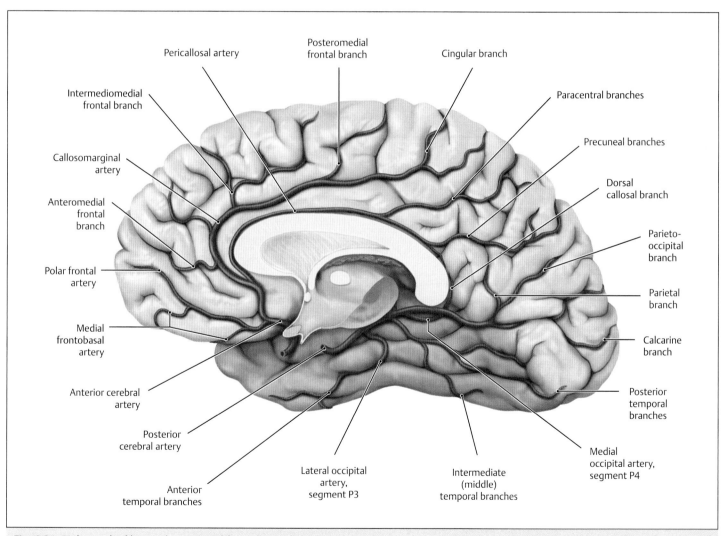

Fig. 6.21 Right cerebral hemisphere viewed from the medial side.

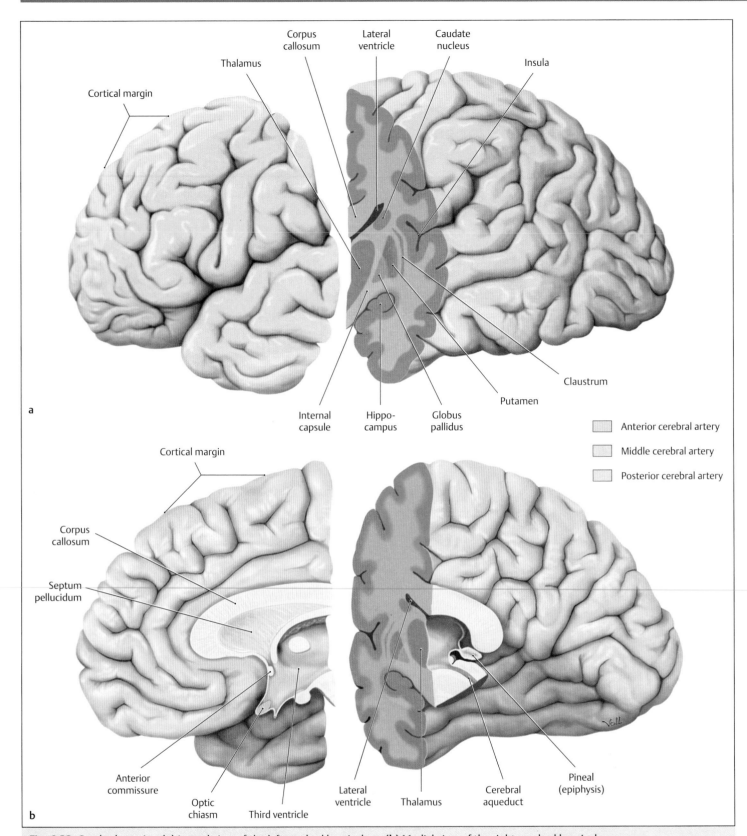

Fig. 6.22 Cerebral arteries. **(a)** Lateral view of the left cerebral hemisphere **(b)** Medial view of the right cerebral hemisphere.

6.6.2 Distribution of the Three Main Cerebral Arteries in Transverse and Coronal Sections

Coronal sections at the level of the mammillary bodies (**Fig. 6.23a,b**). Transverse section at the level of the internal capsule (**Fig. 6.23c**). The internal capsule, basal ganglia, and thalamus derive most of their blood supply from perforating branches of the following vessels at the base of the brain:

- Anterior choroidal artery (from the internal carotid artery)
- Anterolateral central arteries (lenticulostriate arteries and striate branches) with their terminal branches (from the MCA)
- Posteromedial central arteries (from the posterior cerebral artery)
- Perforating branches (from the posterior communicating artery)

The internal capsule, which is traversed by the pyramidal tract and other structures, receives most of its blood supply from the MCA (anterior crus and genu) and from the anterior choroidal artery (posterior crus). If these vessels become occluded, the pyramidal tract and other structures will be interrupted, causing paralysis on the contralateral side of the body.

6.6.3 Functional Centers on the Surface of the Cerebrum

- Lateral view of the left cerebral hemisphere (**Fig. 6.24a**). Regions supplied by branches of the MCA are shaded orange. Specific functions can be assigned to well-defined areas of the cerebrum. These areas are supplied by branches of the three main cerebral arteries. The sensorimotor cortex (pre- and post-central gyrus) and the motor and sensory speech centers (Broca and Wernicke areas) are supplied by branches of the MCA (see **Fig. 6.24b**). These areas of distribution of the MCA (in green) of the dominant hemisphere (usually left) are the most likely to be involved in aphasia and the variety of language problems that the term encompasses. Therefore, a language deficit (aphasia) or the loss of motor or sensory function on one side of the body suggests an occlusion of the MCA.
- Medial view of the right cerebral hemisphere (**Fig. 6.24b**). The "margin" of the sensorimotor cortex may be deprived of blood (clinically manifested by paralysis and sensory disturbances mainly affecting the lower limb) by an occlusion of the *anterior* cerebral artery. The visual cortex may lose its blood supply (causing blindness) through an occlusion of the *posterior* cerebral artery.

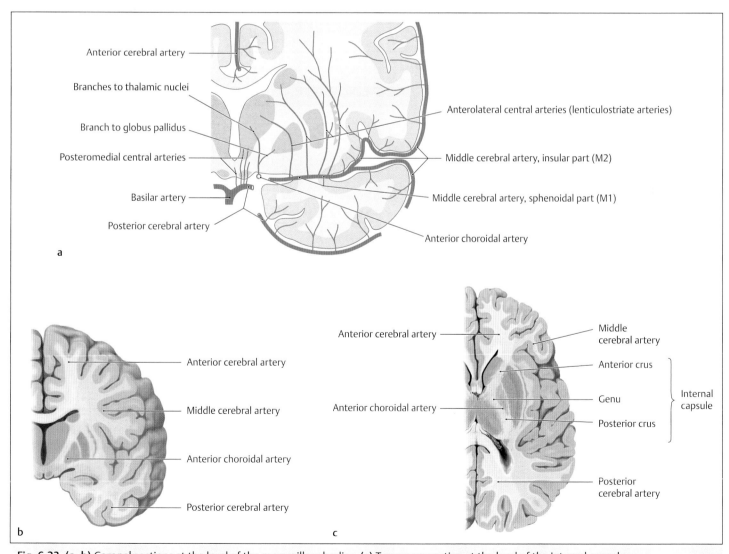

Fig. 6.23 (a, b) Coronal sections at the level of the mammillary bodies. **(c)** Transverse section at the level of the internal capsule.

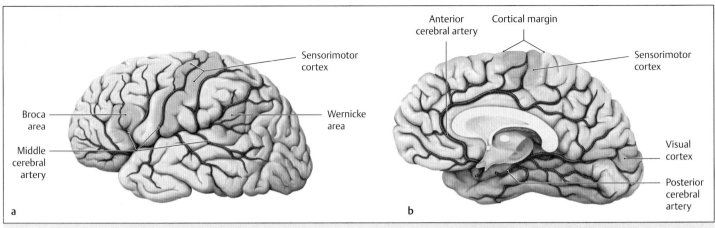

Fig. 6.24 **(a)** Lateral view of the left cerebral hemisphere. **(b)** Medial view of the right cerebral hemisphere.

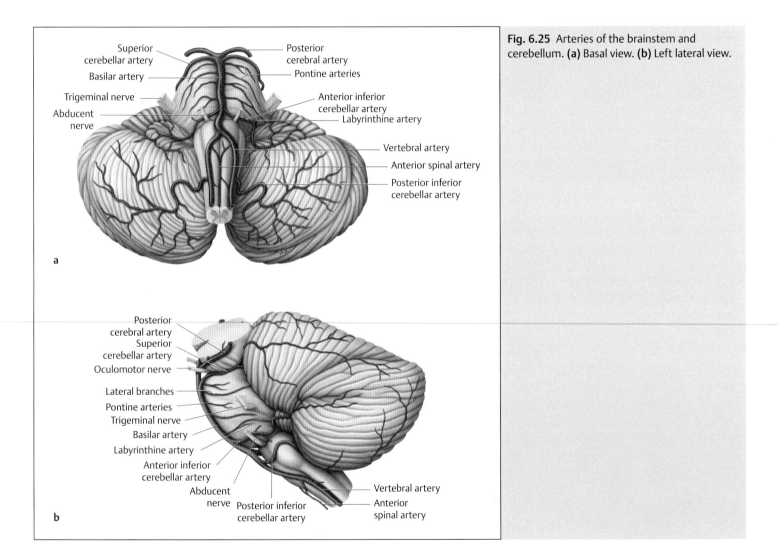

Fig. 6.25 Arteries of the brainstem and cerebellum. **(a)** Basal view. **(b)** Left lateral view.

6.7 Arteries of the Brainstem and Cerebellum

6.7.1 Origin and Distribution of Arteries of Brainstem and Cerebellum

The brainstem and cerebellum are supplied by the basilar and cerebellar arteries. Because the basilar artery is formed by the union of the two vertebral arteries, blood supplied by the basilar artery is said to come from the *vertebrobasilar complex* (**Fig. 6.25**). The vessels that supply the **brainstem** (mesencephalon, pons, and medulla oblongata) arise either directly from the basilar artery (e.g., the pontine arteries) and vertebral arteries or from their branches. The branches are classified by their sites of entry and distribution as medial, mediolateral, or lateral (paramedian branches; short and long circumferential branches). Decreased perfusion in or occlusion of these vessels leads to transient or permanent impairment of blood flow (brainstem syndrome) and may produce a great variety of clinical symptoms, given the many nuclei and tract systems that exist in the brainstem. The **spinal cord** receives a portion of its blood supply from the anterior spinal artery (see **Fig. 6.25b**), which arises from the vertebral artery. The **cerebellum** is supplied by three large arteries:

- Posterior inferior cerebellar artery (PICA), the largest branch of the vertebral artery. This vessel is usually referred to by its acronym, PICA.
- Anterior inferior cerebellar artery (AICA), the first major branch of the basilar artery.
- Superior cerebellar artery (SCA), the last major branch of the basilar artery before it divides into the posterior cerebral arteries.

Note: The labyrinthine artery which supplies the inner ear usually arises from the anterior inferior cerebellar artery, as pictured here, although it may also spring directly from the basilar artery. Impaired blood flow in the labyrinthine artery leads to an acute loss of hearing (sudden sensorineural hearing loss), frequently accompanied by tinnitus.

6.7.2 Distribution of the Arteries of the Brainstem and Cerebellum in Midsagittal Section

All of the brain sections shown here and below are supplied by the vertebrobasilar complex. The transverse sections are presented in a caudal-to-cranial series corresponding to the direction of the vertebrobasilar blood supply (**Fig. 6.26**).

6.7.3 Distribution of the Arteries of the Mesencephalon (Midbrain) in Transverse Section

Besides branches from the superior cerebellar artery, the mesencephalon is supplied chiefly by branches of the posterior cerebral artery and posterior communicating artery (**Fig. 6.27**).

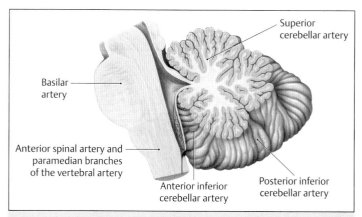

Fig. 6.27 Distribution of the arteries of the mesencephalon (midbrain).

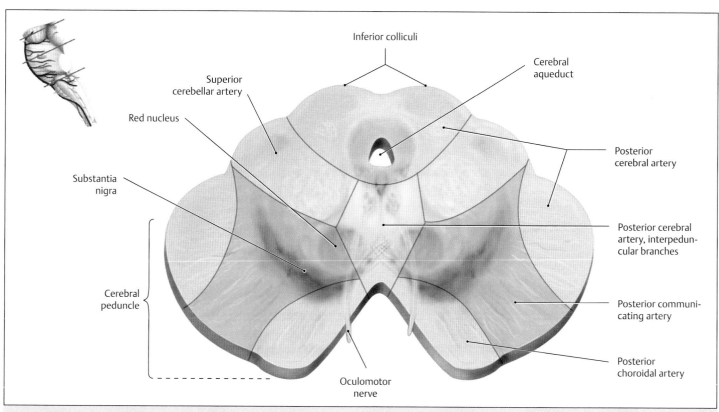

Fig. 6.26 Distribution of the arteries of the brainstem and cerebellum in midsagittal section.

6.7.4 Distribution of the Arteries of the Pons in Transverse Section

The pons derives its blood supply from short and long branches of the basilar artery (**Fig. 6.28**).

6.7.5 Distribution of the Arteries of the Medulla Oblongata in Transverse Section

The medulla oblongata is supplied by branches of the anterior spinal artery, and posterior inferior cerebellar artery (both arising from the vertebral artery), as well as the anterior inferior cerebellar artery (first large branch of the basilar artery) (**Fig. 6.29**).

6.8 Dural Sinuses, Overview

6.8.1 Relationship of the Principal Dural Sinuses to the Skull

Oblique posterior view from the right side (brain removed and tentorium windowed on the right side) (**Fig. 6.30**). The dural sinuses are stiff-walled venous channels that receive blood from the internal and external cerebral veins, orbits, and calvaria (the upper domelike portion of the skull) and convey it to the internal jugular veins on both sides. With few exceptions (inferior sagittal sinus, straight sinus), the walls of the dural sinuses are formed by both the periosteal and meningeal layers of the dura mater. The valveless dural sinuses are lined internally by endothelium (flat layer of cells that line blood vessels and other body surfaces) and are expanded at some sites (particularly in the superior sagittal sinus) to form "lateral lacunae" (see Chapter 6.8.2). These expansions contain the arachnoid villi through which cerebrospinal fluid (CSF) is absorbed into the venous blood. The dural

sinuses are endothelial-lined spaces between the outer periosteal and inner meningeal layers of the dura mater into which empty the cerebral veins, the cerebellar veins, and the veins draining the brainstem and that lead to the internal jugular veins. This system of veins then returns the blood in the circulatory system back to the heart to get oxygenated. The system of dural sinuses is divided into an upper group and a lower group:

- **Upper group:** Superior and inferior sagittal sinuses, straight sinus, occipital sinus, transverse sinus, sigmoid sinus, and the confluence of the sinuses.
- **Lower group:** Cavernous sinus with anterior and posterior intercavernous sinuses, sphenoparietal sinus, superior and inferior petrosal sinuses.

The upper and lower groups of dural sinuses communicate with the venous plexuses of the vertebral canal through the marginal sinus at the inlet to the foramen magnum and through the basilar plexus on the clivus (see Chapter 6.8.3).

6.8.2 Structure of a Dural Sinus, Shown Here for the Superior Sagittal Sinus

Transverse section, occipital view (detail from Chapter 6.8.1) (**Fig. 6.31**). The sinus wall is composed of endothelium and tough, collagenous dural connective tissue with a periosteal and meningeal layer. Between the two layers is the sinus lumen.

Note: The lateral lacunae, where the arachnoid villi open into the venous system. Superficial cerebral veins (superior cerebral veins, bridging veins) open into the sinus itself along with diploic veins from the adjacent cranial bone. The sinus also receives emissary veins—valveless veins that establish connections among the sinuses, the diploic veins, and the extracranial veins (the veins serving the spongy part of the skull), of the scalp.

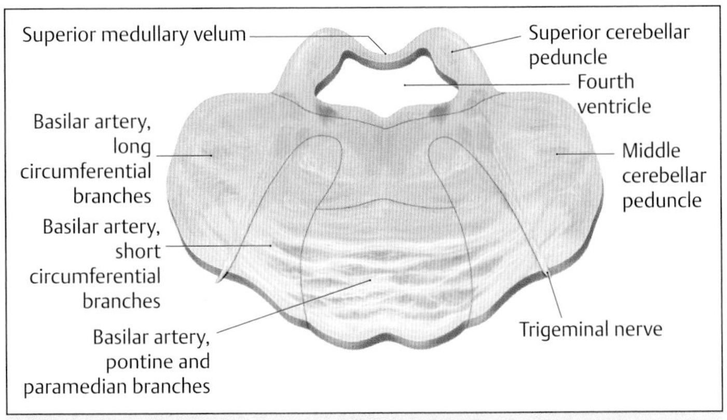

Fig. 6.28 Distribution of the arteries of the pons.

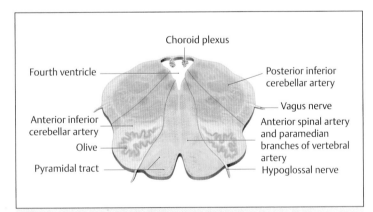

Fig. 6.29 Distribution of the arteries of the medulla oblongata.

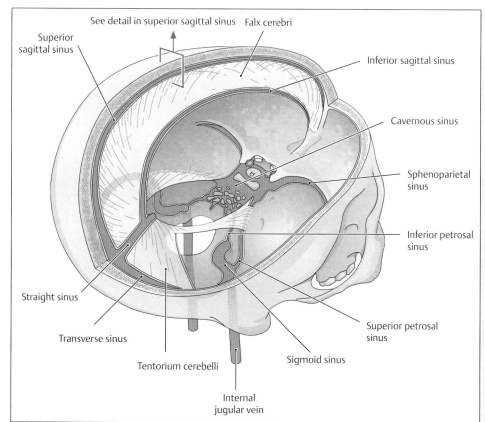

Superior sagittal sinus

See detail in superior sagittal sinus

Falx cerebri

Inferior sagittal sinus

Cavernous sinus

Sphenoparietal sinus

Inferior petrosal sinus

Straight sinus

Transverse sinus

Tentorium cerebelli

Sigmoid sinus

Superior petrosal sinus

Internal jugular vein

Fig. 6.30 Dural sinuses (oblique posterior view from the right side).

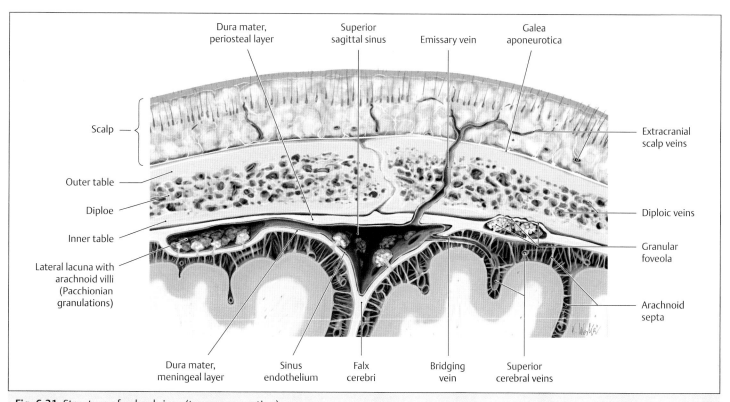

Dura mater, periosteal layer

Superior sagittal sinus

Emissary vein

Galea aponeurotica

Scalp

Extracranial scalp veins

Outer table

Diploe

Inner table

Lateral lacuna with arachnoid villi (Pacchionian granulations)

Diploic veins

Granular foveola

Arachnoid septa

Dura mater, meningeal layer

Sinus endothelium

Falx cerebri

Bridging vein

Superior cerebral veins

Fig. 6.31 Structure of a dural sinus (transverse section).

6.8.3 Dural Sinuses at the Skull Base

Transverse section at the level of the tentorium cerebelli, viewed from above (brain removed, orbital roof and tentorium windowed on the right side) (**Fig. 6.32**). The cavernous sinus forms a ring around the sella turcica, its left and right parts being interconnected at the front and behind by an anterior and a posterior intercavernous sinus. Behind the posterior intercavernous sinus, on the clivus (bony surface in the posterior cranial fossa sloping upward), is the basilar plexus. This plexus also contributes to the drainage of the cavernous sinus.

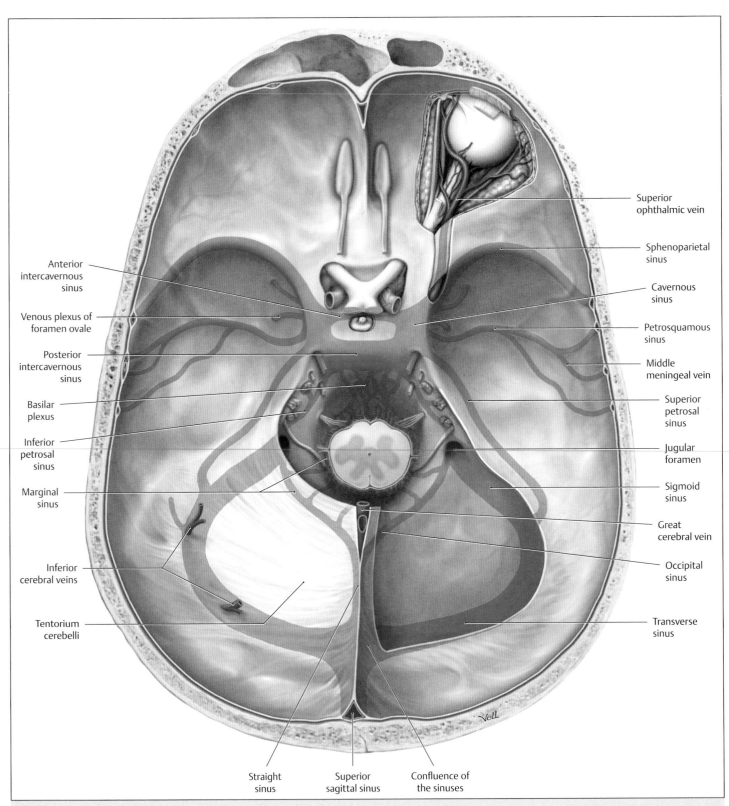

Anterior intercavernous sinus

Venous plexus of foramen ovale

Posterior intercavernous sinus

Basilar plexus

Inferior petrosal sinus

Marginal sinus

Inferior cerebral veins

Tentorium cerebelli

Superior ophthalmic vein

Sphenoparietal sinus

Cavernous sinus

Petrosquamous sinus

Middle meningeal vein

Superior petrosal sinus

Jugular foramen

Sigmoid sinus

Great cerebral vein

Occipital sinus

Transverse sinus

Straight sinus

Superior sagittal sinus

Confluence of the sinuses

Fig. 6.32 Transverse section at the level of the tentorium cerebelli.

6.9 Blood Vessels of the Brain: Intracranial Hemorrhage

Intracranial hemorrhages may be extracerebral (see Chapter 6.9.1) or intracerebral (see Chapter 6.9.3).

6.9.1 Extracerebral Hemorrhages

Extracerebral hemorrhages are defined as bleeding between the calvaria and brain. Because the bony calvaria is immobile, the developing hematoma exerts pressure on the soft brain. Depending on the source of the hemorrhage (arterial or venous), this may produce a rapidly or slowly developing incompressible mass with a rise of intracranial pressure that may damage not only the brain tissue at the bleeding site but also in more remote brain areas. Three types of intracranial hemorrhage can be distinguished based on their relationship to the dura mater (**Fig. 6.33**):

(a) **Epidural hematoma** (epidural = above the dura). This type generally develops after a head injury involving a skull fracture. The bleeding most commonly occurs from a ruptured middle meningeal artery (due to the close proximity of the middle meningeal artery to the calvaria, a sharp bone fragment may lacerate the artery). The hematoma forms between the calvaria and the periosteal layer of the dura mater. Pressure from the hematoma separates the dura from the calvaria and displaces the brain. Typically, there is an initial transient loss of consciousness caused by the impact, followed 1 to 5 hours later by a second decline in the level of consciousness, this time due to compression of the brain by the arterial hemorrhage. The interval between the first and second loss of consciousness is called the *lucid interval* (occurs in approximately 30–40% of all epidural hematomas). Detection of the hemorrhage (computed tomography [CT] scanning of the head) and prompt evacuation of the hematoma are lifesaving.

(b) **Subdural hematoma** (subdural = below the dura). Trauma to the head causes the rupture of a *bridging vein* (see p. 160) that bleeds between the dura mater and arachnoid. The bleeding occurs into a potential "subdural space," which exists only when extravasated blood has dissected the arachnoid membrane from the dura. Because the bleeding source is venous, the increased intracranial pressure and mass effect develop more slowly than with an arterial epidural hemorrhage. Consequently, a subdural hematoma may develop *chronically* over a period of weeks, even after a relatively mild head injury.

(c) **Subarachnoid hemorrhage** is an arterial bleed caused by the rupture of an aneurysm (abnormal outpouching) of an artery at the base of the brain (see Chapter 6.9.2). It is typically caused by a brief, sudden rise in blood pressure, like that produced by a sudden rise of intra-abdominal pressure (straining at stool or urine, lifting a heavy object, etc.). Because the hemorrhage is into the CSF-fl I led subarachnoid space, blood can be detected in the CSF by means of lumbar

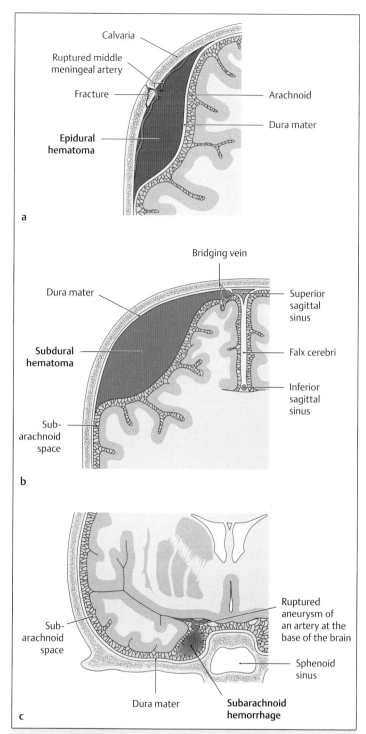

Fig. 6.33 (a) Epidural hematoma. **(b)** Subdural hematoma. **(c)** Subarachnoid hemorrhage.

puncture. The cardinal symptom of a subarachnoid hemorrhage is a sudden, excruciating headache accompanied by a stiff neck caused by meningeal irritation. Signs and symptoms of these cerebral bleeds include aphasia, confusion, difficulty with balance or walking, headache, lethargy or confusion, loss of consciousness, nausea and vomiting, sensory loss or numbness in the face or limbs, seizures, dysarthria (imprecise speech due to movement impairment of the articulators), visual disturbances, or limb weakness or paralysis.

6.9.2 Sites of Berry Aneurysms at the Base of the Brain

Aneurysms are a bulging or ballooning of a weakened portion of the blood vessel wall (**Fig. 6.34**). The rupture of congenital or acquired arterial aneurysms at the base of the brain is the most frequent cause of subarachnoid hemorrhage and accounts for approximately 5% of all strokes. These are abnormal saccular dilations of the circle of Willis and are especially common at the site of branching. When one of these thin-walled aneurysms ruptures, arterial blood escapes into the subarachnoid space. The most common site is the junction between the anterior cerebral and anterior communicating arteries (1); the second most likely site is the branching of the posterior communicating artery from the internal carotid artery (2).

6.9.3 Intracerebral Hemorrhage

Coronal section at the level of the thalamus (**Fig. 6.35**). Unlike the intracranial *extracerebral* hemorrhages described above, *intracerebral* hemorrhage occurs when damaged arteries bleed directly *into the substance of the brain*. This distinction is of very great clinical importance because extracerebral hemorrhages can be controlled by surgical hemostasis (clipping or clamping) of the bleeding vessel, whereas intracerebral hemorrhages cannot. (Hemostasis is a complex process that causes the bleeding process to stop. It refers to the process of keeping blood within a damaged blood vessel; the opposite of hemostasis is "bleeding" or hemorrhage.) The most frequent cause of intracerebral hemorrhage (hemorrhagic stroke) is high blood pressure. Because the soft brain tissue offers very little resistance, a large hematoma may form within the brain. The most common sources of intracerebral bleeding are specific branches of the middle cerebral artery—the lenticulostriate arteries pictured here (known also as the "stroke arteries"). The hemorrhage causes a cerebral infarction in the region of the internal capsule, one effect of which is to disrupt the pyramidal tract and cause paralysis or weakness, which passes through the capsule. The loss of pyramidal tract function below the lesion is manifested clinically by spastic paralysis of the limbs on the side of the body *opposite* to the injury (the pyramidal tracts cross below the level of the lesion at the decussation of the pyramids in the medulla). The hemorrhage is not always massive, and smaller bleeds may occur in the territories of the three main cerebral arteries, producing a typical clinical presentation (see clinical manifestations above).

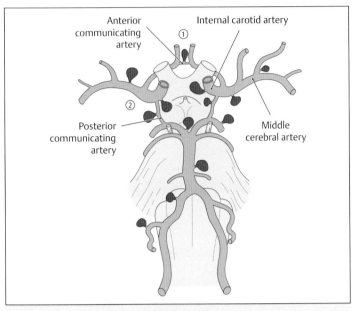

Fig. 6.34 Sites of berry aneurysms at the base of the brain.

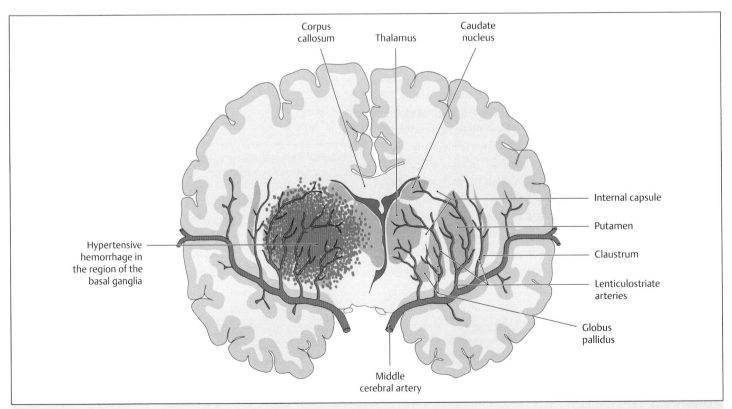

Fig. 6.35 Intracerebral hemorrhage (coronal section at the level of the thalamus).

6.10 Blood Vessels of the Brain: Cerebrovascular Disease

6.10.1 Frequent Causes of Cerebrovascular Disease

Disturbances of cerebral blood flow that deprive the brain of oxygen (cerebral ischemia) are the most frequent cause of central neurological deficits. The most serious complication is cerebrovascular accident or stroke: the vast majority of all strokes are caused by cerebral *ischemic* disease. Stroke has become the third leading cause of death in western industrialized countries (approximately 700,000 strokes occur in the United States each year). Cerebral ischemia is caused by a prolonged diminution or interruption of blood flow and involves *the distribution area of the internal carotid artery* in up to 90% of cases. Much less commonly,

cerebral ischemia is caused by an obstruction of venous outflow due to cerebral venous thrombosis (see Chapter 6.10.2). A decrease of arterial blood flow in the carotid system most commonly results from an embolic or local thrombotic occlusion. Most emboli originate from atheromatous (plaque buildup inside vessels) lesions at the carotid bifurcation (arterioarterial emboli) or from the expulsion of thrombotic material from the left ventricle (cardiac emboli). Blood clots (thrombi) may be dislodged from the heart as a result of valvular disease or atrial fibrillation. This produces emboli that may be carried by the bloodstream to the brain, where they may cause the functional occlusion of an artery supplying the brain. The most common example of this involves all of the distribution region of the MCA, which is a direct continuation of the internal carotid artery, and the artery that supplies the language and speech areas of the dominant cerebral hemisphere (**Fig. 6.36**).

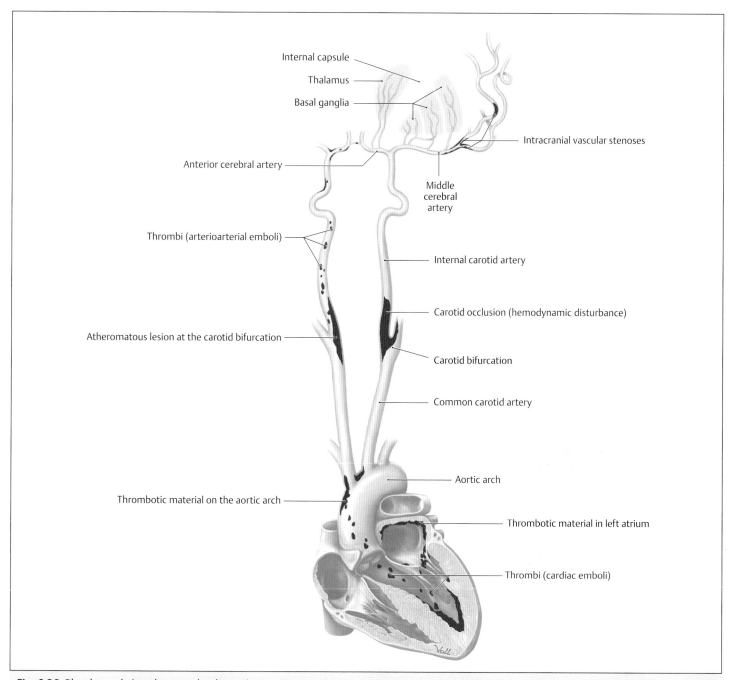

Fig. 6.36 Blood vessels (cerebrovascular disease).

6.10.2 Cerebral Venous Thrombosis

Coronal section, anterior view (**Fig. 6.37**). The cerebral veins, like the cerebral arteries, serve specific territories. Though much less common than decreased arterial flow, the obstruction of venous outflow is an important potential cause of ischemia and infarction (death or necrosis of tissue or cells due to reduced or loss of blood supply). With a thrombotic occlusion, for example, the quantity of blood and thus the venous pressure are increased in the tributary region of the occluded vein. This causes a drop in the capillary pressure gradient, with an increased extravasation of fluid from the capillary bed into the brain tissue (edema or swelling). There is a concomitant reduction of arterial inflow into the affected region, depriving it of oxygen. The occlusion of specific cerebral veins (e.g., due to cerebral venous thrombosis) leads to brain infarctions at characteristic locations:

(a) **Superior cerebral veins:** Thrombosis and infarction in the areas drained by the:

- Medial superior cerebral veins (right, *symptoms:* contralateral lower limb weakness)
- Posterior superior cerebral veins (left, *symptoms:* contralateral hemiparesis)

Aphasia in many of its forms occurs if the infarction involves the dominant hemisphere language areas (Broca's area, Wernicke's area, parietal–temporal–occipital (PTO) cortex).

(b) **Inferior cerebral veins:** Thrombosis of the right inferior cerebral veins leads to infarction of the right temporal lobe *(symptoms:* visual construction tasks, contralateral hemianopia, prosopagnosia or difficulty recognizing faces, and a variety of other right hemisphere signs and symptoms as detailed in LaPointe et al[2]).

(c) **Internal cerebral veins:** Bilateral thrombosis leads to a symmetrical infarction affecting the thalamus and basal ganglia. This is characterized by a rapid deterioration of consciousness ranging to coma.

6.10.3 Cardinal Symptoms of Occlusion of the Three Main Cerebral Arteries

When the *anterior, middle,* or *posterior cerebral artery* becomes occluded, characteristic functional deficits occur in the oxygen-deprived brain areas supplied by the occluded vessel. In many cases the affected artery can be identified based on the associated neurological deficit (**Fig. 6.38**):

- Bladder weakness (cortical bladder center) and paralysis of the lower limb (hemiplegia with or without hemisensory deficit, predominantly affecting the leg) on the side opposite the occlusion indicate an infarction in the territory of the **anterior cerebral artery**.
- Contralateral hemiplegia affecting the arm and face more than the leg indicates an infarction in the territory of the **MCA**. If the dominant hemisphere is affected, aphasia also occurs (the patient cannot name objects, may have reduced comprehension of speech, and reading and writing may be impaired, for example).

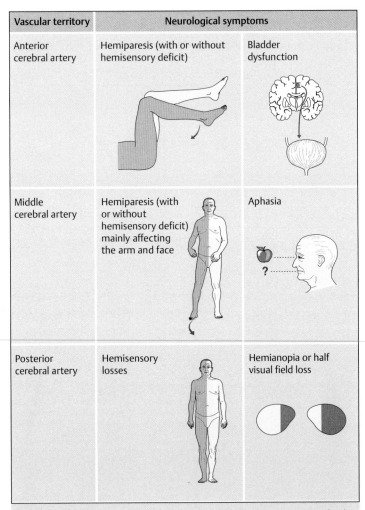

Vascular territory	Neurological symptoms	
Anterior cerebral artery	Hemiparesis (with or without hemisensory deficit)	Bladder dysfunction
Middle cerebral artery	Hemiparesis (with or without hemisensory deficit) mainly affecting the arm and face	Aphasia
Posterior cerebral artery	Hemisensory losses	Hemianopia or half visual field loss

Fig. 6.38 Cardinal symptoms of occlusion of the three main cerebral arteries.

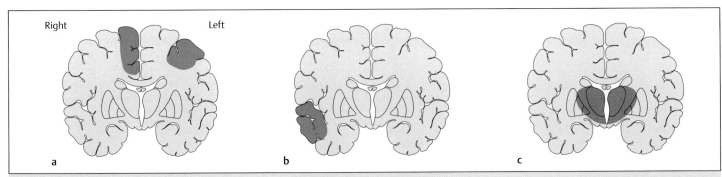

Fig. 6.37 **(a)** Superior cerebral veins. **(b)** Inferior cerebral veins. **(c)** Internal cerebral veins.

- Visual disturbances affecting the contralateral visual field (hemianopia) may signify an infarction in the territory of the **posterior cerebral artery**, because the structures supplied by this artery include the visual cortex in the calcarine sulcus of the occipital lobe.

The extent of the infarction depends partly on whether the occlusion is proximal or distal. Generally, a proximal occlusion will cause a much more extensive infarction than a distal occlusion. MCA infarctions are the most common because the middle cerebral artery is essentially a direct continuation of the internal carotid artery.

Summary of clinical manifestations of neuropathology and brain damage: Any brain function can be disrupted by neuropathology: excessive sleepiness, inattention, difficulty concentrating, impaired memory, faulty judgment, depression, irritability, emotional outbursts, disturbed sleep, diminished libido, difficulty switching between two tasks, and slowed thinking all can be part of the equation. The extent and the severity of cognitive neurological dysfunction can be measured with the aid of neuropsychological, cognitive, and speech and language testing by certified and licensed professionals. Cognitive and speech and language tests can be used to clarify and highlight dysfunction to specific areas of the brain. The ability to plan properly and execute those plans is known as "executive function."

7 Functional and Dysfunctional Systems

7.1 Brain: Functional Organization

7.1.1 Functional Organization of the Neocortex

Left lateral view (**Fig. 7.1**). The primary sensory and motor areas are shown in red, and the areas of the association cortex are shown in different shades of green. Projection tracts begin or end, respectively, in the primary motor or sensory areas. More than 80% of the cortical surface area is association cortex, which is secondarily connected to the primary sensory or primary motor areas. The neuronal processing of differentiated behavior and intellectual performance takes place in the association cortex, which has increased greatly in size over the course of human evolution. The functional organization pattern shown here, such as the localization of the primary motor cortex in the precentral gyri (both hemispheres), can be demonstrated in living subjects with modern imaging techniques. The results of such studies are illustrated in the figures below. Interestingly, the correlations described in these studies correspond reasonably well with the cortical areas defined by Brodmann. As detailed earlier in the section that views the cortex according to Brodmann's areas (4.10), the primary language areas in the dominant cortical hemisphere (the left hemisphere in most cases) include the Broca area (44 , 45), Wernicke's area (22), and the PTO cortex (39, 19).

Recent improvements in neural imaging suggest that the primary speech/language areas are more widely distributed than previously reported and rich interconnections exist between the traditional primary language areas and other cortical and subcortical areas involved in specific linguistic tasks. No doubt future research will continue to refine the demarcations of the traditionally appreciated speech and language zones of the human nervous system.

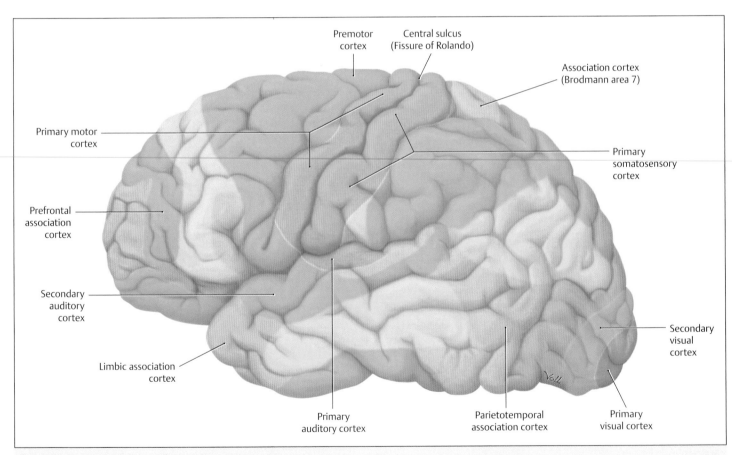

Fig. 7.1 Neocortex (left lateral view).

7.1.2 Analysis of Brain Function Based on Studies of Regional Cerebral Blood Flow

Left lateral view of the brain. When neurons are activated they consume more glucose and oxygen, which must be delivered to them via the bloodstream. This may produce a detectable increase in regional blood flow. These brain maps illustrate the local patterns of cerebral blood flow at rest (**Fig. 7.2a**) and during movement of the right hand (**Fig. 7.2b**). When the right hand is moved, increased blood flow is recorded in the left precentral gyrus, which contains the motor representation of the right hand (see motor homunculus in Chapter 7.9.2). Simultaneous activation is noted in the sensory cortex of the postcentral region, showing that the sensory cortex is also active during motor function (feedback loop).

7.1.3 Sex Differences in Neuronal Processing

Patterns of brain activity can also be demonstrated by functional magnetic resonance imaging (fMRI). This provides a noninvasive method for investigating the metabolic activity of the brain. Because no human brain is identical to any other, a comparison of several brains will show slight variations in the distribution of specific functions. By superimposing the results of examinations in different brains, we can produce a generalized map that shows the approximate distribution of brain functions. Compare the summation map for female brains (**Fig. 7.3a**) with a map for male brains (**Fig. 7.3b**). Both groups of subjects were given phonological tasks based on recognizing differences in the meaning of spoken sounds. While the female subjects activated both sides of their brain when solving the tasks, the male subjects activated only the left side (the sectional images are viewed from below, as are many neural images, so beware of confusing the left and right sides).

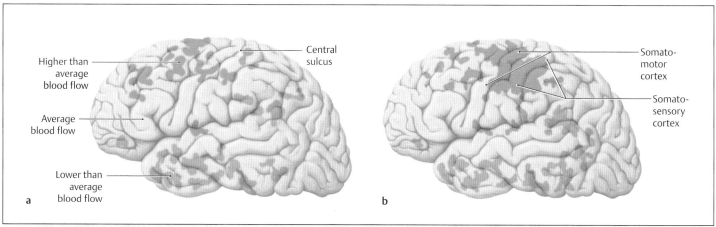

Fig. 7.2 Local patterns of cerebral blood flow at rest (**a**) and during movement of the right hand (**b**).

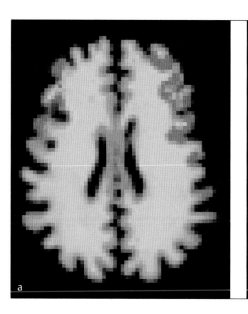
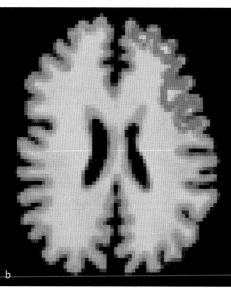

Fig. 7.3 Patterns of brain activity. (**a**) Female brain. (**b**) Male brain.

7.1.4 Modulating Subcortical Centers

The cerebral cortex, the seat of our conscious thoughts and actions, is influenced by various subcortical centers (**Fig. 7.4**). The parts of the limbic system that are crucial for learning and memory are indicated in light red.

7.2 Brain: Fiber Tracts

7.2.1 Fiber Tracts

Fiber tracts are the "information highways" of the white matter of the brain and spinal cord. The most important terms pertaining to central nervous system (CNS) fiber tracts are listed in **Table 7.1**.

Table 7.1 Fiber tracts

Projection fibers	Connect the cerebral cortex to subcortical centers, either ascending or descending
• Ascending fibers • Descending fibers	
Association fibers	
Commissural fibers	Connect like cortical areas in both hemispheres (= interhemispheric association fibers)
Fornix	

7.2.2 Brain Specimen Prepared to Show the Structure of the Projection Fibers

Medial view of the right hemisphere (**Fig. 7.5**). This type of specimen is prepared by fixing the brain in formaldehyde and then freezing it. The gray matter, which has a high water content, is destroyed by ice crystal formation, while the lipid-containing white matter remains relatively intact. The frozen brain is then thawed, and the tissue is dissected and teased with a spatula to bring out the fiber architecture of the white matter. A more contemporary strategy of revealing white matter and myelinated tracts is diffusion tensor imaging (DTI). This is a magnetic resonance imaging (MRI) technique that allows measurement of restricted diffusion of water through tissue of myelinated white matter tracts. Clinical applications include the following:

- Tract-specific localization of white matter lesions
- Localization of tumors in relation to the white matter tracts (infiltration, deflection)
- Localization of the main white matter tracts for neurosurgical planning
- Assessment of the white matter maturation
- Determination of changed neuroconnectivity among brain regions in studies of experiential (therapy) influence on brain plasticity

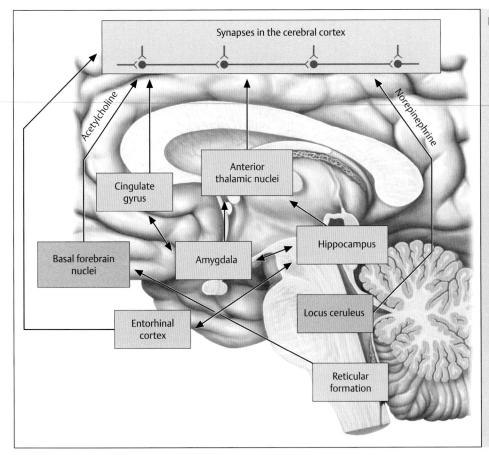

Fig. 7.4 The cerebral cortex.

The fibers represent bundled axons that pass collectively from their site of origination to their destination. Because the brain has a topographic organization, many equidirectional axons pass through the white matter as fasciculi (for the designations of different fiber types, see Chapter 7.2.1, above). The projection fibers shown here connect the cerebral cortex to subcortical structures (e.g., basal ganglia, spinal cord). A distinction is drawn between ascending and descending fibers and their systems. In descending systems, the cell bodies of the neurons are located in the cerebral cortex and their axons terminate in subcortical structures (e.g., the

corticospinal tract). In ascending systems, the neurons from subcortical structures terminate in the cerebral cortex (e.g., sensory tracts from the spinal cord).

7.2.3 Association Fibers

Long association fibers interconnect different brain areas that are located in different lobes, whereas short association fibers interconnect cortical areas within the same lobe. Adjacent cortical areas are interconnected by short, U-shaped arcuate fibers, which run just below the cortex (**Fig.7.6**).

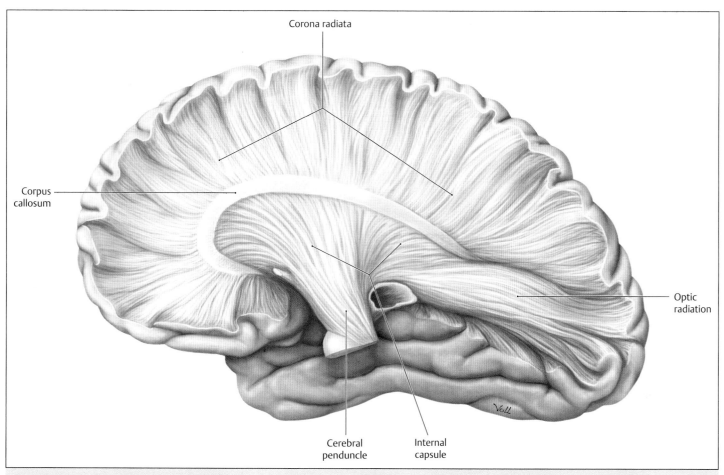

Fig. 7.5 Medial view of the right hemisphere.

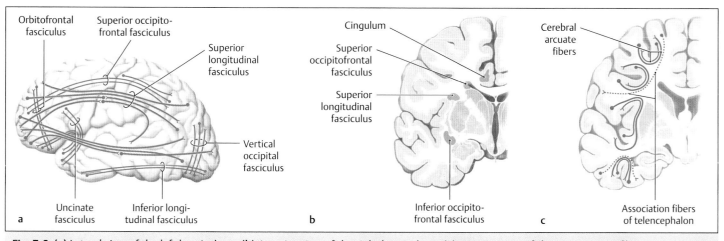

Fig. 7.6 **(a)** Lateral view of the left hemisphere. **(b)** Anterior view of the right hemisphere. **(c)** Anterior view of short association fibers.

7.2.4 Commissural Fibers

Commissural fibers interconnect the two hemispheres of the brain (**Fig. 7.7**). The most important connecting structure between the hemispheres is the corpus callosum. If the corpus callosum is intentionally divided, as in a neurosurgical procedure, the two halves of the brain can no longer communicate with each other ("split-brain" patient, see Chapter 7.3.1). There are other, smaller commissural tracts besides the corpus callosum (anterior commissure, fornical commissure).

7.2.5 Somatotopic Organization of the Internal Capsule

Transverse section (**Fig. 7.8**). Both ascending and descending projection fibers pass through the internal capsule. If blood flow to the internal capsule is interrupted, as by a stroke, these ascending and descending tracts undergo irreversible damage. The figure of the child shows how the sites where the pyramidal tract fibers pass through the internal capsule can be assigned to peripheral areas of the human body (notice that the genu or bend of the internal capsule is where fibers that innervate the head and neck are located. This is important to communication disorders since we deal primarily with disorders that affect the head and neck). Thus, we see that smaller lesions of the internal capsule may cause a loss of central innervation (= spastic paralysis) in certain areas of the body. This accounts for the great clinical importance of this structure. The internal capsule is bounded medially by the thalamus and the head of the caudate nucleus, and laterally by the globus pallidus and

putamen. The internal capsule consists of an anterior limb, a genu, and a posterior limb, which are traversed by specific tracts (**Table 7.2**).

Table 7.2 Fiber tracts of the internal capsule	
Anterior limb	• Frontopontine tracts (red dashes) • Anterior thalamic peduncle (blue dashes)
Genu of internal capsule	• Corticobulbar (corticonuclear) fibers (red dots)
Posterior limb	• Corticospinal fibers (red dots) • Posterior thalamic peduncle (blue dots) • Temporopontine tract (orange dots) • Posterior thalamic peduncle (light blue dots)

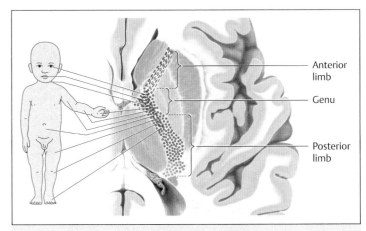

Fig. 7.8 Internal capsule (transverse section).

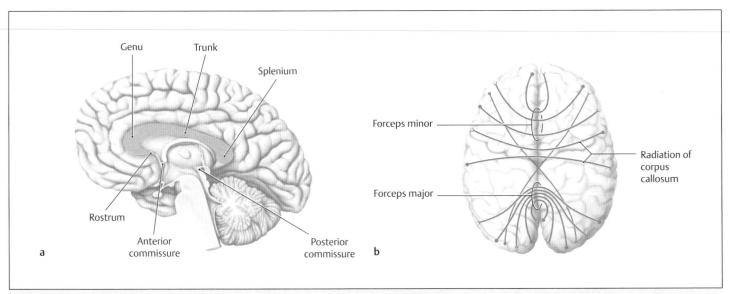

Fig. 7.7 (a) Medial view of the right hemisphere. (b) Superior view of the transparent brain.

7.3 Brain: Hemispheric Dominance

7.3.1 Demonstration of Hemispheric Dominance for Language in Split-Brain Patients

The corpus callosum is by far the most important commissural tract, interconnecting areas of like function in both hemispheres of the brain. Because lesions of the corpus callosum were once considered to have no clinical effects, surgical division of the corpus callosum was commonly performed at one time in epileptic patients to keep epileptic seizures from spreading across the brain. This operation interrupts the connections in the *upper telencephalon* while leaving intact the more deeply situated *diencephalon*, which contains the optic tract. Patients who have undergone this operation are referred to in the older, pre-person first literature as "split-brain patients." They have no obvious clinical abnormalities, but special neuropsychological tests reveal deficits, the study of which has improved our understanding of brain function. In one test, the patient sits in front of a screen on which words are projected. Meanwhile, the patient can grasp objects behind the screen without being able to see them. When the word "Ball" is flashed briefly on the left side of the screen, the patient perceives it in the visual cortex on the right side (the optic tract has not been cut). Because language production resides in the *left* hemisphere in 97% of the population, the patient cannot verbalize the projected word out loud because communication between the hemispheres has been interrupted at the level of the telencephalon (seat of speech production). However, the patient is still able to feel the ball manually and pick it out from other objects. The function of the corpus callosum is to enable both hemispheres (which can function independently to a degree) to communicate with each other when the need arises (**Fig. 7.9**). Because of the phenomenon of hemispheric dominance, the corpus callosum in humans is more elaborately developed than in other animal species.

Split-brain functioning refers to how the two cerebral hemispheres of the brain are involved to different degrees in certain psychological and behavioral functions. In the popular literature, the functions of the "right brain" and "left brain" have been quite oversimplified. In the normal brain the two hemispheres work together in a coordinated manner and these differences in functioning complement one another. Certain functions can be lateralized to a certain degree but no one is totally "right-brained" or "left-brained." We need both hemispheres, although interesting clusters of behavioral impairment have been associated with lesions to the right versus the left cerebral hemisphere. The division of psychological and behavioral functions between the two cerebral hemispheres can be referred to as functional lateralization, asymmetry, or brain laterality. See Chapter 17 on Right Hemisphere Damage in *Aphasia and Related Neurogenic Language Disorders, 4th ed.*[3]

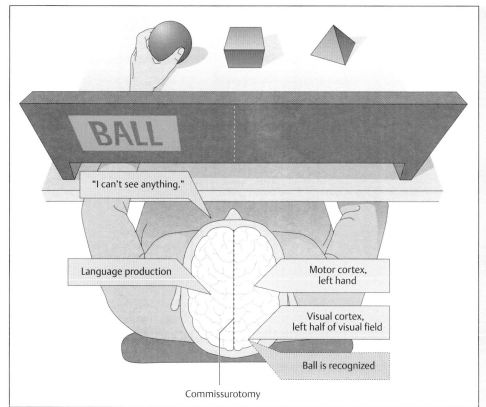

Fig. 7.9 Demonstration of hemispheric dominance for language in split-brain patients.

7.3.2 Hemispheric Asymmetry

Superior view of the temporal lobe of a brain that has been taken apart (i.e., the frontal lobes have been removed) along the lateral fissure (**Fig. 7.10**). The *planum temporale*, located on the posterior and superior surface of the temporal lobe, has different contours on the two sides of the brain, being more pronounced on the left side than on the right in two-thirds of individuals. The functional significance of this asymmetry is uncertain. We cannot explain it simply by noting that the Wernicke speech area is located in that part of the temporal lobe, because while temporal asymmetry is present in only 67% of the population, the speech area is located on the left side in 97%.

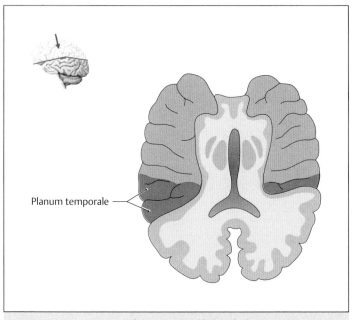

Fig. 7.10 Superior view of the temporal lobe of a brain.

7.3.3 Language Areas in the Normally Dominant Left Hemisphere

Lateral view (**Fig. 7.11**). The brain contains several language areas whose loss is associated with typical clinical symptoms. The *Wernicke area* (the posterior part of area 22) is necessary for language comprehension, while the *Broca area* (area 44 and 45) is concerned with language production. The two areas are interconnected by the superior longitudinal (arcuate) fasciculus. The Broca area activates the mouth and tongue region of the motor cortex for the production of speech. The angular gyrus coordinates the inputs from the visual, acoustic, and somatosensory cortices and relays them onward to the Wernicke area. As noted earlier, recent improvements in neural imaging suggest that the primary speech/language areas are more widely distributed than previously reported and rich interconnections exist between the traditional primary language areas and other cortical and subcortical areas involved in specific linguistic tasks. No doubt future research will continue to refine the demarcations of the traditionally appreciated speech and language zones of the human nervous system. The old days of the oversimplified brain diagrams with boxes and arrows have gone to the historical resting place of black and white television, carbon paper, and rotary phones. Sophisticated neural imaging and linguistic measurement techniques will continue to advance the evolution of our knowledge of the nervous system's role in speech and language.

7.4 The Autonomic Nervous System

7.4.1 Structure of the Autonomic Nervous System

The system of motor innervation of skeletal muscle is complemented by the *autonomic nervous system*, with two divisions: sympathetic (red) and parasympathetic (blue) (**Fig. 7.12**). Both

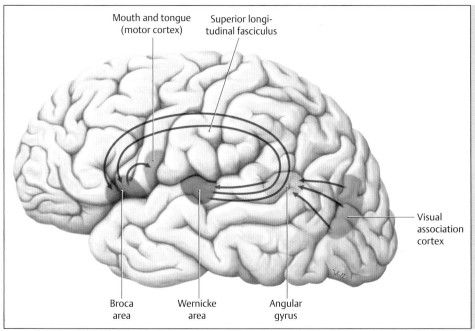

Fig. 7.11 Language areas in the normally dominant left hemisphere (lateral view).

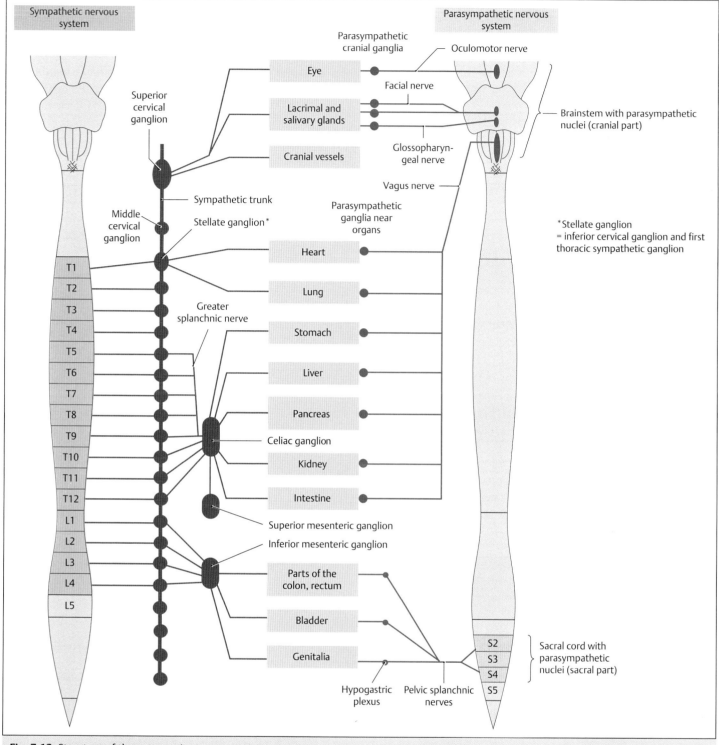

Fig. 7.12 Structure of the autonomic nervous system.

divides have a two-neuron path between the CNS and their targets: a *preganglionic* CNS neuron, and a ganglion cell in the peripheral nervous system (PNS) that is close to the target. The preganglionic neurons of the sympathetic system are in the lateral horns of the cervical, thoracic, and lumbar spinal cord. Their axons exit the CNS via the ventral roots and synapse in sympathetic ganglia in bilateral *paravertebral* chains *(sympathetic trunks)*, or as single midline *prevertebral ganglia* (see Chapter 7.4.5). Axons from these ganglion cells course in unmyelinated bundles on blood vessels or in peripheral nerves to their targets. The preganglionic neurons of the parasympathetic system are located in the brainstem and sacral spinal cord. Their

axons exit the CNS via cranial and pelvic splanchnic (pertaining to viscera or vital organs) nerves to synapse with parasympathetic ganglion cells. In the head, these cells are in discrete ganglia associated with the cranial nerves. In other locations the parasympathetic ganglion cells are in tiny clusters embedded in their target tissues. The sympathetic and parasympathetic systems regulate blood flow, secretions, and organ function; the two divisions often act in antagonistic ways on the same target (see Chapter 7.4.2). Although this basic dichotomy of visceral motor activity was identified early, it has been shown more recently that autonomic control of various organs, particularly in the gastrointestinal and urogenital tracts, is highly sophisticated, dependent on feedback from local visceral afferents that relay pain and stretch information, etc., through complex local circuits.

7.4.2 Synopsis of the Sympathetic and Parasympathetic Nervous Systems

1. The sympathetic nervous system can be considered the excitatory part of the autonomic nervous system that prepares the body for a "fight or flight" response.
2. The parasympathetic nervous system is the part of the autonomic nervous system that coordinates the "rest and digest" responses of the body.
3. Although there are separate control centers for the two divisions in the brainstem and spinal cord, they have close anatomical and functional ties in the periphery.
4. The principal transmitter at the target organ is *acetylcholine* in the parasympathetic nervous system and *norepinephrine* in the sympathetic nervous organ.
5. Stimulation of the sympathetic and parasympathetic nervous systems produces the following different effects on specific organs (**Table 7.3**):

7.4.3 Circuit Diagram of the Autonomic Nervous System

The synapse of the central, preganglionic neuron uses *acetylcholine* as a transmitter in both the sympathetic *and* parasympathetic nervous systems (cholinergic neuron, shown in blue). In the sympathetic nervous system, the transmitter changes to

norepinephrine at the synapse of the postganglionic neuron with the target organ (adrenergic neuron, shown in red), while the parasympathetic system continues to use acetylcholine at that level (**Fig. 7.13**).

Note: Various types of receptors for acetylcholine (= neurotransmitter sensors) are located in the membrane of the target cells. As a result, acetylcholine can produce a range of effects depending on the receptor type.

Table 7.3 Different effects on specific organs

Organ	Sympathetic nervous system	Parasympathetic nervous system
Eye	Pupillary dilation	Pupillary constriction and increased curvature of the lens
Salivary glands	Decreased salivation (scant, viscous)	Increased salivation (copious, watery)
Heart	Elevation of the heart rate	Slowing of the heart rate
Lungs	Decreased bronchial secretions and bronchial dilation	Increased bronchial secretions and bronchial constriction
Gastrointestinal tract	Decreased secretions and motor activity	Increased secretions and motor activity
Pancreas	Decreased secretion from the endocrine part of the gland	Increased secretion
Male sex organs	Ejaculation	Erection
Skin	Vasoconstriction, sweat secretion, piloerection ("goose bumps")	No effect

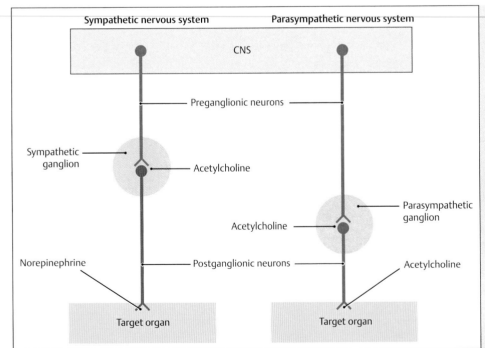

Fig. 7.13 Circuit diagram of the autonomic nervous system.

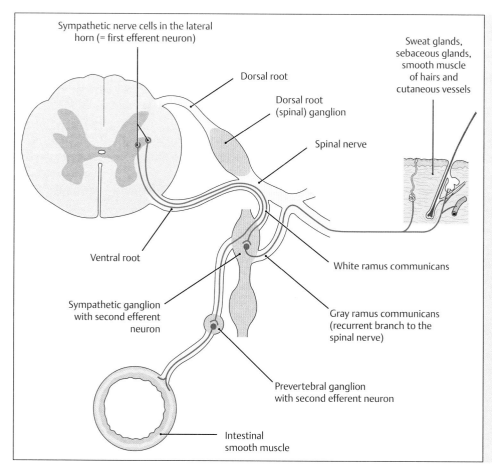

Fig. 7.14 Distribution of sympathetic fibers in the periphery.

7.4.4 Distribution of Sympathetic Fibers in the Periphery

Some sympathetic fibers in the periphery (e.g., in the trunk region) "hitchhike" on spinal nerves to reach their destinations. The synapse of the first with the second efferent neuron (red) may occur at three locations (see Chapter 7.4.5) (**Fig. 7.14**).

7.4.5 Location of Synapses in the Autonomic Nervous System

Acetylcholine is the transmitter for both the first and second neurons in the parasympathetic system, but the sympathetic system switches to norepinephrine for the second neuron. Synapses of the first, preganglionic cholinergic neuron (blue) with the second neuron (red) may be located in three different sites (**Fig. 7.15**):

① In discrete bilateral clusters of postganglionic neurons (autonomic ganglia). In the sympathetic system, these synapses are in the paravertebral ganglia on either side of the vertebral column. In the cranial part of the parasympathetic system, the synapses are in paired cranial parasympathetic ganglia (see Chapter 7.4.1).

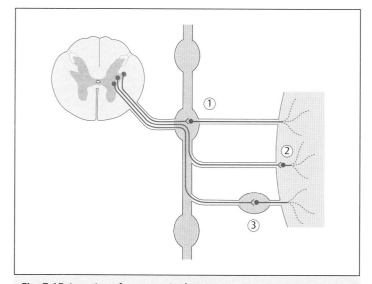

Fig. 7.15 Location of synapses in the autonomic nervous system.

② In the target organ, on small clusters of embedded ganglion cells (parasympathetic system only). In the adrenal gland, preganglionic cholinergic sympathetic fibers synapse directly on adrenal medullary (endocrine) cells.

③ In unpaired prevertebral ganglia (celiac and mesenteric), located in front of the vertebral column, in close proximity to the abdominal aorta (sympathetic system only).

7.5 Sensory System, Overview

7.5.1 Simplified Diagram of the Sensory Pathways of the Spinal Cord

Stimuli generate impulses in various receptors in the periphery of the body that are transmitted to the cerebrum and cerebellum along the sensory (afferent) pathways or tracts shown here (**Fig. 7.16**) (see Chapter 7.5.2 for details). While most of the sensory qualities listed in Chapter 7.5.2 are intuitively clear (e.g., pain and temperature sensation), the concept of proprioception is more difficult to convey and will be explained in more detail. Proprioception is concerned with the position of the limbs and

body in space (= position sense). As noted earlier, kinesthesia is frequently the term used to describe the sensation of movement of the limbs or body. The types of *information* involved in proprioception are complex: position sense (the position of the limbs in relation to one another) is distinguished from motion sense (speed and direction of joint movements) and force sense (the muscular force associated with joint movements).

Accordingly, the receptors for proprioception and kinesthesia (proprioceptors) consist mainly of muscle and tendon spindles and joint receptors. We also distinguish between conscious and unconscious proprioception. Information on **conscious proprioception** travels in the posterior funiculus of the spinal cord (fasciculus gracilis and fasciculus cuneatus) and is relayed through

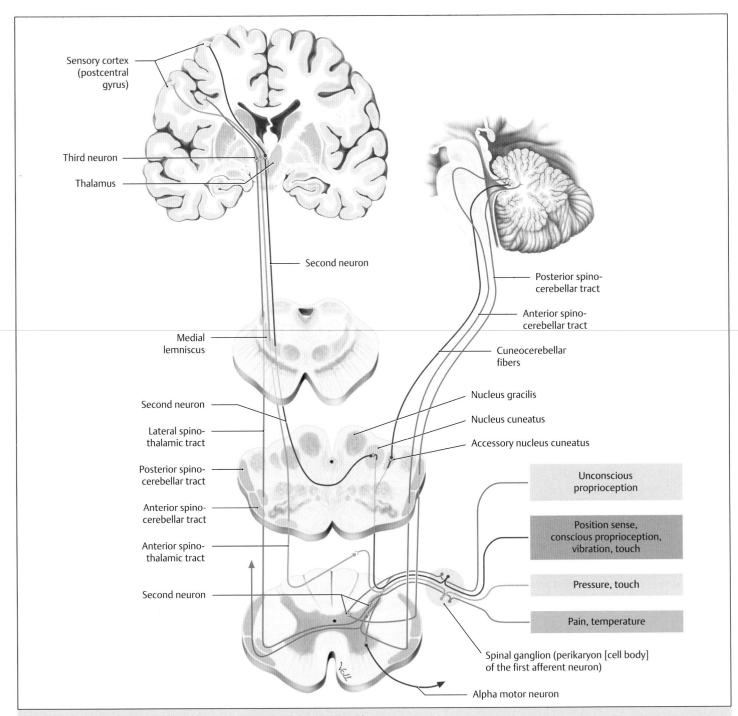

Fig. 7.16 Simplified diagram of the sensory pathways of the spinal cord.

its nuclei (nucleus gracilis and nucleus cuneatus) to the *thalamus*. From there it is conveyed to the *sensory cortex* (postcentral gyrus), where the information presumably rises to consciousness ("I know that my left hand is making a fist, even though my eyes are closed"). **Unconscious proprioception**, which enables us to ride a bicycle and climb stairs without thinking about it, is conveyed by the spinocerebellar tracts to the *cerebellum*, where it remains at the unconscious level. Sensory information from the head is mediated by the trigeminal nerve and is not depicted here (see Chapter 5.2).

7.5.2 Synopsis of Sensory Pathways

The various stimuli generate impulses in different receptors which are transmitted in peripheral nerves to the spinal cord. The perikarya (unmyelinated cell bodies of neurons) of the first afferent neuron (to which the receptors are connected) for all pathways are located in the spinal ganglion. The axons from the ganglion pass along various tracts in the spinal cord to the second neuron. Its axons either pass directly to the cerebellum or are relayed by a third neuron to the cerebrum (**Table 7.4**).

Table 7.4 Name, quality, and course of sensory pathways

Name of pathway	Sensory quality	Receptor	Course in the spinal cord	Central course (above the spinal cord)
Spinothalamic tracts				
Anterior spinothalamic tract	• Crude touch	• Hair follicles • Various skin receptors	The perikaryon (cell body) of the second neuron is located in the posterior (dorsal) horn and may be up to 15 segments above or 2 segments below the entry of the first neuron. Its axons cross in the anterior commissure	The axons of the second neuron (spinal lemniscus) terminate in the ventral posterolateral nucleus of the thalamus. There they synapse onto the third neuron, whose axons project to the postcentral gyrus of the primary sensory strip in the cortex
Lateral spinothalamic tract	• Pain and temperature	• Mostly free nerve endings	The perikaryon of the second neuron is in the substantia gelatinosa (a narrow, dense, vertical band of gelatinous gray matter forming the dorsal part of the posterior column of the spinal cord). Its axon crosses at the same level in the anterior commissure	The axons of the second neuron (spinal lemniscus) terminate in the ventral posterolateral nucleus of the thalamus. There they synapse onto the third neuron, whose axons project to the postcentral gyrus
Tracts of the posterior funiculus				
Fasciculus gracilis	• Fine touch • Conscious proprioception of *lower* limb	• Vater–Pacini corpuscles • Muscle and tendon receptors	The axons of the first neuron pass to the nucleus gracilis in the lower medulla oblongata (second neuron)	The axons of the second neuron cross in the brainstem and traverse the medial lemniscus to the ventral posterolateral nucleus of the thalamus. There they synapse onto the third neuron, whose axons project to the postcentral gyrus of the cortex
Fasciculus cuneatus	• Fine touch • Conscious proprioception of upper limb	• Vater–Pacini corpuscles • Muscle and tendon receptors	The axons of the first neuron pass to the nucleus cuneatus in the lower medulla oblongata (second neuron)	The axons of the second neuron cross in the brainstem and traverse the medial lemniscus to the ventral posterolateral nucleus of the thalamus. There they synapse onto the third neuron, whose axons project to the postcentral gyrus
Spinocerebellar tracts				
Anterior spinocerebellar tract	• Unconscious crossed and uncrossed extero- and proprioception to the cerebellum	• Muscle spindles • Tendon receptors • Joint receptors • Skin receptors	The second neuron is located in the dorsal column in the central part of the gray matter. The axons of the second neuron run directly to the cerebellum, both crossed and uncrossed, without synapsing with a third neuron	The axons of the second neuron pass through the superior cerebellar peduncle to the vermian part of the spinocerebellum (no third neuron)
Posterior spinocerebellar tract	• Unconscious uncrossed extero- and proprioception to the cerebellum	• Muscle spindles • Tendon receptors • Joint receptors • Skin receptors	The second neuron is located in the thoracic nucleus in the gray matter at the base of the posterior (dorsal) horn. The axons of the second neuron run directly to the cerebellum without crossing	The axons of the second neuron pass through the inferior cerebellar peduncle to the vermian part of the spinocerebellum (no third neuron)

7.6 Sensory System: Stimulus Processing

7.6.1 Receptors of the Somatosensory System

See **Fig. 7.17**.

- **Skin receptors:** Various types of stimuli generate impulses in different receptors in the periphery of the body (illustrated here in sections through hair-bearing and hairless skin). These impulses are transmitted through peripheral nerves to the spinal cord, from which they are relayed and carried by specific tracts to the sensory cortex (see previous unit). Sensory qualities cannot always be uniquely assigned to specific receptors. The figure does not indicate the prevalence of the different receptor types. Nociceptors (= pain receptors), like heat and cold receptors, consist of free nerve endings. Nociceptors make up approximately 50% of all receptors.
- **Joint receptors:** Proprioception encompasses position sense, motion sense, and force sense. Proprioceptors include muscle spindles, tendon sensors, and joint sensors (not shown).

7.6.2 Receptive Field Sizes of Cortical Modules in the Upper Limb of a Primate

Sensory information is processed in cortical "modules." This drawing shows the size of the receptive fields supplied by modules (**Fig. 7.18**). In areas where high resolution of sensory information is not required (e.g., the forearm), one module supplies a

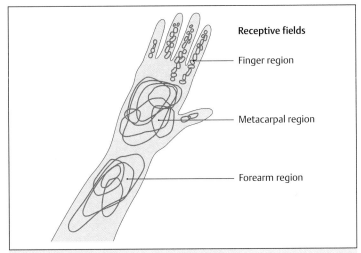

Fig. 7.18 Receptive field sizes of cortical modules.

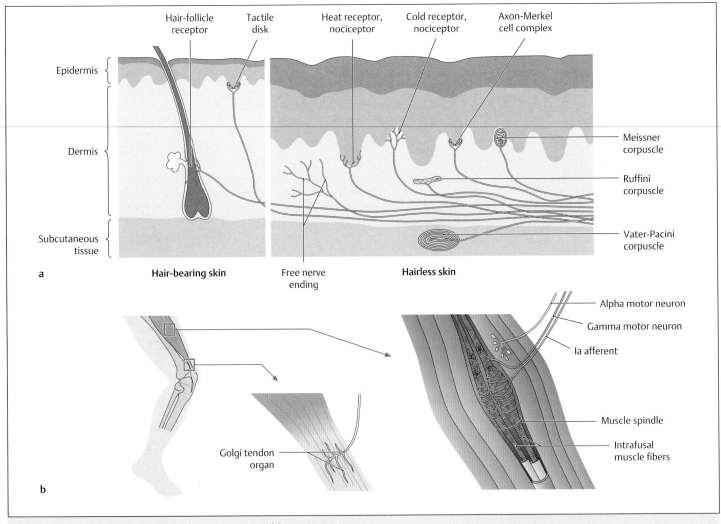

Fig. 7.17 Somatosensory system. **(a)** Skin receptors. **(b)** Joint receptors.

large receptive field. In areas that require finer tactile sensation (e.g., the fingers), one module supplies a much smaller receptive field. The size of these fields determines the overall proportions of the sensory homunculus (see Chapter 7.6.3). Because one skin area may be innervated by several neurons, many of the receptive fields overlap. Information is transmitted from the receptive field to the cortex by a chain of neurons and their axons. These neurons and axons are located at specific sites in the CNS that correspond to the body area that is served (topographical principle).

7.6.3 Arrangement of Sensory Pathways in the Cerebrum

Anterior view of the right postcentral gyrus (**Fig. 7.19**). The perikarya (cell bodies) of the third neurons of the sensory pathways are located in the thalamus. Their axons project to the postcentral gyrus, where the primary somatosensory cortex is located. The postcentral gyrus has a somatotopic organization, meaning that each body region is represented in a particular cortical area. The body regions in the cortex are not represented in proportion to their actual size, but in proportion to the density of their sensory innervation. The fingers and head have abundant sensory receptors, and so their cortical representation is correspondingly large (see Chapter 7.6.2). Conversely, the less dense sensory

innervation of the buttocks and legs results in smaller areas of representation. Based on these varying numbers of peripheral receptors, we can construct a "sensory homunculus" whose parts correspond to the cortical areas concerned with their perception.

Note: The head of the homunculus ("little human") is upright while the trunk is upside down.

The axons of the sensory neurons ascending from the thalamus travel side by side with the axons forming the pyramidal tract (red) in the dorsal part of the internal capsule. Because of this arrangement, a large cerebral hemorrhage involving the internal capsule produces sensory as well as motor deficits.

7.6.4 Primary Somatosensory Cortex and Parietal Association Cortex

(a) Left lateral view. (b) The Brodmann areas are numbered in the sectional view. The contralateral body half is represented in the primary somatosensory cortex (except the perioral region, which is represented bilaterally: related to speech, for example) (**Fig. 7.20a, b**). This area of the cortex is concerned with somatosensory perception. The parietal association cortex (area 5) receives information from both sides of the body. Thus, the processing of stimuli becomes increasingly complex in these cortical areas.

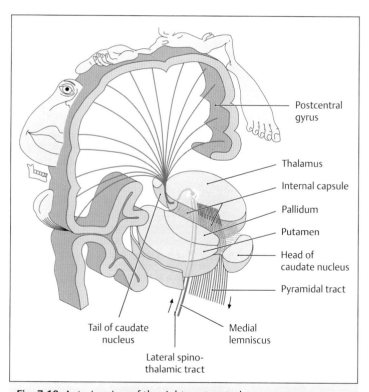

Fig. 7.19 Anterior view of the right postcentral gyrus.

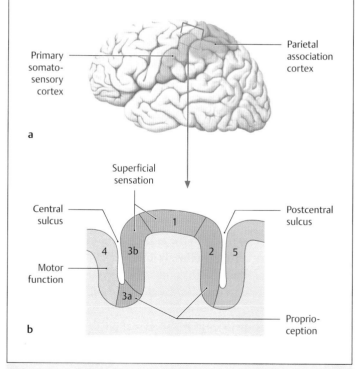

Fig. 7.20 Primary somatosensory cortex and parietal association cortex. **(a)** Left lateral view. **(b)** Sectional view.

7.6.5 Activity of Cortical Cell Columns in the Primary Somatosensory Cortex

Amplitude of the neuronal response in the primary somatosensory cortex to a peripheral pressure stimulus (**Fig. 7.21a**). The intensity of the stimulus is shown in **Fig. 7.21b**. The diagrams illustrate the principle of sensory information processing in the cortex. When approximately 100 intensity detectors in the fingertip are stimulated by pressure, approximately 10,000 neurons in the corresponding cell column in the primary somatosensory cortex respond to the stimulus. Because the intensity of the peripheral pressure stimulus is maximal at the center and fades toward the edges, it is processed in the cortex accordingly. Cortical processing amplifies the contrast between the greater and lesser stimulus intensities, resulting in a sharper peak (**Fig. 7.21a**). While the stimulated area on the fingertip measures approximately 100 mm², the information is processed in only a 1-mm² area of the primary somatosensory cortex.

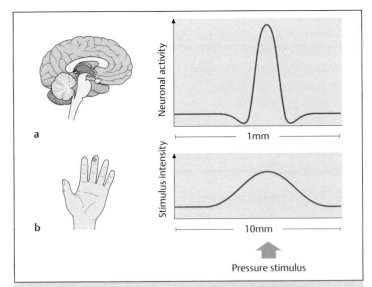

Fig. 7.21 (a) Amplitude of the neuronal response in the primary somatosensory cortex to a peripheral pressure stimulus. **(b)** The intensity of the stimulus.

7.7 Sensory System: Lesions

7.7.1 Sites of Occurrence of Lesions in the Sensory Pathways

The central portions of the sensory pathways may be damaged at various sites from the spinal root to the somatosensory cortex as a result of trauma, tumor mass effect, hemorrhage, or infarction. The signs and symptoms are helpful in determining the location of the lesion. This unit deals strictly with lesions in conscious sensory pathways. The innervation of the trunk and limbs is mediated by the spinal nerves (**Fig. 7.22**). The innervation of the head is mediated by the trigeminal nerve, which has its own nuclei (see below).

Cortical or subcortical lesion (1, 2): A lesion at this level is manifested by paresthesia (tingling) and numbness in the corresponding regions of the trunk and limbs on the *opposite* side of the body. The symptoms may be most pronounced distally because of the large receptive fields on the fingers and the relatively small receptive fields on the trunk (see previous unit). The motor and sensory cortex are closely interlinked because fibers in the sensory tracts from the thalamus also terminate in the motor cortex, and because the cortical areas are adjacent (pre- and postcentral gyrus).

Subthalamic lesion (3): All sensation is abolished in the *contralateral* half of the body (thalamus = "gateway to consciousness"). A partial lesion that spares the pain and temperature pathways (**4**) is characterized by hypoesthesia (decreased tactile sensation) on the *contralateral* face and body. Pain and temperature sensation are unaffected.

Lesion of the trigeminal lemniscus and lateral spinothalamic tract (5): Damage to these pathways in the brainstem causes a loss of pain and temperature sensation in the *contralateral* half of the face and body. Other sensory qualities are unaffected.

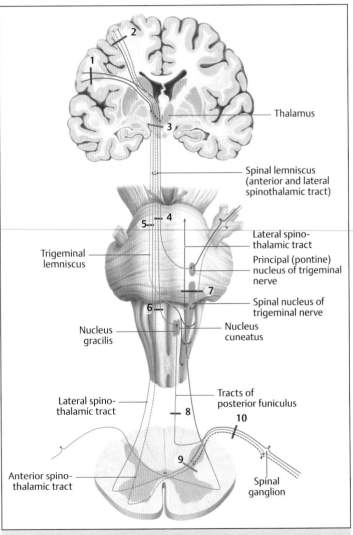

Fig. 7.22 Sites of occurrence of lesions in the sensory pathways.

Lesion of the medial lemniscus and anterior spinothalamic tract (6): All sensory qualities on the *opposite* side of the body are abolished except for pain and temperature.

The medial lemniscus transmits the axons of the second neurons of the anterior spinothalamic tract and both tracts of the posterior funiculus.

Lesion of the trigeminal nucleus, spinal tract of the trigeminal nerve, and lateral spinothalamic tract (7): Pain and temperature sensation are abolished on the *ipsilateral* side of the face (uncrossed axons of the first neuron in the trigeminal ganglion) and on the *contralateral* side of the body (axons of the crossed second neuron in the lateral spinothalamic tract).

Lesion of the posterior funiculi (8): This lesion causes an *ipsilateral* loss of position sense, vibration sense, and two-point discrimination. Because coordinated motor function relies on sensory input that operates in a feedback loop, the lack of sensory input leads to ipsilateral sensory ataxia.

Posterior horn lesion (9): A circumscribed lesion involving one or a few segments causes an *ipsilateral* loss of pain and temperature sensation in the affected body segment(s), because pain and temperature sensation are relayed to the second neuron within the posterior horn. Other sensory qualities including crude touch are transmitted in the posterior funiculus and relayed in the dorsal column nuclei; hence they are unaffected. The effects of a posterior horn lesion are called a "dissociated sensory deficit."

Dorsal root lesion (10): This lesion causes *ipsilateral*, radicular sensory disturbances that may range from pain in the corresponding dermatome to a complete loss of sensation. Concomitant involvement of the ventral root leads to segmental weakness. This clinical situation may be caused by a herniated intervertebral disk. Radicular pain, or radiculitis, is pain "radiated" along the dermatome (sensory distribution) of a nerve due to inflammation or other irritation of the nerve root at its connection to the spinal column. A common form of radiculitis is sciatica—radicular pain that radiates along the sciatic nerve from the lower spine to the lower back, gluteal muscles, back of the upper thigh, calf, and foot as often secondary to nerve root irritation from a spinal disc herniation or from osteophytes (bone spurs) in the lumbar region of the spine.

Lesions of *unconscious* cerebellar tracts that lead to sensorimotor deficits are not considered here. The volume on *General Anatomy and Musculoskeletal System* may be consulted for information on peripheral sensory nerve lesions.

7.8 Motor System, Overview

7.8.1 Simplified Representation of the Anatomical Structures Involved in a Voluntary Movement (Pyramidal Motor System)

The first step in performing a voluntary movement is to plan the movement in the association cortex of the cerebrum (e.g.,

goal: "I want to pick up my venti caramel macchiato coffee"). The cerebellar hemispheres and basal ganglia work in parallel to program the movement and inform the premotor cortex of the result of this planning. The premotor cortex passes the information to the primary motor cortex (M1), which relays the information through the *pyramidal tract* to the alpha motor neuron *(pyramidal motor system)*. The alpha motor neuron then initiates the process whereby the skeletal muscle transforms the program into a specific voluntary movement. Sensorimotor functions supply important feedback during this process (How far has the movement progressed? How strong is my grip on the cup handle? —different from gripping an eggshell or a pet monkey's earlobe for example). Although some of the later figures portray the primary motor cortex as the starting point for a voluntary movement, this diagram shows that many motor centers are involved in the execution of a voluntary movement (including the *extrapyramidal motor system*, see Chapters 7.8.3 and 7.8.4; cerebellum). For practical reasons, however, the discussion commonly begins at the primary motor cortex (M1) (**Fig. 7.23**).

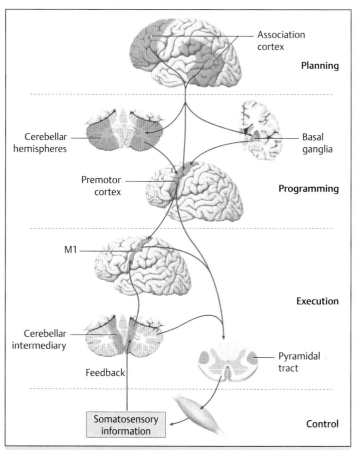

Fig. 7.23 Simplified representation of the anatomical structures involved in a voluntary movement (pyramidal motor system).

7.8.2 Cortical Areas with Motor Function: Initiating a Movement

Lateral view of the left hemisphere (**Fig. 7.24**). The initiation of a voluntary movement (reaching for a coffee cup) results from the interaction of various cortical areas. The *primary motor cortex* (M1, Brodmann's area 4) is located in the precentral gyrus (execution of a movement). The rostrally adjacent area 6 consists of the lateral premotor cortex and medial supplementary motor cortex (initiation of a movement). Association fibers establish close functional connections with sensory areas 1, 2, and 3 (postcentral gyrus with primary somatosensory cortex, S1) and with areas 5 and 7 (= posterior parietal cortex), which have an associative motor function. These areas provide the cortical representation of space, which is important in precision grasping movements, eye movements, and perhaps the precise time–space coordinates that need to be realized for the rapid sequences of movements necessary for speech.

7.8.3 Connections of the Cortex with the Basal Ganglia and Cerebellum: Programming Complex Movements

The pyramidal motor system (the primary motor cortex and the pyramidal tract arising from it) is assisted by the basal ganglia and cerebellum in the planning and programming of complex movements. While afferent fibers of the motor nuclei (green) project directly to the basal ganglia (left) without synapsing, the cerebellum is indirectly controlled via pontine nuclei (right) (**Fig. 7.25**). The motor thalamus provides a feedback loop for both structures. The efferent fibers of the basal nuclei and cerebellum are distributed to lower structures including the spinal cord. The importance of the basal ganglia and cerebellum in voluntary movements can be appreciated by noting the effects of lesions in these structures. While diseases of the basal ganglia impair

the initiation and execution of movements (e.g., in Parkinson's disease), cerebellar lesions are characterized by uncoordinated writhing (athetoid) and irregularly spaced movements (e.g., the reeling, unbalanced, uncoordinated movements of inebriation, caused by a temporary toxic insult to the cerebellum).

7.8.4 Simplified Block Diagram of the Sensorimotor System in Movement Control

Voluntary movements require constant feedback from the periphery (muscle spindles, tendon organs) in order to remain within the desired limits (**Fig. 7.26**). Because the motor and sensory systems are so closely interrelated functionally, they are often described jointly as the sensorimotor system. The spinal cord, brainstem, cerebellum, and cerebral cortex are the three control levels of the sensorimotor system. All information from periphery, cerebellum, and the basal ganglia passes through the thalamus on its way to the cerebral cortex. The clinical importance of the sensory system in movement is illustrated by the sensory ataxia that may occur when sensory function is lost. The oculomotor component of the sensorimotor system is not shown.

Speech note: Skilled motor movements are so interconnected with the basal ganglia, cerebellum, and other subcortical and cortical regions, that determining the source and explanation for motor planning, motor programming, and motor execution deficits can be a formidable task. This may be the reason that such motor planning and programming deficits such as apraxia of speech have eluded consensus on location and nature of the damage that causes it. Even agreement on the differential salient characteristics of such movement—phonological–linguistic clusters of deviant dimensions has avoided consensus, especially against the backdrop of a developing linguistic and nervous system in children.

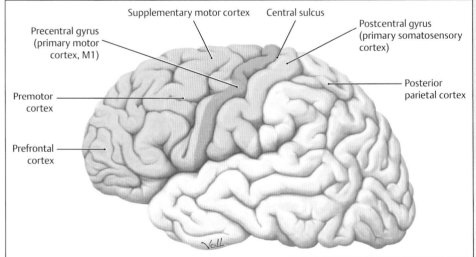

Fig. 7.24 Cortical areas (lateral view of the left hemisphere).

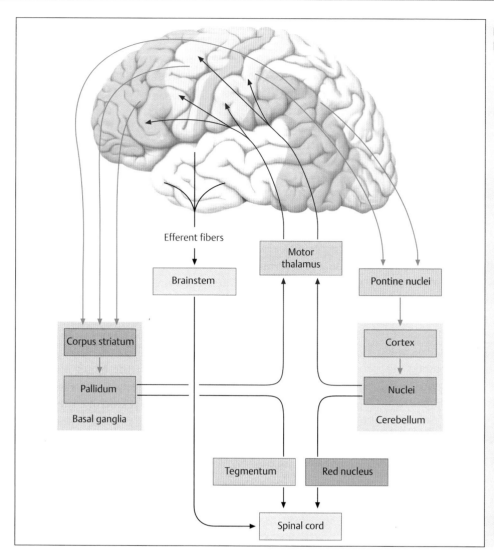

Fig. 7.25 Connections of the cortex with the basal ganglia and cerebellum.

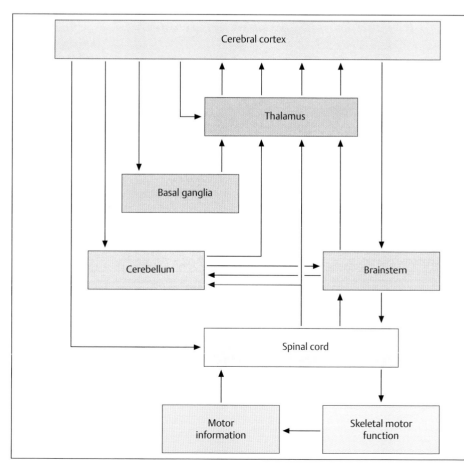

Fig. 7.26 Simplified block diagram of the sensorimotor system in movement control.

7.9 Motor System: Pyramidal (Corticospinal) Tract

7.9.1 Course of the Pyramidal (Corticospinal) Tract

The pyramidal tract consists of three fiber systems: corticospinal fibers, corticobulbar (corticonuclear) fibers, and corticoreticular fibers (the latter are not shown here; they pass to the gigantocellular nucleus of the reticular formation in the brainstem) (**Fig. 7.27**). The gigantocellular nucleus, as the name indicates, is mainly composed of the so-called giant neuronal cells. This nucleus has been known to innervate the caudal hypoglossal nucleus. This nucleus is related to all functions of the hypoglossal nerve, which is most important for tongue movement in speech, mastication (chewing), and swallowing. The dorsal rostral section of the nucleus reticularis gigantocellularis is also involved in mediating expiration (or outbreathing, including breathing for speech). These groups of fibers (corticospinal, corticobulbar, corticoreticular) constitute the descending motor pathways from the primary motor cortex. The corticospinal fibers pass to the motor anterior horn cells in the spinal cord, while the corticonuclear fibers pass to the motor nuclei of the cranial nerves.

Corticospinal fibers: Only a small percentage of the axons of the corticospinal fibers originate from the large pyramidal neurons in lamina (layer) V of the precentral gyrus (the laminar structure of the motor cortex is described in Chapter 7.9.4). Most of the axons arise from small pyramidal cells and other neurons in laminae V and VI. Other axons originate from adjacent brain regions. All of them descend through the internal capsule. Eighty to 90% of the fibers *cross the midline* at the level of the medulla oblongata (decussation of the pyramids) and descend in the spinal cord as the *lateral corticospinal (pyramidal) tract.* The *uncrossed* fibers descend in the cord as the *anterior corticospinal (pyramidal) tract* and cross later at the segmental level. Most of the axons terminate on intercalated ("between layers") cells whose synapses end on motor neurons.

Note: The basic pattern of somatotopic organization described earlier at the spinal cord level is found at all levels of the pyramidal tract. This facilitates localization of the lesion in the pyramidal tract.

Corticobulbar (corticonuclear) fibers: The motor nuclei and motor segments of the cranial nerves receive their axons from pyramidal cells in the facial region of the premotor cortex. These

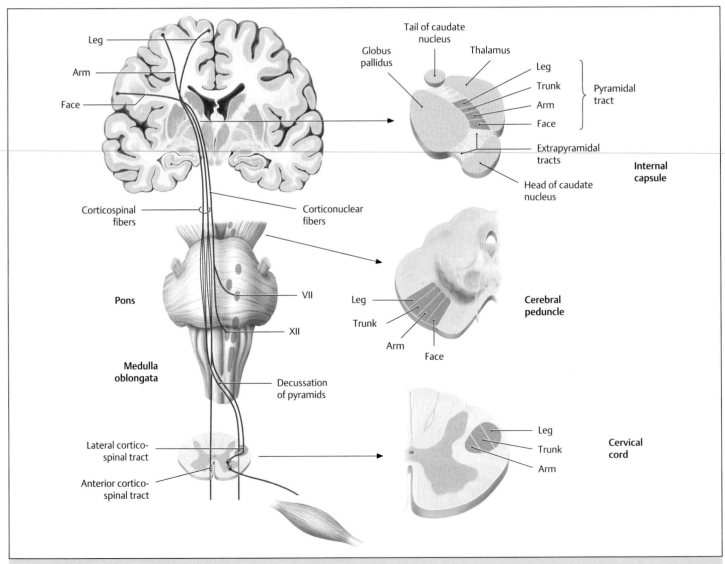

Fig. 7.27 The pyramidal (corticospinal) tract.

corticobulbar fibers terminate in the contralateral motor nuclei of cranial nerves III to VII and IX to XII in the brainstem (the fibers to other brainstem nuclei are described in Chapter 7.9.3). Besides this contralateral supply, axons also pass to several cranial nerve nuclei on the same (ipsilateral) side, resulting in a bilateral innervation pattern (not shown here). This dual supply is clinically important in lesions of the frontal branch of the facial nerve.

Notes on the "pyramidal tract": Some authors interpret this term as applying strictly to the portion of the tract below the decussation of the pyramids, while other authors apply the term to the entire tract. Most publications, including this atlas, use "pyramidal tract" as a collective term for all of the fiber tracts described here. Some authors derive the term not from the decussation of the pyramids but from the giant pyramidal cells (Betz's cells) in the cerebral cortex.

7.9.2 Somatotopic Representation of the Skeletal Muscle in the Precentral Gyrus (Motor Homunculus)

Anterior view (**Fig. 7.28**). Regions in which the muscles are very densely innervated (e.g., the hand, fingers, tongue) must be supplied by many neurons in the precentral gyrus. As a result, they require a larger representation area in the cortex than regions supplied by fewer neurons (e.g., the trunk). This cortical representation is analogous to that in sensory innervation, where areas of varying size are also represented in the cortex (postcentral gyrus; compare with the sensory homunculus).

One cortical area is devoted to the trunk and limbs and another to the head. The axons for the head area are the corticobulbar fibers, and the axons for the trunk and limbs are the corticospinal fibers. The latter fibers split into two groups below the telencephalon, forming the lateral and anterior corticospinal tracts.

7.9.3 Variety of Cortical Efferent Fibers

Anterior view (**Fig. 7.29**). Besides the corticospinal and corticobulbar fibers described above, a variety of axons descends from the cortex to various subcortical regions and into the spinal cord. The following subcortical regions also receive cortical efferent fibers: the corpus striatum, thalamus, red nucleus, pontine nuclei, reticular formation, inferior olive, dorsal column nuclei (these nuclear regions are described subsequently), and spinal cord. The supraspinal efferent fibers listed above consist partially of axon collaterals from pyramidal tract neurons and partially of separate axons.

7.9.4 Laminar Structure of the Motor Cortex (= Area 4 in the Precentral Gyrus)

The axons from giant pyramidal cells (Betz's cells) in lamina V account for only a small percentage (< 4%) of the axons that

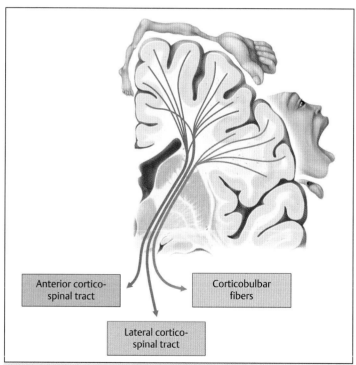

Fig. 7.28 Somatotopic representation of the skeletal muscle in the precentral gyrus (motor homunculus).

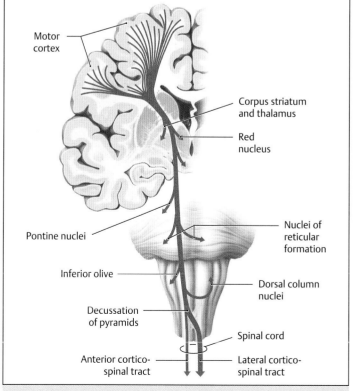

Fig. 7.29 Cortical efferent fibers (anterior view).

make up the corticospinal tract (**Fig. 7.30**). Small pyramidal cells and other neurons from laminae V and VI contribute the rest. In all, however, only about 40% of the axons of the pyramidal tract originate in area 4. The remaining 60% come from neurons in the supplementary motor fields.

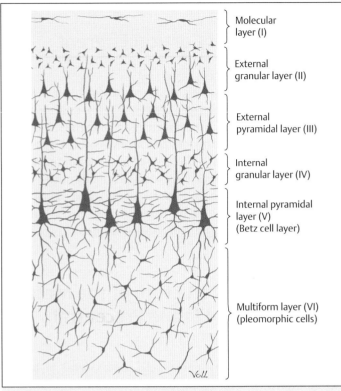

Molecular layer (I)

External granular layer (II)

External pyramidal layer (III)

Internal granular layer (IV)

Internal pyramidal layer (V) (Betz cell layer)

Multiform layer (VI) (pleomorphic cells)

Fig. 7.30 Laminar structure of the motor cortex.

7.10 Motor System: Motor Nuclei

7.10.1 Motor Nuclei

Coronal section (**Fig. 7.31**). The basal ganglia (more accurately called basal nuclei, but tradition is entrenched) are subcortical nuclei of the telencephalon that have a role in the planning and execution of movements (including speech and swallowing). They are particularly related to the variety of movement disorders that are seen clinically and play a role in several different types of dysarthria. They are the central relay station of the extrapyramidal motor system and make up almost all the central gray matter of the cerebrum. The only other central gray matter structure is the thalamus, which is primarily sensory ("gateway to consciousness") but is involved secondarily, through feedback mechanisms, in motor sequences. The three largest motor nuclei are as follows:

- Caudate nucleus.
- Putamen.
- Globus pallidus (developmentally, part of the diencephalon).

These three nuclei are sometimes known by varying collective designations:

- The *lentiform nucleus* is formed by the putamen, globus pallidus, and intervening fiber tracts.
- The *corpus striatum consists* of the putamen, caudate nucleus, and intervening streaks of gray matter. In addition to these three nuclei, there are other nuclei that are considered functional components of the motor system (also shown here).

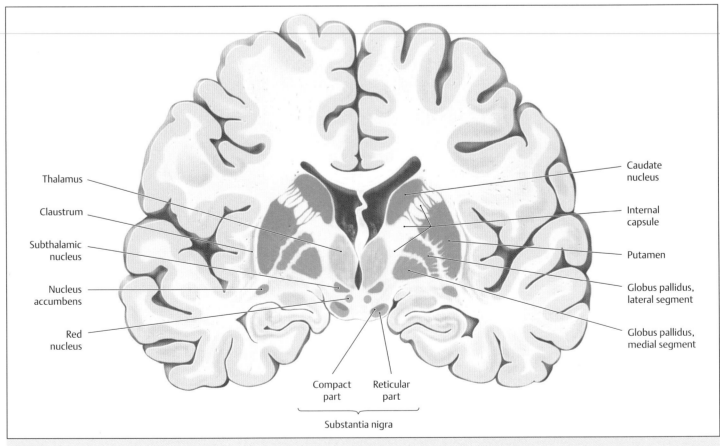

Thalamus

Claustrum

Subthalamic nucleus

Nucleus accumbens

Red nucleus

Caudate nucleus

Internal capsule

Putamen

Globus pallidus, lateral segment

Globus pallidus, medial segment

Compact part   Reticular part

Substantia nigra

Fig. 7.31 Motor nuclei (coronal section).

In a strictly anatomical sense, only the telencephalic structures listed above are constituents of the basal ganglia (nuclei). Some textbooks include the *subthalamic nucleus* of the diencephalon and the *substantia nigra* of the mesencephalon among the basal ganglia because of their close functional relationship to nuclei. Functional disturbances of the basal nuclei are characterized by movement disorders. There are a variety of movement disorders that are related to basal ganglia and extrapyramidal system disorders. These include Parkinson's disease; Huntington's disease and other choreic disorders (rapid, jerky, involuntary movements); Tourette's and other tic-related disorders; dystonia; tremor; myoclonus; and ataxia.

7.10.2 Flow of Information between Motor Cortical Areas and Basal Ganglia: Motor Loop

The basal ganglia are concerned with the controlled, purposeful execution of fine voluntary movements (e.g., picking up an egg or a waffle without breaking it). They integrate information from the cortex and subcortical regions, which they process in parallel and then return to motor cortical areas via the thalamus (feedback). Neurons from the premotor, primary motor, supplementary motor, and somatosensory cortex and from the parietal lobe send their axons to the putamen (**Fig. 7.32**). Initially, there is a direct (yellow)

and indirect (green) pathway for relaying the information out of the putamen. Both pathways ultimately lead to the motor cortex by way of the thalamus. In the *direct* pathway (yellow), the neurons of the putamen project to the medial globus pallidus and to the reticular part of the substantia nigra. Both nuclei then return feedback signals to the motor thalamus, which projects back to motor areas of the cortex. The *indirect* pathway (green) leads from the putamen through the lateral globus pallidus and subthalamic nucleus back to the medial globus pallidus, which then projects to the thalamus. An alternate indirect route leads from the subthalamic nucleus to the reticular part of the substantia nigra, which in turn projects to the thalamus. When inhibitory dopaminergic neurons in the compact part of the substantia nigra cease to function, the indirect pathway is suppressed and the direct pathway is no longer facilitated. Both effects lead to the increased inhibition of thalamocortical neurons, resulting in decreased movements (= *hypokinetic disorder,* e.g., in Parkinson's disease. This reveals why the inadequate loudness, light articulatory contacts, and short phrases in Parkinson's disease is called *hypokinetic dysarthria*). Conversely, reduced activation of the internal part of the globus pallidus and the reticular part of the substantia nigra leads to increased activation of the thalamocortical neurons, resulting in abnormal spontaneous movements (= *hyperkinetic disorder*, e.g., Huntington's disease; dystonia).

The diagram at lower left shows a close-up view of the boxed area (thalamus).

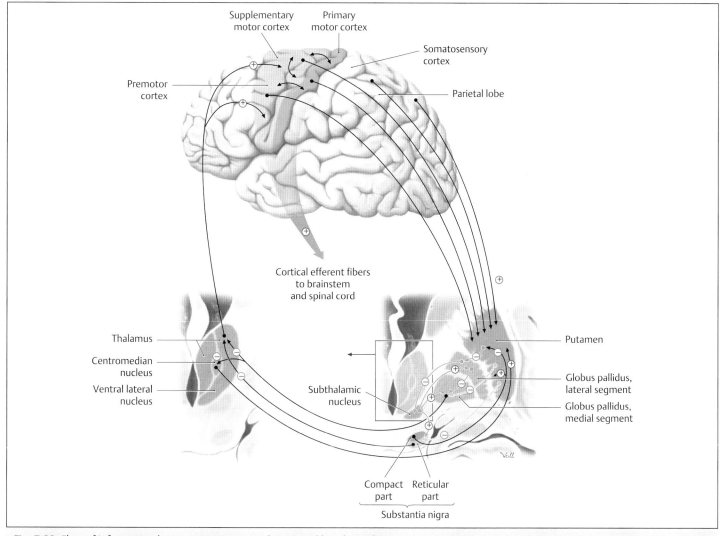

Fig. 7.32 Flow of information between motor cortical areas and basal ganglia.

Speech note: Basal ganglia and extrapyramidal damage, as well as cortical and subcortical lesions, can cause disorders of swallowing and movement-related speech as seen and heard in the many types of dysarthria. Dysarthria is a sensorimotor speech disorder that results from abnormalities in speed, strength, range, steadiness, tone, or accuracy of movements. It can affect the control of the respiratory, phonatory, resonatory, articulatory, and prosodic aspects of speech production. Central or PNS lesions are responsible for the deficits. The most frequent results are weakness, spasticity, involuntary movements, incoordination, or excessive, reduced, and variable muscle tone.

7.11 Motor System: Extrapyramidal Motor System and Lesions

7.11.1 Descending Tracts of the Extrapyramidal Motor System

The neurons of origin of the descending tracts of the extrapyramidal motor system* arise from a heterogeneous group of nuclei that includes the basal ganglia (putamen, globus pallidus, and caudate nucleus), the red nucleus, the substantia nigra, and even

motor cortical areas (e.g., area 6) (**Fig. 7.33**). The following descending tracts are part of the extrapyramidal motor system:

- Rubrospinal tract.
- Olivospinal tract.
- Vestibulospinal tract.
- Reticulospinal tract.
- Tectospinal tract.

These long descending tracts terminate on interneurons which then form synapses onto alpha and gamma motor neurons, which they control. Besides these long descending motor tracts, the motor neurons additionally receive sensory input (blue). The stretch reflexes (frequently called deep tendon reflexes) provide information on the integrity of the central and PNSs. In general, decreased reflexes (hyporeflexia) reflect a peripheral problem, and exaggerated reflexive responses (hyperreflexia) indicate a problem in the CNS. Types of reflexes, which are usually tested in a clinical neurological examination, include the knee-jerk or patellar reflex, the Achilles reflex, the cremasteric reflex (retraction of the testicle in males upon lightly stroking the thigh; thought to be protective since extreme pressure or pounding on a testicle can elicit a howler monkey cry of pain), and the plantar (Babinski) reflex. Abnormal Babinski's reflexes may indicate problems with the corticospinal tract. It is not necessary, but this reflex may be set to music in what some might regard as a choreographed, reflexive dance.

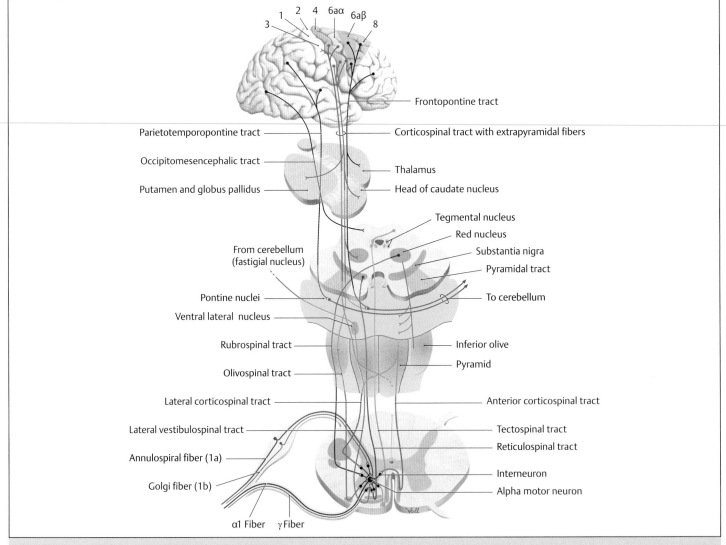

Fig. 7.33 Descending tracts of the extrapyramidal motor system.

7.11.2 Lesions of The Central Motor Pathways and Their Effects

See **Fig. 7.34**.

Lesion near the cortex (1): Paralysis of the muscles innervated by the damaged cortical area. Because the face and hand are represented by particularly large areas in the motor cortex, paralysis often affects primarily the arm and face ("brachiofacial" paralysis). The paralysis invariably affects the side opposite the lesion (decussation of the pyramids) and is flaccid and partial *(paresis)* rather than complete because the extrapyramidal fibers are not damaged. If the extrapyramidal fibers were also damaged, the result would be *complete spastic paralysis* (see below). Spasticity refers to a muscular hyperclonic state or state of hypercontractivity.

Lesion at the level of the internal capsule (2): This leads to chronic, contralateral, spastic *hemiplegia* (= complete paralysis) because the lesion affects both the pyramidal tract and the extrapyramidal motor pathways,[a] which mix with pyramidal tract fibers in front of the internal capsule. Stroke is a frequent cause of lesions at this level.

Lesion at the level of the cerebral peduncles (crura cerebri) (3): Contralateral spastic hemi*paresis*.

Lesion at the level of the pons (4): Contralateral hemiparesis or bilateral paresis, depending on the size of the lesion. Because the fibers of the pyramidal tract occupy a larger cross-sectional area in the pons than in the internal capsule, not all of the fibers are damaged in many cases. For example, the fibers for the facial nerve and hypoglossal nerve are usually unaffected because of their dorsal location.

Damage to the abducent nucleus may cause ipsilateral damage to the trigeminal nucleus (not shown).

Lesion at the level of the pyramid (5): Flaccid (floppy, weakened) contralateral paresis occurs because the fibers of the extrapyramidal motor pathways (e.g., the rubrospinal and tectospinal tract) are more dorsal than the pyramidal tract fibers and are therefore unaffected by an isolated lesion of the pyramid.

Lesion at the level of the spinal cord (6, 7): A lesion at the level of the cervical cord (6) leads to ipsilateral spastic hemiplegia because the fibers of the pyramidal and extrapyramidal system are closely interwoven at this level and have already crossed to the opposite side. A lesion at the level of the thoracic cord (7) leads to spastic paralysis of the ipsilateral leg.

Lesion at the level of the peripheral nerve (8): This lesion damages the axon of the alpha motor neuron, resulting in flaccid paralysis.

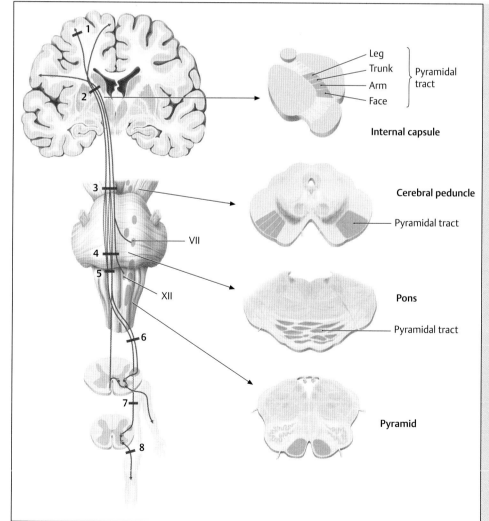

Fig. 7.34 Lesions of the central motor pathways.

---

[a] Thus, spastic paralysis is actually a sign of extrapyramidal motor damage. This fact was unknown when pyramidal tract lesions were first described, however, and it was assumed that a *pyramidal tract lesion* led to spastic paralysis. Because this fact has few practical implications, spasticity is still described in some textbooks as the classic sign of a pyramidal tract lesion. It would be better simply to regard spastic paralysis as a form of central paralysis.

7.12 Lesions of the Brachial Plexus

7.12.1 Brachial Plexus Paralysis

Anterior view of the right side (**Fig. 7.35**). Lesions are circled. By definition, two forms of brachial plexus paralysis are distinguished: *upper brachial plexus paralysis*, which is caused by a lesion of the C5 and C6 ventral rami (see Chapter 7.12.3), and *lower brachial plexus paralysis*, which is caused by a lesion of the C8 and T1 ventral rami (see Chapter 7.12.4). C7 forms a "watershed"

between the two forms of paralysis and is typically unaffected by either form. A complete lesion of the brachial plexus may also occur in severe trauma.

7.12.2 Site of Lesion in Brachial Plexus Paralysis

A brachial plexus lesion affects the ventral rami of several spinal nerves, which transmit afferent signals to the plexus (**Fig. 7.36**). Because the ventral rami (branches) carry both motor and

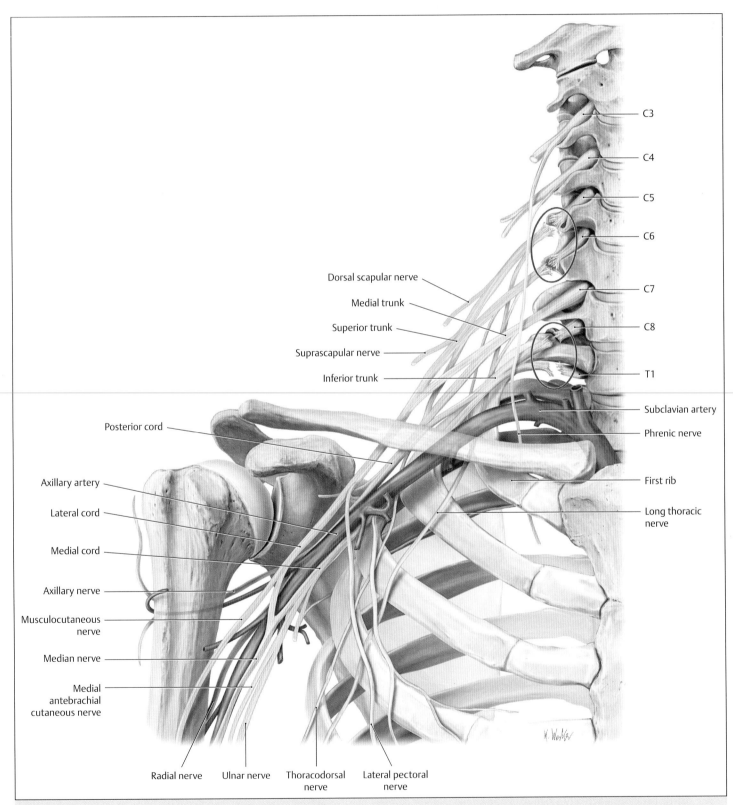

Fig. 7.35 Brachial plexus paralysis (anterior view of the right side).

sensory fibers, a brachial plexus lesion always causes a combination of motor and sensory deficits. The resulting paralysis (see Chapter 7.12.3) is always of the flaccid type because of its peripheral nature (= lesion of the second motor neuron).

7.12.3 Example: Upper Brachial Plexus Paralysis (Erb's Palsy)

This condition results from a lesion of the ventral rami of the C5 and C6 spinal nerves, causing paralysis of the abductors and external rotators of the shoulder joint and of the upper arm flexors and supinator (**Fig. 7.37**). The arm hangs limply at the side (loss of the upper arm flexors), and the palm faces backward (loss of the supinator with dominance of the pronators). There may also be partial paralysis of the extensor muscles of the elbow joint and hand. Typical cases present with sensory disturbances on the lateral surface of the upper arm and forearm, but these signs may be absent. A frequent cause of upper brachial plexus paralysis is obstetric trauma.

7.12.4 Example: Lower Brachial Plexus Paralysis (Dejerine–Klumpke Palsy)

This paralysis results from a lesion of the ventral rami of the C8 and T1 spinal nerves (see Chapter 7.12.1). It affects the hand muscles, the long digital flexors, and the flexor muscles in the wrist (claw hand with atrophy of the small hand muscles, (**Fig. 7.38a**). Sensory disturbances affect the ulnar surfaces of the forearm and hand. (Augusta Dejerine–Klumpke was an American born physician who moved to France, married the famous French neurologist Dejerine, became one of the first women who served a medical internship at hospitals in Paris, and was a member of several scientific societies, including the Société de Biologie and the Société de Neurologie de Paris). Because the sympathetic fibers for the head leave the spinal cord at T1 (**Fig. 7.38b**), the sympathetic innervation of the head is also lost. This is manifested by a *unilateral Horner syndrome*, characterized by miosis (contracted pupil due to paralysis of the dilator pupillae) and

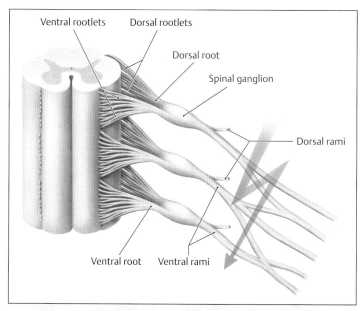

Fig. 7.36 Site of lesion in brachial plexus paralysis.

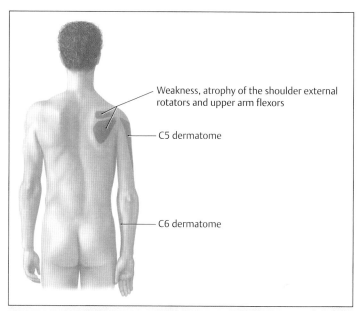

Fig. 7.37 Upper brachial plexus paralysis (Erb palsy).

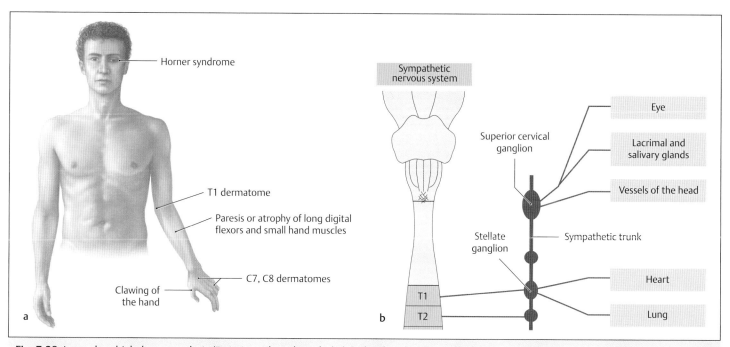

Fig. 7.38 Lower brachial plexus paralysis (Dejerine–Klumpke palsy). **(a)** Claw hand with atrophy of the small hand muscles. **(b)** Sympathetic fibers.

narrowing of the palpebral fissure (not ptosis or drooping of the eyelid) due to a loss of sympathetic innervation to the superior and inferior tarsal muscles. The narrowed palpebral fissure mimics enophthalmos (sinking of the eyeball into the orbit). These examples are presented to reveal the complexity and clarity of a careful neurological examination and how the site and extent of a lesion or disorder of the nervous system can be revealed by judicious examination of sensation, movements, behavior, and characteristics of abnormality.

7.13 Auditory Pathway

7.13.1 Afferent Auditory Pathway of the Left Ear

The receptors of the auditory pathway are the inner hair cells of the organ of Corti. Because they lack neural processes, they are called *secondary sensory cells*. They are located in the cochlear duct of the basilar membrane and are studded with stereocilia, which are exposed to shearing forces from the tectorial membrane in response to a traveling wave (**Fig. 7.39**). This causes

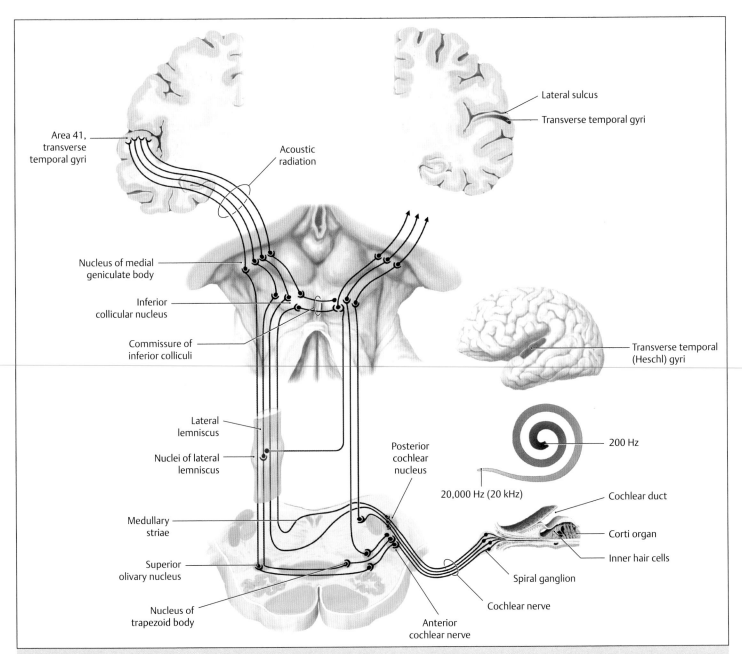

Fig. 7.39 Afferent auditory pathway of the left ear.

waves and bowing of the stereocilia. These bowing movements act as a stimulus to evoke cascades of neural signals. Dendritic processes of the bipolar neurons in the spiral ganglion pick up the stimulus. The bipolar neurons then transmit impulses via their axons, which are collected to form the cochlear nerve, to the anterior and posterior cochlear nuclei. In these nuclei, the signals are relayed to the second neuron of the auditory pathway. Information from the cochlear nuclei is then transmitted via 4 to 6 nuclei to the primary auditory cortex, where the auditory information is consciously perceived (analogous to the visual cortex). The primary auditory cortex is located in the transverse temporal gyri (Heschl's gyri, Brodmann's area 41). The auditory pathway thus contains the following key stations:

- Inner hair cells in the organ of Corti.
- Spiral ganglion.
- Anterior and posterior cochlear nuclei.
- Nucleus of the trapezoid body and superior olivary nucleus.
- Nucleus of the lateral lemniscus.
- Inferior collicular nucleus.
- Nucleus of medial geniculate body.
- Primary auditory cortex in the temporal lobe (transverse temporal gyri = Heschl's gyri or Brodmann's area 41).

The individual parts of the cochlea are correlated with specific areas in the auditory cortex and its relay stations. This is known as the *tonotopic organization of the auditory pathway*. This organizational principle is similar to that in the visual pathway. Binaural processing of the auditory information (binaural or stereo hearing) first occurs at the level of the superior olivary nucleus. This is important for sound localization (i.e., where a sound is coming from). At all further stages of the auditory pathway there are also interconnections between the right and left sides of the auditory pathway. Conductive hearing loss involves damage to the outer or middle ear. Sensorineural hearing loss involves damage to the hair cells, the auditory nerve, or central auditory pathways. Because of the neural damage, both air conduction and bone conduction of sound are diminished.

7.13.2 The Stapedius Reflex

When the volume of an acoustic signal reaches a certain threshold, the stapedius reflex triggers a contraction of the stapedius muscle. This reflex can be utilized to test hearing without the patient's cooperation ("objective" auditory testing) (**Fig. 7.40**). The test is done by introducing a sonic probe into the ear canal and presenting a test noise to the tympanic membrane. When the noise volume reaches a certain threshold, it evokes the stapedius reflex and the tympanic membrane stiffens. The change in the resistance of the tympanic membrane is then measured and recorded. The *afferent* limb of this reflex is in the cochlear nerve. Information is conveyed to the facial nucleus on each side by way of the superior olivary nucleus. The *efferent* limb of this reflex is formed by special visceromotor fibers of the facial nerve.

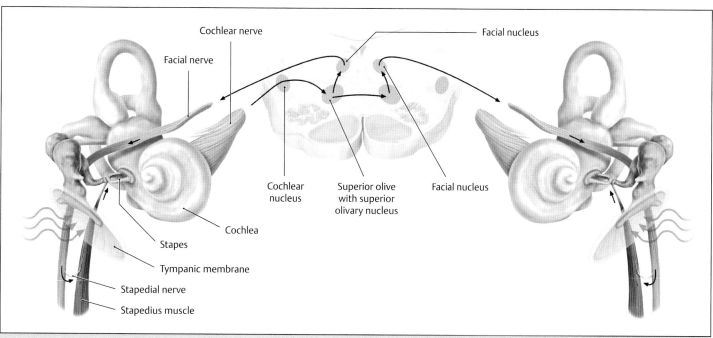

Fig. 7.40 The stapedius reflex.

7.13.3 Efferent Fibers from the Olive to the Corti Organ

Besides the afferent fibers from the organ of Corti (see Chapter 7.13.1, shown here in blue), which form the vestibulocochlear nerve, there are also efferent fibers (red) that pass to the organ of Corti in the inner ear and are concerned with the active preprocessing of sound ("cochlear amplifier") and acoustic protection (**Fig. 7.41**). The efferent fibers arise from neurons that are located in either the lateral or medial part of the superior olive and project from there to the cochlea (lateral or medial olivocochlear bundle). The fibers of the lateral neurons pass *uncrossed* to the dendrites of the *inner* hair cells, while the fibers of the medial neurons *cross* to the opposite side and terminate at the base of the outer hair cells, whose activity they influence. When stimulated, the outer hair cells can actively amplify the traveling wave. This increases the sensitivity of the inner hair cells (the actual receptor cells). The activity of the efferents from the olive can be recorded as otoacoustic emissions (OAE). This test can be used to screen for hearing abnormalities in newborns.

7.14 Vestibular System

7.14.1 Central Connections of the Vestibular Nerve

Three systems are involved in the regulation of human balance:

- Vestibular system.
- Proprioceptive system.
- Visual system.

The peripheral receptors of the *vestibular system* are located in the membranous labyrinth, which consists of the utricle and saccule and the ampullae of the three semicircular ducts (**Fig. 7.42**). The maculae of the utricle and saccule respond to linear acceleration, while the semicircular duct organs in the ampullary crests respond to angular (rotational) acceleration. Like the hair cells of the inner ear, the receptors of the vestibular system are *secondary* sensory cells. The basal portions of the secondary sensory cells are surrounded by dendritic processes of bipolar neurons. Their cell bodies or perikarya are located in the vestibular ganglion. The axons from these neurons form the vestibular nerve and terminate in the four vestibular nuclei (see Chapter 7.14.3). Besides input from the vestibular apparatus, these nuclei also receive sensory input (see Chapter 7.14.2). The vestibular nuclei show a topographical organization (see Chapter 7.14.3) and distribute their efferent fibers to three targets:

- Motor neurons in the spinal cord via the lateral vestibulospinal tract. These motor neurons help to maintain upright stance, mainly by increasing the tone of extensor muscles.
- Flocculonodular lobe of the cerebellum (archicerebellum) via vestibulocerebellar fibers.
- Ipsilateral and contralateral oculomotor nuclei via the ascending part of the medial longitudinal fasciculus.

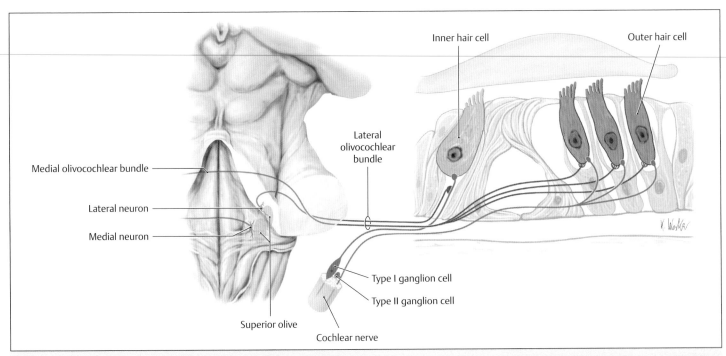

Labels: Inner hair cell, Outer hair cell, Lateral olivocochlear bundle, Medial olivocochlear bundle, Lateral neuron, Medial neuron, Type I ganglion cell, Type II ganglion cell, Superior olive, Cochlear nerve

Fig. 7.41 Efferent fibers from the olive to the Corti orga.

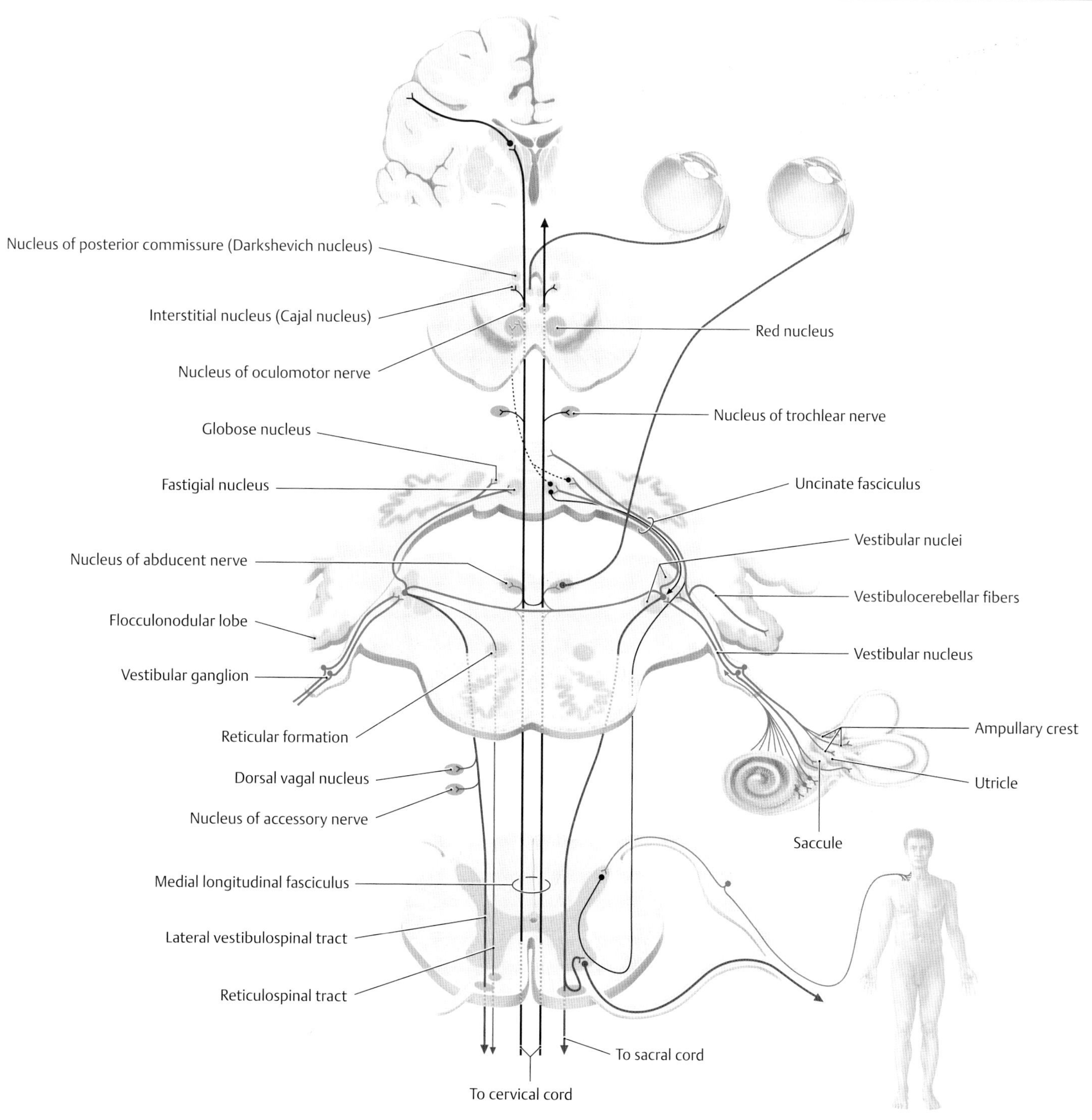
Nucleus of posterior commissure (Darkshevich nucleus)
Interstitial nucleus (Cajal nucleus)
Nucleus of oculomotor nerve
Globose nucleus
Fastigial nucleus
Nucleus of abducent nerve
Flocculonodular lobe
Vestibular ganglion
Reticular formation
Dorsal vagal nucleus
Nucleus of accessory nerve
Medial longitudinal fasciculus
Lateral vestibulospinal tract
Reticulospinal tract
To cervical cord
To sacral cord
Red nucleus
Nucleus of trochlear nerve
Uncinate fasciculus
Vestibular nuclei
Vestibulocerebellar fibers
Vestibular nucleus
Ampullary crest
Utricle
Saccule

Fig. 7.42 Central connections of the vestibular nerve.

7.14.2 Central Role of the Vestibular Nuclei in the Maintenance of Balance

The afferent fibers that pass to the vestibular nuclei and the efferent fibers that emerge from them demonstrate the central role of these nuclei in maintaining balance (**Fig. 7.43**). The vestibular nuclei receive afferent input from the vestibular system, proprioceptive system (position sense, muscles, and joints), and visual system. They then distribute efferent fibers to nuclei that control the motor systems important for balance. These nuclei are located in the following regions:

- Spinal cord (motor support).
- Cerebellum (fine control of motor function).
- Brainstem (oculomotor nuclei for oculomotor function).

Efferents from the vestibular nuclei are also distributed to the following regions:

- Thalamus and cortex (spatial sense).
- Hypothalamus (autonomic regulation: vomiting in response to vertigo).

Note: Acute failure of the vestibular system is manifested by rotary vertigo. Vertigo is the feeling that you or your environment is moving or spinning. It differs from dizziness in that vertigo describes an illusion of movement. When you feel as if you yourself are moving, it's called subjective vertigo, and the perception that your surroundings are moving is called objective vertigo. Vertigo can be caused by problems in the brain or the inner ear, including benign paroxysmal position vertigo (the sensation of motion caused by sudden head movements), viral or bacterial labyrinthitis (inner ear infection), Meniere's disease (vertigo, tinnitus, hearing loss), acoustic neuroma, cerebellar damage, multiple sclerosis, and traumatic brain injury.

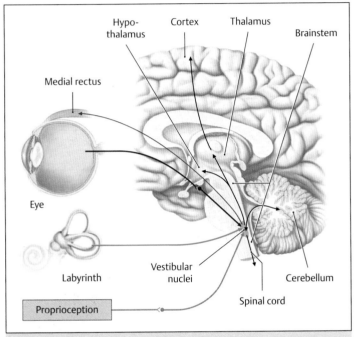

Fig. 7.43 Central role of the vestibular nuclei.

7.14.3 Vestibular Nuclei: Topographic Organization and Central Connections

Four nuclei are distinguished:

- Superior vestibular nucleus (of Bechterew).
- Lateral vestibular nucleus (of Deiters).
- Medial vestibular nucleus (of Schwalbe).
- Inferior vestibular nucleus (of Roller).

The vestibular system has a topographic organization:

- The afferent fibers of the saccular macula terminate in the inferior vestibular nucleus and lateral vestibular nucleus.
- The afferent fibers of the utricular macula terminate in the medial part of the inferior vestibular nucleus, the lateral part of the medial vestibular nucleus, and the lateral vestibular nucleus.
- The afferent fibers from the ampullary crests of the semicircular canals terminate in the superior vestibular nucleus, the upper part of the inferior vestibular nucleus, and the lateral vestibular nucleus.

The efferent fibers from the lateral vestibular nucleus pass to the lateral vestibulospinal tract. This tract extends to the sacral part of the spinal cord, its axons terminating on motor neurons (**Fig. 7.44**). Functionally it is concerned with keeping the body upright, chiefly by increasing the tone of the extensor muscles. The vestibulocerebellar fibers from the other three nuclei act through the cerebellum to modulate muscular tone. All four vestibular nuclei distribute ipsilateral and contralateral axons via the medial longitudinal fasciculus to the three motor nuclei of the nerves to the extraocular muscles (i.e., the nuclei of the abducent, trochlear, and oculomotor nerves).

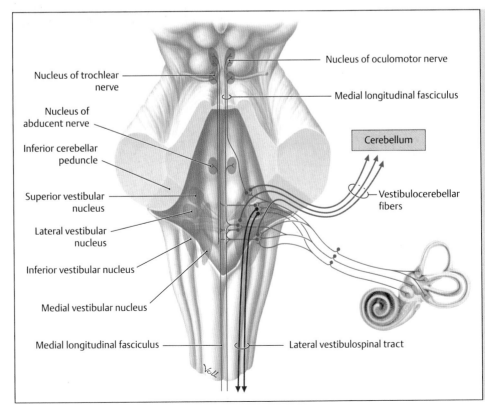

Fig. 7.44 Vestibular nuclei (topographic organization and central connections).

7.15 Gustatory System (Taste)

7.15.1 Gustatory Pathway

The receptors for the sense of taste are the taste buds of the tongue (see Chapter 7.15.2). Unlike other receptor cells, the receptor cells of the taste buds are specialized epithelial cells (secondary sensory cells, as they do not have an axon). When these epithelial cells are chemically stimulated, the base of the cells releases glutamate, which stimulates the peripheral processes of afferent cranial nerves. These different cranial nerves serve different areas of the tongue. It is rare, therefore, for a complete loss of taste (ageusia) to occur (**Fig. 7.45**).

- The *anterior two-thirds* of the tongue are supplied by the facial nerve (CN VII), the afferent fibers first passing in the lingual nerve (branch of the trigeminal nerve) and then in the chorda tympani to the geniculate ganglion of the facial nerve.
- The *posterior third of the tongue* and the *vallate papillae* are supplied by the glossopharyngeal nerve (CN IX).
- The *epiglottis* is supplied by the vagus nerve (CN X).

Peripheral processes from pseudounipolar ganglion cells (which correspond to pseudounipolar spinal ganglion cells) terminate on the taste buds. The central portions of these processes convey taste information to the gustatory part of the nucleus of the solitary tract. Thus, they function as the first afferent neuron of the gustatory pathway. Their perikarya (cell bodies) are located in the geniculate ganglion for the facial nerve, in the inferior (petrosal) ganglion for the glossopharyngeal nerve, and in the inferior (nodose) ganglion for the vagus nerve. After synapsing in the gustatory part of the nucleus of the solitary tract, the axons from the second neuron are believed to terminate in the medial parabrachial nucleus, where they are relayed to the third neuron. Most of the axons from the third neuron cross to the opposite side and pass in the dorsal trigeminothalamic tract to the contralateral ventral posteromedial nucleus of the thalamus. Some of the axons travel uncrossed in the same structures. The fourth neurons of the gustatory pathway, located in the thalamus, project to the postcentral gyrus and insular cortex, where the fifth neuron is located. Collaterals from the first and second neurons of the gustatory afferent pathway are distributed to the superior and inferior salivatory nuclei. Afferent impulses in these fibers induce the secretion of saliva during eating ("salivary reflex"). Besides this purely gustatory pathway, spicy foods (5-alarm, burn-your-tongue-off, fish curry) may also stimulate trigeminal fibers (not shown), which

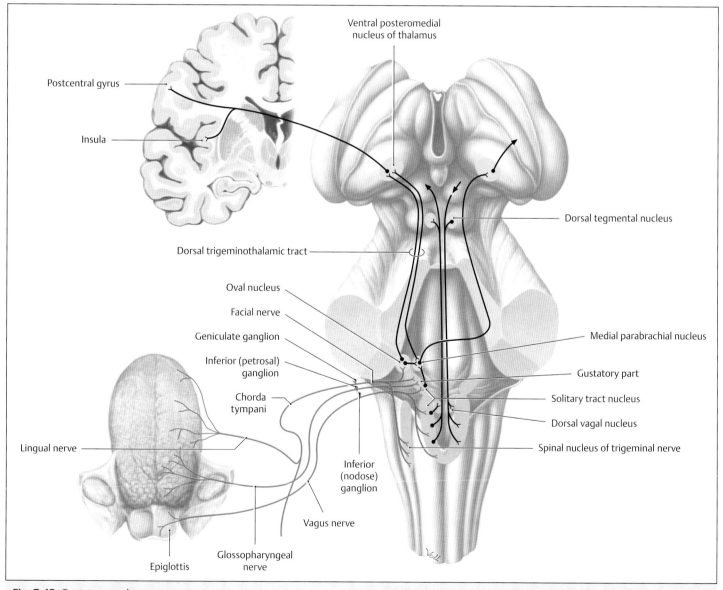

Fig. 7.45 Gustatory pathway.

contribute to the sensation of taste. Finally, olfaction (the sense of smell), too, is a major component of the sense of taste as it is subjectively perceived: patients who cannot smell (anosmia) report that their food tastes abnormally bland. Although often discounted and overlooked in a basic examination, deficiencies in taste and smell can cause anxiety, depression, and even nutritional deficiencies due to decreased enjoyment of food. Overall, the most common causes of primary olfactory deficits are nasal and/or sinus disease, prior viral upper respiratory infections (URIs), and head trauma.

7.15.2 Organization of the Taste Receptors in the Tongue

The human tongue contains approximately 4,600 taste buds in which the secondary sensory cells for taste perception are collected (**Fig. 7.46**). The taste buds (see Chapter 7.15.3) are embedded in the epithelium of the lingual mucosa and are located on the surface expansions of the lingual mucosa—the vallate papillae (principal site, **Fig. 7.46b**), the fungiform papillae (**Fig. 7.46c**), and the foliate papillae (**Fig. 7.46d**). Additionally, isolated taste buds are located in the mucous membranes of the soft palate and pharynx. The surrounding serous glands of the tongue (Ebner's glands), which are most closely associated with the vallate papillae, constantly wash the taste buds clean to allow for new tasting. Humans can perceive five basic taste qualities: sweet, sour, salty, bitter, and a fifth "savory" quality, called umami, which is activated by glutamate (a taste enhancer). Taking its name from Japanese, umami is a pleasant savory taste imparted by glutamate, a type of amino acid and other chemical components that occur naturally in many foods including meat, fish, vegetables, and dairy products. As the taste of umami itself is subtle and blends well with other tastes to expand and round out flavors, most people don't recognize umami when they encounter it, but it plays an important role making food taste delicious. Foods rich in umami include seaweed, oysters, shrimp, mushrooms, truffles, Parmesan cheese, green tea, and soy sauce.

7.15.3 Microscopic Structure of a Taste Bud

Nerves induce the formation of taste buds in the oral mucosa (**Fig. 7.47**). Axons of cranial nerves VII, IX, and X grow into the oral mucosa from the basal side and induce the epithelium to differentiate into the light and dark taste cells (= modified epithelial cells). Both types of taste cell have microvilli that extend to the gustatory pore. For sour and salty, the taste cell is stimulated by hydrogen ions. The other taste qualities are mediated by receptor proteins to which the low-molecular-weight flavored substances bind (details may be found in textbooks of physiology). When the low-molecular-weight flavored substances bind to the receptor proteins, they induce signal transduction that causes the release of glutamate, which excites the peripheral processes of the pseudounipolar neurons of the three cranial nerve ganglia. The taste cells have a life span of approximately 12 days and regenerate from cells at the base of the taste buds, which differentiate into new taste cells.

Note: The old notion that particular areas of the tongue are sensitive to specific taste qualities has been found to be oversimplified and for the most part false.

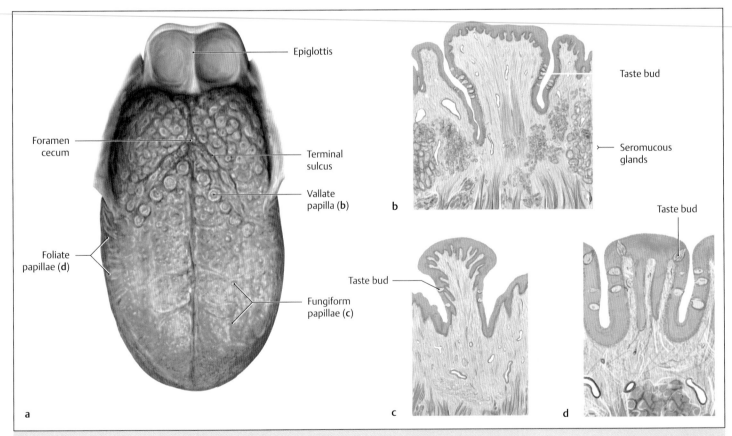

Fig. 7.46 (a) The human tongue. (b) Vallate papillae (principal site. (c) Fungiform papillae. (d) Foliate papillae.

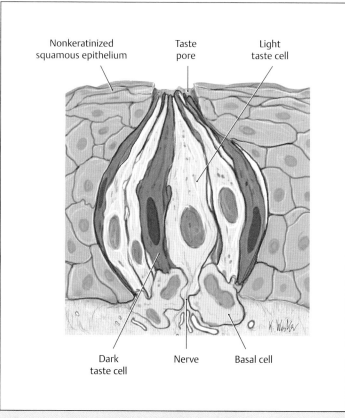

Fig. 7.47 Microscopic structure of a taste bud.

7.16 Olfactory System (Smell)

7.16.1 Olfactory System: the Olfactory Mucosa and Its Central Connections

Olfactory tract viewed in midsagittal section (**Fig. 7.48a**) and from below (**Fig. 7.48b**). The olfactory mucosa is located in the roof of the nasal cavity. The olfactory cells (= primary sensory cells) are bipolar neurons. Their peripheral receptor–bearing processes terminate in the epithelium of the nasal mucosa, while their central processes pass to the olfactory bulb (see Chapter 7.16.2 for details). The olfactory bulb, where the second neurons of the olfactory pathway (mitral and tufted cells) are located, is considered an extension of the telencephalon. The axons of these second neurons pass centrally as the *olfactory tract*. In front of the anterior perforated substance, the olfactory tract widens to form the olfactory trigone and splits into the lateral and medial olfactory striae.

- Some **of the axons** of the olfactory tract run in the **lateral olfactory stria** to the olfactory centers: the amygdala, semilunar gyrus, and ambient gyrus. The prepiriform area (Brodmann's area 28) is considered to be the primary olfactory cortex in the strict sense. It contains the third neurons of the olfactory pathway.

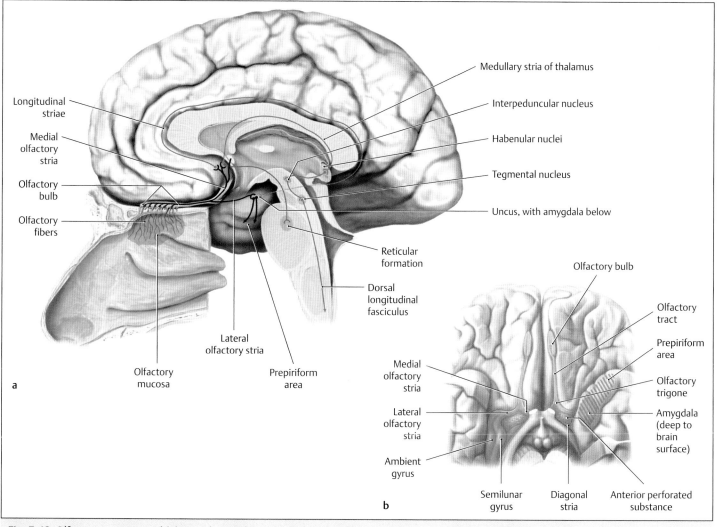

Fig. 7.48 Olfactory tract viewed (a) in midsagittal section and (b) from below.

Note: The prepiriform area is shaded in **Fig. 7.48b**, lying at the junction of the basal side of the frontal lobe and the medial side of the temporal lobe.

- **Other axons** of the olfactory tract run in the **medial olfactory stria** to nuclei in the septal (subcallosal) area, which is part of the limbic system, and to the olfactory tubercle, a small elevation in the anterior perforated substance.
- **Yet other axons** of the olfactory tract terminate in the **anterior olfactory nucleus**, where the fibers that cross to the opposite side branch off and are relayed. This nucleus is located in the olfactory trigone, which lies between the two olfactory striae and in front of the anterior perforated substance.

Note: None of these three tracts are routed through the thalamus. Thus, *the olfactory system is the only sensory system that is not relayed in the thalamus* before reaching the cortex. There is, however, an indirect route from the primary olfactory cortex to the neocortex passing through the thalamus and terminating in the basal forebrain.

The olfactory signals are further analyzed in these basal portions of the forebrain (not shown).

The olfactory system is linked to other brain areas well beyond the primary olfactory cortical areas, with the result that olfactory stimuli can evoke complex emotional and behavioral responses. Smell is also associated with the memory. The smell of a madeleine (small cake or cookie) dipped in tea triggered a flood of memories in Proust's *Remembrance of Things Past*. The relationship between smell and memory is sometimes referred to as a "Proustian moment." Noxious smells may induce nausea, while appetizing smells evoke watering of the mouth. Presumably these sensations are processed by the hypothalamus, thalamus, and limbic system (see next unit) via connections established mainly by the medial forebrain bundle and the medullary striae of the thalamus. The medial forebrain bundle distributes axons to the following structures:

- Hypothalamic nuclei.
- Reticular formation.
- Salivatory nuclei.
- Dorsal vagal nucleus.

The axons that run in the medullary striae of the thalamus terminate in the habenular nuclei. This tract also continues to the brainstem, where it stimulates salivation in response to smell.

7.16.2 Olfactory Mucosa and Vomeronasal Organ

The **olfactory mucosa** occupies an area of approximately 2 cm² on the roof of each nasal cavity, and 10^7 primary sensory cells are concentrated in each of these areas (**Fig. 7.49a**). At the molecular level, the olfactory receptor proteins are located in the cilia of the sensory cells (**Fig. 7.49b**). Each sensory cell has only one specialized receptor protein that mediates signal transduction when an odorant molecule binds to it. Although humans are microsmatic, having a sense of smell that is feeble compared with other mammals, the olfactory receptor proteins still make up 2% of the human genome. This underscores the importance of olfaction in humans. The primary olfactory sensory cells have a life span of approximately 60 days and regenerate from the basal cells (lifelong division of

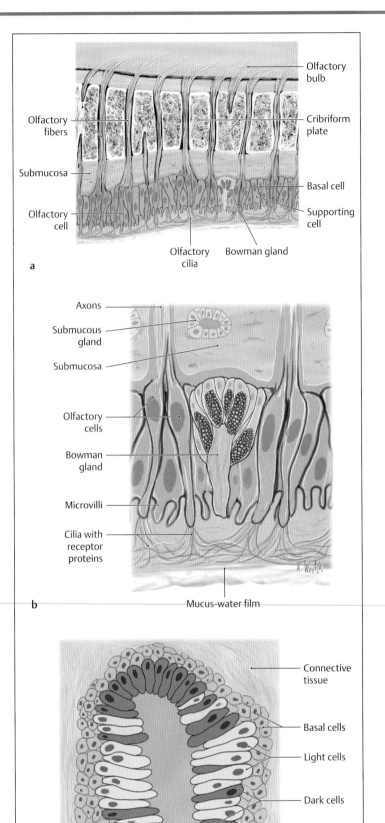

Fig. 7.49 (a) Olfactory fibers. (b) Cilia of the sensory cells. (c) The vomeronasal organ.

neurons). The bundled central processes (axons) from hundreds of olfactory cells form olfactory fibers (**Fig. 7.49a**) that pass through the *cribriform plate* of the ethmoid bone and terminate in the *olfactory bulb* (see Chapter 7.16.3), which lies above the cribriform plate. The vomeronasal organ (**Fig. 7.49c**) is located on both sides of the anterior nasal septum. Its central connections in humans are unknown. It responds to steroids and evokes unconscious reactions in subjects (possibly influences the choice of a mate). Mate selection in many animal species is known to be mediated by olfactory impulses that are perceived in the vomeronasal organ (VNO).

7.16.3 Synaptic Patterns in an Olfactory Bulb

Specialized neurons in the olfactory bulb, called mitral cells, form apical dendrites that receive synaptic contact from the axons of thousands of primary sensory cells (**Fig. 7.50**). The dendrite plus

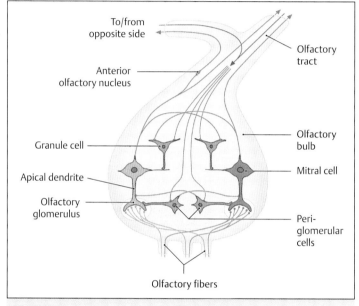

Fig. 7.50 Synaptic patterns in an olfactory bulb.

the synapses make up the *olfactory glomeruli*. Axons from sensory cells with the same receptor protein form glomeruli with only one or a small number of mitral cells. The basal axons of the mitral cells form the olfactory tract. The axons that run in the olfactory tract project primarily to the olfactory cortex but are also distributed to other nuclei in the CNS. The axon collaterals of the mitral cells pass to granule cells: both granule cells and periglomerular cells inhibit the activity of the mitral cells, causing less sensory information to reach higher centers. These inhibitory processes are believed to heighten olfactory contrast, which aids in the more accurate perception of smells. The tufted cells, which also project to the primary olfactory cortex, are not shown.

Clinical note: In 2009, the U.S. Food and Drug Administration warned consumers to stop using several popular cold remedies because they could result in the loss of smell. Smoking also can interfere with our sense of smell. Problems with our chemical senses (taste and smell) may be a sign of other serious health conditions. A smell disorder can be an early sign of Parkinson's disease, Alzheimer's disease, or multiple sclerosis. It can also accompany or be a sign of diabetes, hypertension, and malnutrition. We cannot smell like our dog, but our smell structure can be an early warning system.

7.17 Limbic System

7.17.1 Limbic System Viewed through the Partially Transparent Cortex

Medial view of the right hemisphere (**Fig. 7.51**). The term "limbic system" (Latin limbus = "border" or "fringe") was first used by Broca in 1878 (the same Paul Broca who presented the landmark papers on the relationship between speech and language and the cortical areas of the frontal lobe in 1861), who collectively

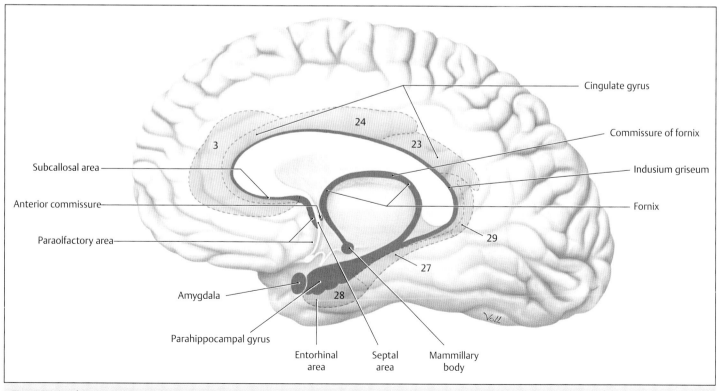

Fig. 7.51 Limbic system viewed through the partially transparent cortex.

described the gyri surrounding the corpus callosum, diencephalon, and basal ganglia as the *grand lobe limbique*. The limbic system encompasses neo-, archi-, and paleocortical regions as well as subcortical nuclei. The anatomical extent of the limbic system is such that it can exchange and integrate information between the telencephalon (cerebral cortex), diencephalon, and mesencephalon. Viewed from the medial aspect of the cerebral hemispheres, the limbic system is seen to consist of an inner arc and an outer arc. The outer arc is formed by the following regions:

- Parahippocampal gyrus.
- Cingulate gyrus (also called the limbic gyrus).
- Subcallosal area (paraolfactory area).
- Indusium griseum.

The inner arc is formed by the following regions:

- Hippocampal formation.
- Fornix.
- Septal area (also known simply as the septum).
- Diagonal band of Broca (not visible in this view).
- Paraterminal gyrus.

The limbic system also includes the amygdalae and mammillary bodies. The following nuclei are also considered part of the limbic system but are not shown: the anterior thalamic nucleus, habenular nucleus, dorsal tegmental nucleus, and interpeduncular nucleus. The limbic system is concerned with the regulation of drive and affective behavior and plays a crucial role in memory and learning. The numbers in the diagram indicate the Brodmann areas.

7.17.2 Neuronal Circuit (Papez's Circuit)

Several nuclei of the limbic system are interconnected by a *neuronal circuit* called the Papez circuit after the anatomist who first described it. James Papez was an American neuroanatomist educated at the University of Minnesota, where the snow flies free and often. The sequence below indicates the nuclei (normal print) and tracts *(italic print)* that are the successive stations of this neuronal circuit:

Hippocampus → *fornix* → mammillary body → *mammillothalamic tract* (Vicq d'Azyr bundle) → anterior thalamic nuclei → *thalamocingular tract (radiation)* → cingulate gyrus → *cingulohippocampal fibers* → hippocampus.

This neuronal circuit interconnects ontogenically distinct parts of the limbic system. It establishes a connection between information stored in the unconscious and conscious behavior (**Fig. 7.52**).

7.17.3 Cytoarchitecture of the Hippocampal Formation (after Bähr and Frotscher)

View from anterior left (**Fig. 7.53**).

Note: The hippocampal formation has a three-layered allocortex instead of a six-layered isocortex (lower left in diagram). It is a phylogenetically older structure than the isocortex. At the center of the allocortex is a band of neurons that forms the neuronal layer of the hippocampus (= hippocampus proper = Ammon's horn). The neurons in this layer are mainly pyramidal cells. Three regions, designated CA1 to CA3, can be distinguished based

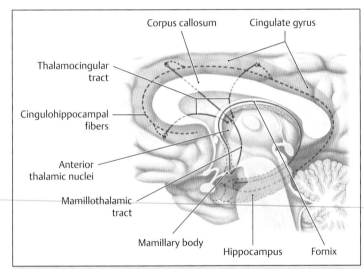

Fig. 7.52 Neuronal circuit (view of the medial surface of the right hemisphere).

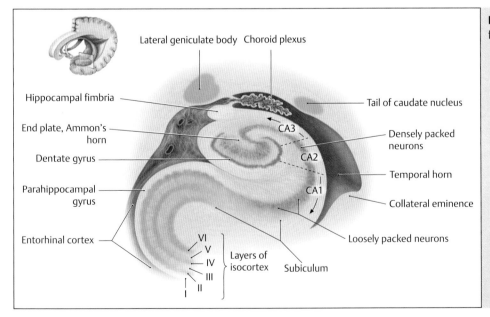

Fig. 7.53 Cytoarchitecture of the hippocampal formation (view from anterior left)

on differences in the density of the pyramidal cells. *Region CA1*, called also the "Sommer sector," is important in neuropathology, as the death of neurons in this sector is the first morphologically detectable sign of cerebral hypoxia. Besides the hippocampus proper, we can also identify the cellular sheet of the dentate gyrus (dentate fascia), which consists mainly of granule cells.

7.17.4 Connections of the Hippocampus

Left anterior view (**Fig. 7.54**). The most important afferent pathway to the hippocampus is the *perforant path* (blue), which extends from the entorhinal region (triangular pyramidal cells of Brodmann area 28) to the hippocampus (where it ends in a synapse). The neurons that project from area 28 into the hippocampus receive afferent input from many brain regions. ***Thus, the entorhinal region is considered the gateway to the hippocampus and helps explain the aforementioned relationship between smell and memory, since the hippocampus is so involved in the consolidation and storage of memory***. Bilateral hippocampal injury results in serious anterograde amnesia. The pyramidal cells of Ammon's horn (triangles) send their axons into the fornix, and the axons transmitted via the fornix continue to the mammillary body (Papez's neuronal circuit) or to the septal nuclei.

Clinical note: The limbic system operates by influencing the endocrine system and the autonomic nervous system. Abnormal activity in the limbic system is also associated with decreased motivation and drive, sleep and appetite problems, and mood disorders.

7.17.5 Important Definitions Pertaining to the Limbic System

Archicortex

Phylogenetically old structures of the cerebral cortex; does not have a six-layered architecture.

Hippocampus (retrocommissural)

Ammon's horn (hippocampus proper), dentate gyrus (dentate fascia), subiculum (some authors consider it part of the hippocampal formation rather than the hippocampus itself).

Hippocampal formation

Hippocampus plus the entorhinal area of the parahippocampal gyrus.

Limbic system

Important coordinating system for memory and emotions. Includes the following telencephalic structures: cingulate gyrus, parahippocampal gyrus, hippocampal formation, septal nuclei, and amygdala. Its diencephalic components include the anterior thalamic nucleus, mammillary bodies, nucleus accumbens, and habenular nucleus. Its brainstem components are the raphe nuclei. The medial forebrain bundle and the dorsal longitudinal fasciculus contribute to the fiber tracts of the limbic system.

Periarchicortex

A broad transitional zone around the hippocampus, consisting of the cingulate gyrus, the isthmus of the cingulate gyrus, and the parahippocampal gyrus.

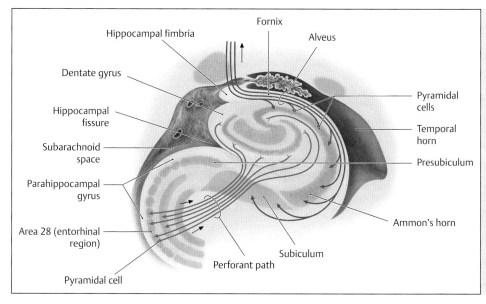

Fig. 7.54 Connections of the hippocampus (left anterior view)

7.18 Sagittal MRIs of the Head

Left lateral view (**Fig. 7.55**). These sections demonstrate the relationship of the nasopharynx to the oropharynx. The optic nerve (CN II) is visible as the optic chiasm in **Fig. 7.55a**. The pituitary gland (hypophysis) can be seen inferior to it, just posterior to the sphenoid sinus. The syphon of the internal carotid artery is beautifully displayed in **Fig. 7.55b**.

Left lateral view (**Fig. 7.56**). This view exposes the superior and inferior rectus muscles within the periorbital fat. The course of the optic nerve (CN II) within the orbit can be seen.

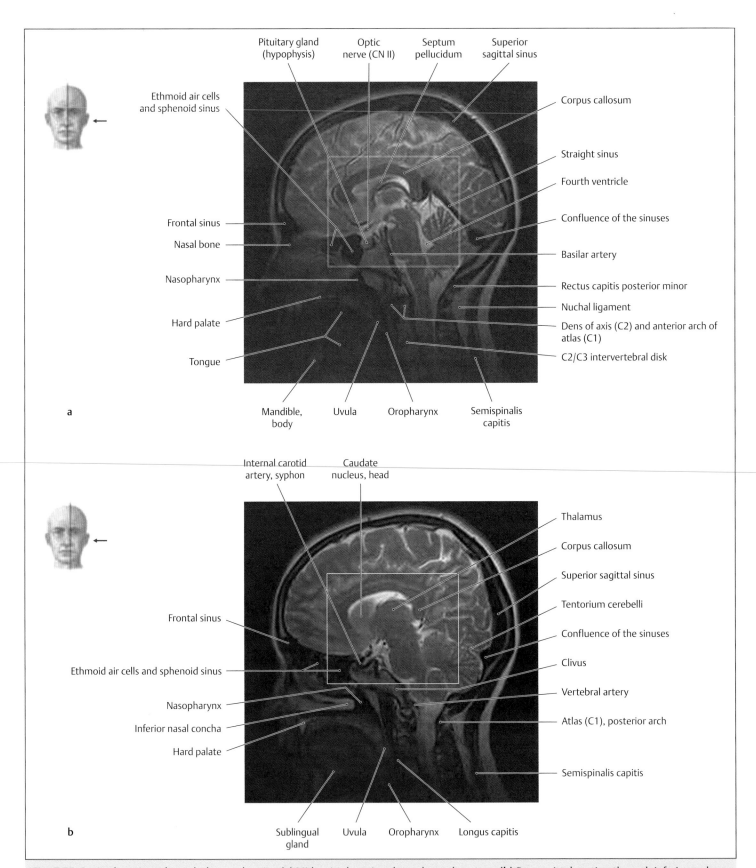

Fig. 7.55 Sagittal sections through the nasal cavity. **(a)** Midsagittal section through nasal septum. **(b)** Parasagittal section through inferior and middle nasal conchae. (Reproduced from Baker, Anatomy for Dental Medicine, 2nd edition, ©2015, Thieme publishers, New York. Illustration by Karl Wesker/Markus Voll.)

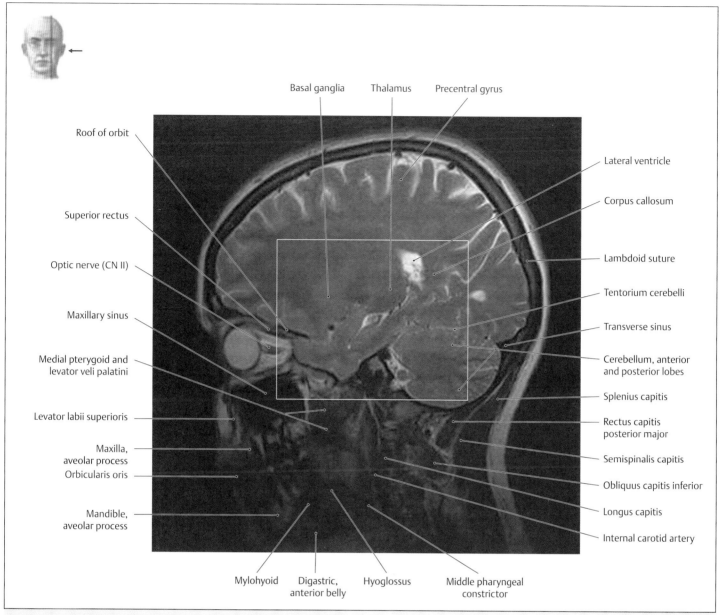

Fig. 7.56 Parasagittal section through the orbit. (Reproduced from Baker, Anatomy for Dental Medicine, 2nd edition, ©2015, Thieme publishers, New York. Illustration by Karl Wesker/Markus Voll.)

Note the proximity of the maxillary teeth to the maxillary sinus. Roots of the maxillary teeth may erupt into the maxillary sinus.

7.19 Principles of the Neurological Examination

In order to conduct a neurological examination and interpret its findings, the examiner has to be knowledgeable about basic neuroanatomy. This learning unit describes selected aspects of the neuroanatomical examination and explains why a neuroanatomical background is essential and indispensable for detecting and analyzing signs and symptoms. The neurological examination as described below is a part of the general examination of a person.

7.19.1 Testing Sensation

Sensation is the perception of different stimuli on the skin, mucosae, muscles, joints and internal organs (**Fig. 7.57**). When assessing sensation, different qualities of sensory are being tested. Different receptors are responsible for different stimuli, which are transmitted to the brain via different pathways. The receptors and their pathways will be discussed in greater detail later on. For now, knowledge about the different sensory qualities and how to test them is sufficient. During all tests described here, the patient should keep the eyes closed in order to prevent a correction of the results by being able to see them. In addition, all tests should be conducted on both sides to detect damage affecting only one side of the body.

Note: All tests described here require the cooperation of the patient. They can only be conducted on a patient who is alert.

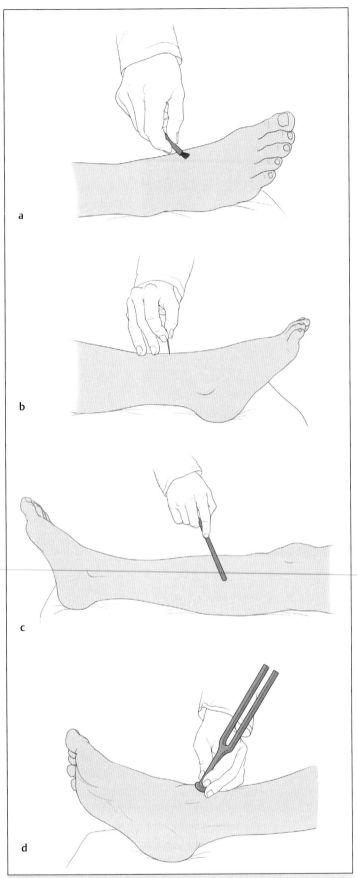

Fig. 7.57 (a) Touch sensation. (b) Sensation of pain. (c) Temperature sensation. (d) The vibratory sensation.

- **Touch sensation** is assessed using a paintbrush, a cotton ball, or the fingertips. The examiner strokes the skin and the patient has to say whether they can feel the touch. A reduced sensation

is referred to as hypoesthesia; a total loss of sensation is referred to as anesthesia.

- **Sensation of pain** is assessed using the pointed tip of an injection needle. A reduced sensation is referred to as hypoalgesia, a total loss of sensation is referred to as analgesia.
- **Temperature sensation** is assessed using a warm or cold metallic object or a test tube filled with either cold or warm water. It is important that the water is not so hot that it generates temperature and in addition, pain sensation. Impaired temperature sensation is referred to as thermohypesthesia; a total loss of sensation is referred to as thermoanesthesia.
- The **vibratory sensation** is assessed using a tuning fork (64 or 128 Hz). A vibrating tuning fork is placed near the patient's ankle or held above the tibia. The patient is asked if they feel a vibration in their bones. A reduced sensation is referred to as pallhypesthesia; a total loss of sensation is referred to as pallesthesia.
- Another sensory quality not described here is the **sense of position** (proprioception). As indicated earlier, it provides information about the spatial position of the limbs. The examiner moves one limb and asks the patient about the its position (e.g., bent or extended). The decisive stimulus is the elongation (tension) of muscles and articular capsules. The stimulus does not come from the body's surface but from deep within (deep sensation). The sensory qualities listed here are found all over the body. In classical neuroanatomy, they are referred to as "sensitivity." The senses perceived by specific sensory organs (the five "classical" senses: olfactory, visual, gustatory, auditory, and vestibular) were initially referred to as "sensation." However, since perception and transmission of impulses are in principle the same for sensibility and sensation, they are both referred to now as sensation.

7.19.2 Testing Motor Function

The efferent systems, which generate movements of the skeletal muscles, are referred to as "motor systems" or "motor function." They are assessed by examining the reflexes. One example listed here is the patellar tendon reflex (**Fig. 7.58a**). When tapping the patellar tendon with a reflex hammer, the quadriceps muscle shortens to such an extent that it causes the knee to extend. If that happens, the reflex arc is intact (**Fig. 7.58b**). By tapping the tendon, the muscle is pulled and elongates. This muscle elongation is perceived by muscle receptors and relayed to the spinal cord. The cell body of the stimulated afferent neuron lies in the spinal ganglion. Its axon releases a transmitter at the α-motoneuron in the spinal cord. This transmitter stimulates the α-motoneuron, which itself releases transmitters at the motor end plate. This transmitter stimulates the muscle which will then contract and the knee extends. The leg kicks forward.

Note: For the α-motoneuron to be stimulated, sensory input pathways must be intact. With regard to reflexes, sensation and motor function are closely related, which is why in physiology the term sensorimotor function is often used. Intact sensation is a precondition for intact motor function, and has been described in a previous chapter in this book.

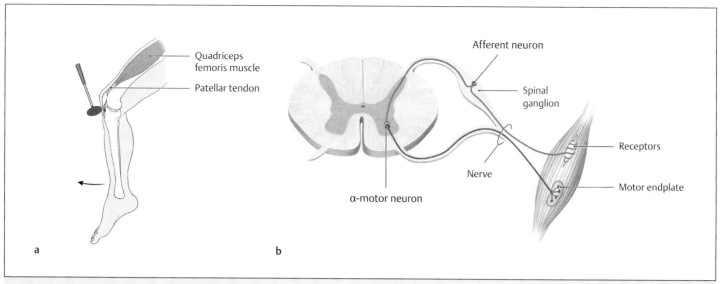

Fig. 7.58 Testing motor function. **(a)** Patellar tendon reflex. **(b)** Reflex arc is intact.

7.19.3 Coordination Assessment

In addition to tests for assessing sensation and reflexes, the neurological examination also includes the assessment of more complex pathways of information processing. One example is Unterberger's stepping test (**Fig. 7.59**). With eyes closed and arms extended forward, the patient is asked to walk on the spot. Performing this task requires the coordination of several sensory systems. It is especially challenging to provide information about the position of the head for which the inner ear is responsible. A malfunctioning of the vestibular parts of the inner ear (the semicircular canals) leads to increased spinning of the affected side. In the example shown here, a turn to the right (illustrated by the arrow) is caused by right inner ear malfunction.

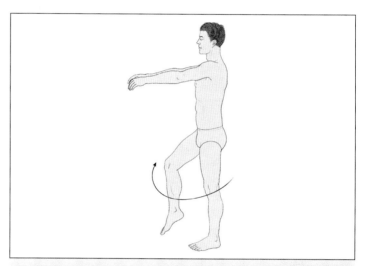

Fig. 7.59 Unterberger's stepping test.

7.19.4 Problems in Neurological–Topical Diagnostics

The figure (**Fig. 7.60**) illustrates a pain pathway extending from the body surface to the sensory cortex. If the pathway is disrupted, the pain information does not reach the sensory cortex. Location of the disruption can be in either the receptive field (1), in the peripheral nerve (2), in the spinal cord (3), or the brain itself (4). Disruption in any of these locations prevents the sensory cortex from perceiving the pain. This explains why the brain always localizes disruption in the receptive field (1) even though the disruption can be located in the spinal cord (3). The physician is confronted with the problem of "tricking" the brain and to identify the location of the disruption, since the therapy differs depending on where the pathway has been damaged. The process of identifying the damaged location is referred to as neurological–topical diagnostics. This is why intimate knowledge of important pathways is essential when examining a patient.

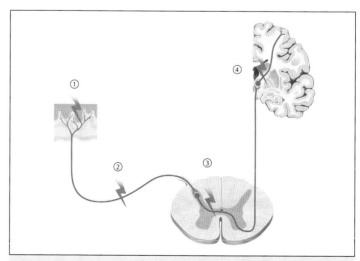

Fig. 7.60 Pain pathway extending from the body surface to the sensory cortex.

7.20 Brain: Clinical Findings

The figures in this unit illustrate the correlations that have been discovered between specific brain areas and clinical findings. Studies of this kind have enabled us to link particular patterns of behavior, some abnormal, and particular clinical signs and symptoms to specific areas in the brain.

7.20.1 Neuroanatomy of Emotions

Emotion is linked to specific regions of the brain (**Fig. 7.61**). The ventromedial prefrontal cortex is connected primarily to the amygdaloid bodies and is believed to modulate emotion, while the dorsolateral prefrontal cortex is connected primarily to the hippocampus. This is the area of the cortex in which memories are stored along with their emotional valence. Abnormalities of this network are believed to play a role in depression.

7.20.2 Spread of Alzheimer's Disease through the Brain

Medial view of the right hemisphere (**Fig. 7.62**). Alzheimer's disease is a relentlessly progressive disease of the cerebral cortex that causes memory loss and, eventually, profound dementia. The progression of the disease can be demonstrated with special staining methods and can be divided into the following stages:

- Stages I–II: The appearance of the nerve cells is altered in the periphery of the entorhinal cortex (= transentorhinal region), which is considered part of the allocortex. These stages are still asymptomatic.
- Stages III–IV: The lesions have spread to involve the limbic system (also part of the allocortex), and initial clinical symptoms appear. These stages may be detectable by imaging studies in some cases.
- Stages V–VI: The entire isocortex is involved, and the clinical manifestations are fully developed.

Thus, the allocortex is important in brain pathophysiology as the site of origin of Alzheimer's dementia, even though it makes up only 5% of the cerebral cortex.

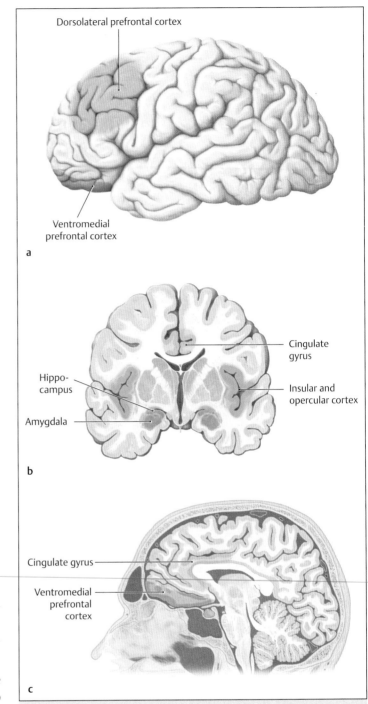

Fig. 7.61 Neuroanatomy of emotions. **(a)** Lateral view of the left hemisphere. **(b)** Anterior view of a coronal section through the amygdala. **(c)** Midsagittal section of the right hemisphere, medial aspect.

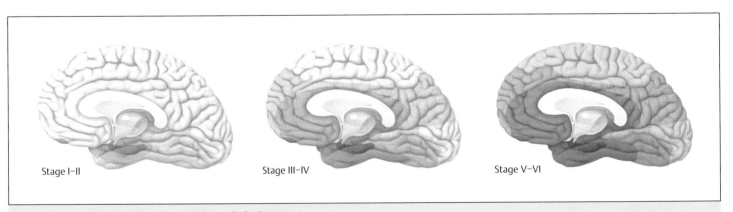

Fig. 7.62 Spread of Alzheimer disease through the brain.

7.20.3 MRI Changes in the Hippocampus in a Patient with Alzheimer's Dementia

Comparing the brain of a healthy subject (**Fig. 7.63a**) with that of a patient with Alzheimer's dementia (**Fig. 7.63b**), we notice that the latter shows atrophy of the hippocampus, a brain region that is part of the allocortex, and very related to memory functions. We notice, too, that the lateral ventricles are enlarged in the patient with Alzheimer's dementia.

7.20.4 Lesions of Certain Brain Areas and Associated Behavioral Changes

Bilateral lesions of the medial temporal lobe and the frontal part of the cingulate gyrus (blue dots) lead to a suppression of drive and affect (**Fig. 7.64**). This structural abnormality in the limbic system produces clinical changes that include apathy, a blank facial expression, monotone speech, and a dull, nonspontaneous mode of behavior. The condition may be caused by tumors, decreased blood flow, or trauma. On the other hand, tumors involving the

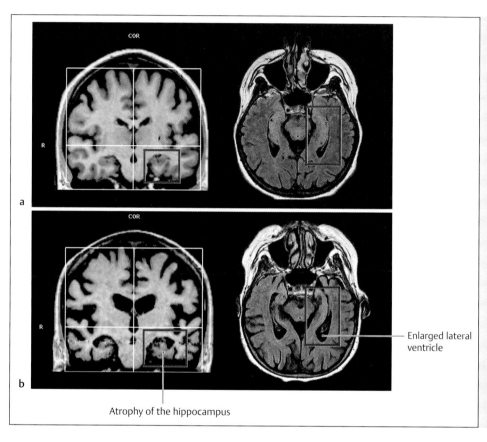

a

b

Atrophy of the hippocampus

Enlarged lateral ventricle

Fig. 7.63 Brain of (**a**) Healthy patient. (**b**) Patient with Alzheimer dementia.

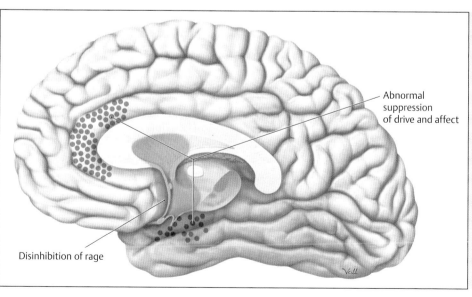

Abnormal suppression of drive and affect

Disinhibition of rage

Fig. 7.64 Lesions of brain areas (medial view of the right hemisphere).

septum pellucidum and hypothalamus (pink-shaded area) and certain forms of epilepsy may cause a disinhibition of anger, and the patient may respond to seemingly trivial events with attacks of "hypothalamic rage" accompanied by screaming and biting. This outburst is not directed against any particular person or object and persists for some time.

7.21 Lesions of the Spinal Cord and Peripheral Nerves: Sensory Deficits

Overview of the next three units (after Bähr and Frotscher).

Two questions should be addressed in the diagnostic evaluation of spinal cord lesions:

1. What structure(s) within the *cross-section* of the spinal cord is (are) affected? This is determined systematically by proceeding from the periphery of the cord toward the center.
2. At what level of the spinal cord (in longitudinal section) is the lesion located?

In these units, we will first correlate various deficit patterns (syndromes) with the structures in the cross-section of the spinal cord. We will then discuss the level of the lesion in the longitudinal or craniocaudal dimension. Since these syndromes present with deficits that result from damage to specific anatomical structures, they can be explained in anatomical terms. Based on the lesions and syndromes described here, the reader can test his or her ability to relate what has already been learned to the locations and effects of spinal cord lesions.

7.21.1 Spinal Ganglion Syndrome Illustrated for an Isolated Lesion of T6

As part of the dorsal roots, the dorsal root (spinal) ganglia are concerned with the transmission of sensory information. (Recall that the ganglia contain the cell bodies of the first sensory neurons.) When only a single spinal ganglion is affected (e.g., by a viral

infection such as herpes zoster), the resulting pain and paresthesia are limited to the sensory distribution (dermatome) of the ganglion. Because the dermatomes show considerable overlap, adjacent dermatomes can assume the function of the affected dermatome. As a result, the area that shows absolute sensory loss, called the "autonomous area" of the dermatome, may be quite small (**Fig. 7.65**).

7.21.2 Dorsal Root Syndrome Illustrated for a Lesion at the C4–T6 Level

When a lesion (trauma, degenerative spinal changes, tumor) affects multiple successive dorsal roots as in this example, complete sensory loss occurs in the affected dermatomes. When this sensory loss affects the afferent limb of a reflex, that reflex will be absent or diminished. If the sensory dorsal roots are irritated but not disrupted, as in the case of a herniated intervertebral disk, severe pain may sometimes be perceived in the affected dermatome. Because pain fibers do not overlap as much as other sensory fibers, the examiner should have no difficulty in identifying the affected dermatome, and thus the corresponding spinal cord segment, from the location of the pain (**Fig. 7.66**).

7.21.3 Posterior Horn Syndrome Illustrated for a Lesion at the C5–C8 Level

This lesion, like a dorsal root lesion of the spinal nerves, is characterized by a segmental pattern of sensory disturbance. However, with a posterior *horn* lesion of the spinal cord, unlike a dorsal root lesion, the resulting sensory deficit is incomplete. Pain and temperature sensation are abolished in the dermatomes on the ipsilateral side because the first peripheral/afferent neuron of the lateral spinothalamic tract arrives to the posterior horn, which is within the damaged area. Position sense and vibration sense

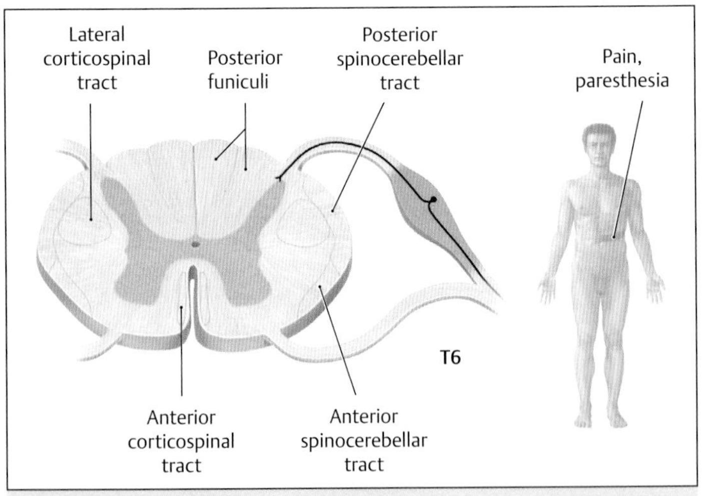

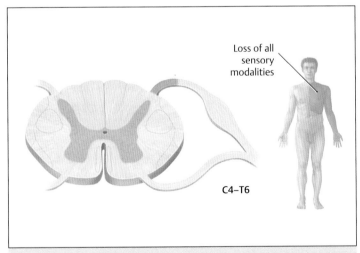

Fig. 7.65 Spinal ganglion syndrome illustrated for an isolated lesion of T6.

Fig. 7.66 Dorsal root syndrome illustrated for a lesion at the C4–T6 level.

are unaffected because the fibers for these sensory modalities are both conveyed in the posterior funiculus. Bypassing the posterior horn, these fibers pass directly via the posterior funiculi and ascend to the nucleus gracilis or nucleus cuneatus where they synapse. A lesion of the anterior spinothalamic tract does not produce striking clinical signs. The deficit (loss of pain and temperature sensation with preservation of position and vibration sense) is called a *dissociated sensory loss*. Pain and temperature sensation are preserved below the lesion because the tracts in the white matter (lateral spinothalamic tract) are undamaged. This type of dissociated sensory loss occurs in syringomyelia, a congenital or acquired condition in which there is an expanded cavity in or near the central canal of the spinal cord. (According to the strictest terminology, expansion of the central canal itself = hydromyelia) (**Fig. 7.67**).

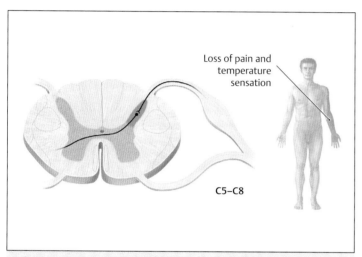

Fig. 7.67 Posterior horn syndrome illustrated for a lesion at the C5–C8 level.

7.21.4 Lesion of the Posterior Funiculi at the T8 Level

A lesion of the posterior funiculi is characterized by a loss of the following:

- Position sense.
- Vibration sense.
- Two-point discrimination.

These deficits occur distal to the lesion; hence, they involve the legs and lower trunk when the lesion is at the T8 level. When the legs are affected, as in the present example, the loss of position sense (mediated by proprioception) leads to an unsteady gait (ataxia). When the arm is affected (not shown here), the only clinical finding is sensory impairment. The lack of feedback to the motor system also prevents the precise interaction of different muscle groups during fine movements (asynergy). Ataxia results from the fact that information on body position is essential for carrying out movements. Vision can (partly) compensate for this loss of information when the eyes are open, and so the ataxia worsens when the eyes are closed (Romberg's sign). This *sensory ataxia* differs from *cerebellar ataxia* in that the latter cannot be compensated by visual control (**Fig. 7.68**).

7.21.5 Gray Matter Syndrome Illustrated for a Lesion at the C4–T4 Level

This syndrome results from a pathological process (e.g., a tumor) in and around the central canal. All tracts that cross through the gray matter are damaged, that is, the anterior and lateral spinothalamic tracts. The result is a dissociated sensory loss (loss

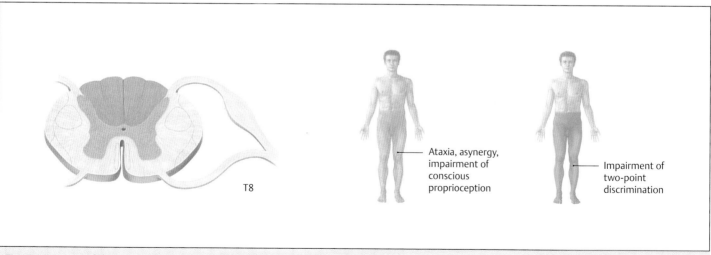

Fig. 7.68 Lesion of the posterior funiculi at the T8 level.

of pain and temperature sensation with preservation of position, vibration, and touch), in this case involving the arms and upper chest (compare with Chapter 7.21.3). A relatively large lesion may additionally affect the anterior horns, which contain the alpha motor neuron, causing a flaccid paralysis in the distal portions of the upper limb. An even larger lesion may concomitantly affect the pyramidal tract, causing spastic paralysis of the distal muscles (here in the legs). This syndrome may result from syringomyelia (see Chapter 7.21.3) or tumors located near the central canal (**Fig. 7.69**).

7.21.6 Combined Disease of the Posterior Funiculi and Pyramidal Tract Illustrated for a Lesion at the T6 Level

A *lesion of the posterior funiculi* leads to loss of position and vibration sense. A concomitant *pyramidal tract lesion* additionally leads to spastic paralysis of the legs and abdominal muscles below the affected dermatome (i.e., below T6 in the example). This predominantly cervicothoracic lesion typically occurs in funicular myelosis (vitamin B₁₂ deficiency), in which the posterior funiculi are affected initially, followed by the pyramidal tract. This disease is characterized by degeneration of the myelin sheaths (**Fig. 7.70**).

7.22 Lesions of the Spinal Cord and Peripheral Nerves: Motor Deficits

7.22.1 Anterior Horn Syndrome Illustrated for a Lesion at the C7–C8 Level

Damage to the motor anterior horn cells leads to ipsilateral paralysis, in this case involving the hands and forearm muscles because the lesion is at C7–C8 and these segments innervate the muscles in this region. The paralysis is flaccid because the alpha motor neuron that supplies the muscles (lower motor neuron) has ceased to function. Because larger muscles are supplied by motor neurons from more than one segment, damage to a single segment may lead only to muscular weakness (paresis) rather than complete paralysis of the affected muscle group. When the lateral horns are additionally involved, decreased sweating and vasomotor function will also be noted because the lateral horns contain the cell bodies of the sympathetic neurons that subserve these functions. This type of lesion may occur in poliomyelitis or in spinal muscular atrophy, for example. These relatively rare diseases are relentlessly progressive (**Fig. 7.71**).

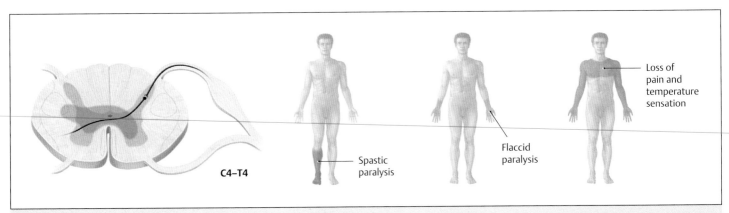

Fig. 7.69 Gray matter syndrome illustrated for a lesion at the C4–T4 level.

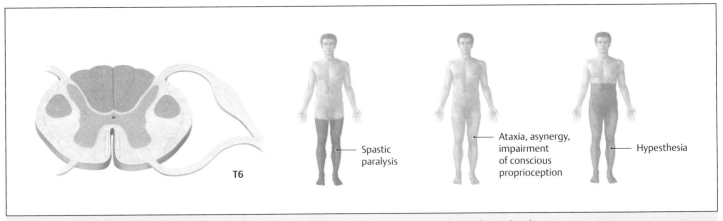

Fig. 7.70 Combined disease of the posterior funiculi and pyramidal tract illustrated for a lesion at the T6 level.

7.22.2 Combined Lesions of the Anterior Horn and Lateral Corticospinal Tract

These lesions produce a combination of flaccid and spastic paralysis. Damage to the motor anterior horns or lower motor neuron causes flaccid paralysis, while a lesion of the lateral corticospinal tract or upper motor neuron causes spastic paralysis. The degree of injury to both types of neuron may be highly variable. In the example shown, an anterior horn lesion at the C7–C8 level has caused flaccid paralysis of the forearm and hand. By contrast, a lesion of the lateral corticospinal tract at the T5 level would cause spastic paralysis of the abdominal and leg muscles (**Fig. 7.72**).

Note: When the second motor neuron in the anterior horn is already damaged (flaccid paralysis), an additional lesion of the lateral corticospinal tract at the level of the same segment will not produce any noticeable effects. This lesion pattern occurs in amyotrophic lateral sclerosis (ALS), in which the first cortical motor neuron (pyramidal tract lesion) and second spinal motor neuron (anterior horn lesion) both undergo progressive degeneration (etiology unclear). The end stage is marked by additional involvement of the motor cranial nerve nuclei, with swallowing and speaking difficulties (bulbar paralysis). The speech–language pathologist may be involved with ALS by assisting in communication of end-of-life wishes.

7.22.3 Corticospinal Tract Syndrome

Progressive spastic spinal paralysis (Erb–Charcot disease) is characterized by a progressive degeneration of the cortical neurons in the motor cortex with increasing failure of the corticospinal pathways (axonal degeneration of the first motor neuron). The course of the disease is marked by a progressive spastic paralysis of the limbs that begins in the legs and eventually reaches the arms (**Fig. 7.73**).

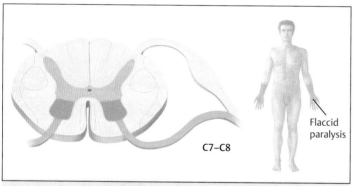

Fig. 7.71 Anterior horn syndrome illustrated for a lesion at the C7–C8 level.

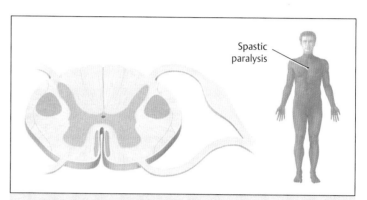

Fig. 7.73 Corticospinal tract syndrome.

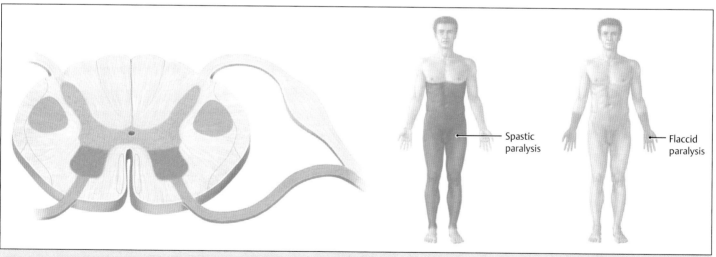

Fig. 7.72 Combined lesions of the anterior horn and lateral corticospinal tract.

7.22.4 Combined Lesions of the Posterior Funiculus, Spinocerebellar Tracts, and Pyramidal Tract

This syndrome begins with destruction of the neurons in the dorsal root (spinal) ganglia, which transmit information on conscious position sense (loss: ataxia, asynergy), vibration sense, and two-point discrimination. This neuronal destruction leads to atrophy of the posterior funiculi. There is little or no impairment of pain and temperature sensation, which are still transmitted to higher centers in the unaffected lateral spinothalamic tract. The loss of conscious proprioception alone is sufficient to cause sensory ataxia (lack of feedback to the motor system. However, the lesions additionally affect the spinocerebellar tracts (unconscious proprioception), injury to which suffices to cause ataxia, and so this dual injury causes a particularly severe loss of conscious and unconscious proprioception. This is the main clinical feature of the disease. Spastic paralysis also develops as a result of pyramidal tract dysfunction. The prototype of this disease is hereditary Friedreich's ataxia, which has several variants. The gene has been localized on chromosome 19 (**Fig. 7.74**).

7.22.5 Spinal Hemisection Syndrome (Brown–Séquard Syndrome) Illustrated for a Lesion at the T10 Level on the Left Side

Hemisection of the spinal cord, though uncommon (e.g., in stab injuries), is an excellent model for testing our understanding of the function and course of the nerve tracts in the spinal cord (**Fig. 7.75**). Spastic paralysis due to interruption of the lateral corticospinal tract occurs on the side of the lesion (and below

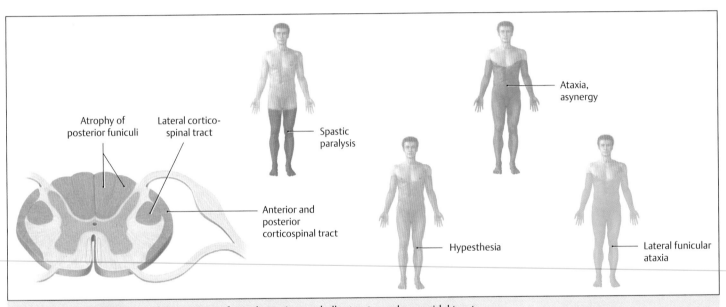

Fig. 7.74 Combined lesions of the posterior funiculus, spinocerebellar tracts, and pyramidal tract.

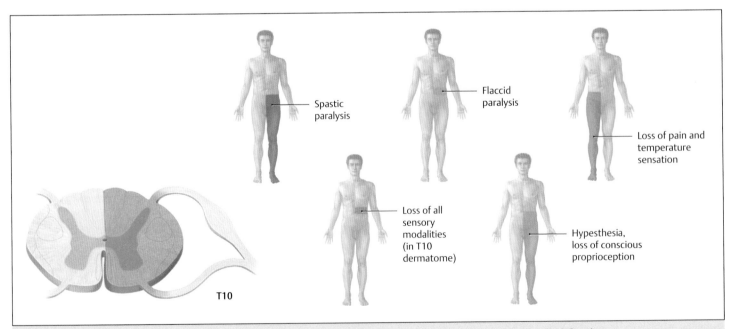

Fig. 7.75 Spinal hemisection syndrome (Brown–Séquard syndrome) illustrated for a lesion at the T10 level on the left side.

the level of the lesion). The interruption of the posterior funiculi (pathways for conscious proprioception) causes a loss of position and vibration sense and two-point discrimination on the side of the lesion. After spinal shock has subsided, spastic paralysis develops below the level of the lesion (here affecting the left leg). Of course, this paralysis does not produce an ataxia like that described following interruption of the posterior funiculi. Destruction of the alpha motor neurons in the locally damaged segment (in this case T10) leads to ipsilateral flaccid paralysis associated with this segment. Because the axons of the lateral spinothalamic tract have already crossed to the unaffected side below the lesion, pain and temperature sensation is preserved on the *ipsilateral* side below the lesion. These two types of sensation are lost on the *contralateral* side, however, because the crossed axons on the opposite side have been interrupted at the level of the lesion. If spinal root irritation occurs at the level of the lesion, radicular pain may occur because of the descending course of the sensory (and motor) roots in the segment above the lesion.

7.23 Lesions of the Spinal Cord, Assessment

7.23.1 Deficits Caused by Complete Cord Lesions at Various Levels

Having explored the manifestations of lesions at different sites in the cross-section of the spinal cord, we will now consider the effects of lesions at various levels of the cord. An example is the paralysis caused by a *complete spinal cord lesion*, which occurs acutely after a severe injury and is considerably more common than the incomplete lesions described earlier (see Chapter 7.22.5). A complete cord lesion following acute trauma is initially manifested by *spinal shock*, the pathophysiology of which is not yet fully understood. This condition is marked by complete flaccid paralysis below the site of the lesion, with a loss of all sensory modalities from the level of the lesion downward. Loss of bladder and rectal function and impotence are also present. Because the lesion also interrupts the sympathetic fibers, sweating and thermoregulation are impaired. The gray matter of the spinal cord recovers over a period ranging from a few days to 8 weeks. The spinal reflexes return, and the flaccid paralysis changes to a spastic paralysis. There is a recovery of bladder and rectal function, but only at a reflex level since voluntary control has been permanently lost. Impotence is permanent. **Lesions of the cervical cord** above C3 are swiftly fatal because they disrupt the efferent supply of the phrenic nerve (main root at C4), which innervates the diaphragm and

maintains abdominal respiration, while innervation to the intercostal muscles is also lost, causing a failure of thoracic respiration. A complete lesion of the lower cervical cord causes paralysis of all four limbs (quadriplegia), and respiration is precarious because of paralysis of the intercostal muscles. **Lesions of the upper thoracic cord** (T2 downward) spare the arms but respiration is compromised because of paralysis of the abdominal muscles. A lesion of the **lower thoracic cord** (the exact site is unimportant) has little or no effect on the abdominal muscles, and respiration is not impaired. If the sympathetic splanchnic nerves are also damaged, there may be compromise of visceral motor function ranging to paralytic ileus. With **lesions of the lumbar cord**, a distinction is drawn between epiconus syndrome (L4–S2) and conus (conus medullaris) syndrome (S3 downward). *Epiconus syndrome* is characterized by a flaccid paralysis of the legs (only the roots are affected, causing peripheral paralysis), and reflex but not conscious emptying of the bladder and rectum is preserved. Sexual potency is lost. In *conus syndrome*, the legs are not paralyzed and only the foregoing autonomic disturbances are present. The motor deficits described here are also associated with sensory deficits (see **Fig. 7.76** and **Table 7.5**).

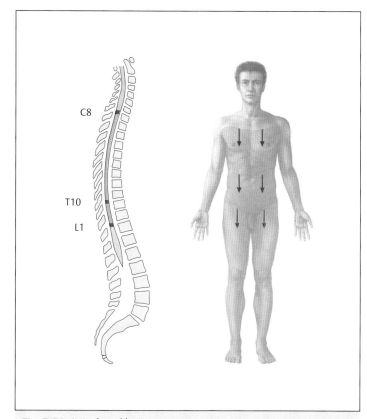

Fig. 7.76 Spinal cord lesion.

Table 7.5 Deficits associated with complete spinal cord lesions at various levels (after Rohkamm)

Level of lesion	Motor deficits	Sensory deficits	Autonomic deficits
C1–C3 (high cervical cord lesion)	• Quadriplegia • Paralysis of nuchal muscles • Spasticity • Respiratory paralysis (immediate death if not artificially ventilated)	• Sensory loss from occiput or mandibular border downward • Pain in occipital region, back of neck, and shoulder region	• Reflex visceral functions (bladder, bowel) with no voluntary control • Horner syndrome
C4–C5	• Quadriplegia • Diaphragmatic respiration only	• Sensory loss from clavicle or shoulder downward	• See above
C6–C8 (lower cervical cord lesion)	• Quadriplegia • Diaphragmatic respiration • Spasticity	• Sensory loss from upper chest wall and back downward, and on the arms (sparing the shoulders)	• See above
T1–T5	• Paraplegia • Decreased respiratory volume	• Sensory loss from inside of forearm, upper chest wall and back	• Reflex function of bladder and rectum • Erection without voluntary control
T5–T10	• Paraplegia, spasticity	• Sensory loss from affected level in chest wall and back	• See above
T11–L3	• Paraplegia	• Sensory loss from groin region or front of thigh, depending on site of lesion	• See above
L4–S2 (epiconus, spinal nerve roots paralyzed)	• Distal paraplegia	• Sensory loss from front of thigh, dorsum of foot, sole of foot, or back of thigh, depending on site of lesion	• Flaccid paralysis of bladder and rectum • Impotence
S3–S5 (conus)	• No deficit	• Sensory loss in perianal region and inside of thigh	• See above

7.23.2 Determining the Level of Spinal Cord Lesions

- **Muscles and the spinal cord segments** that innervate them (**Fig. 7.77a**). Most muscles are multisegmental, that is they receive innervation from several spinal cord segments. Thus, for example, a lesion at the C7 level will not necessarily cause complete paralysis of the latissimus dorsi, because that muscle is also innervated by C6. This is not the case with the "indicator muscles," which are supplied almost exclusively by a single segment. A lesion at the L3 level, for example, will cause almost complete paralysis of the quadriceps femoris because that muscle is innervated almost entirely by L3.
- **The degree of disability varies**, depending on the level of the complete cord lesion (**Fig. 7.77b**).

7.24 Neuropathology of Brain-Based Communication and Cognitive Disorders[2]

Sometimes that mouse-gray parliament of cells, that dream factory, creates a nightmare. When the brain goes bad, there is misery to pay. Although many diseases or conditions that affect the brain do not result in communication systems disorders, there is a vast array of disturbances of speech, voice, and language that are a direct consequence of brain damage. Thus, a communication disorder can be the consequence and is many times one of the very first signs of brain dysfunction.

Aphasia is always caused by injury to the brain, most commonly from a stroke, particularly in older individuals. Although stroke is the most common cause of brain injury resulting in aphasia, it also may occur from head trauma, brain tumors, or brain infections. Not every stroke or brain injury results in aphasia, but the condition of aphasia is never present without some sort of brain damage. This is equally true of motor speech disorders. By definition, these disruptions of speech are the result of underlying movement changes in range, direction, velocity, or coordination of movement.

Cerebrovascular accident (CVA), or stroke, is by far the leading cause of brain-based communication disorders. A stroke takes place when a blood clot blocks a blood vessel or artery, or when a cerebral artery breaks, interrupting blood flow to a portion of the brain. The stroke kills or weakens brain cells in the immediate area. The neurons, or brain cells, that are affected by a direct hit usually die within minutes to a few hours after the stroke begins. When neurons die, the abilities that they controlled are lost or impaired. This includes functions such as speech, language, movement, sensation, and memory. The specific abilities lost or affected depend on where in the brain the stroke occurs and on the size of the stroke (i.e., the extent of brain cell death). Because the left cerebral hemisphere is the area that controls language in upward of 90% of people who are right-handed (the ratio of language dominance is less, but still favors the left hemisphere in left-handed people), nearly all cases of aphasia can be traced to damage in the left cerebral cortex. This does not mean that the right cerebral hemisphere is not involved in any language or language-related activities, but certainly the mighty left controls most of language. Three areas of the left cerebral cortex are critical language zones. The area around the sylvian fissure (the perisylvian zone) is an important neighborhood for human language. In that zone of language resides the Broca area, which is important for the production

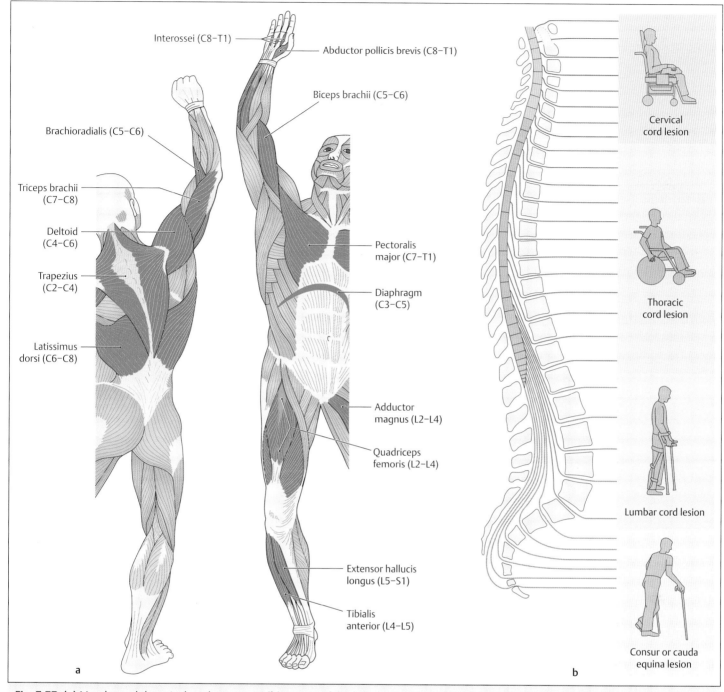

Fig. 7.77 (a) Muscles and the spinal cord segments. (b) Degree of disability varies depending on level of complete cord lesion.

of speech; the Wernicke area, which is important for the processing and comprehension of speech; and the PTO cortex (the area of juncture of the parietal, temporal, and occipital lobes of the cerebral cortex), which is important for reading and word retrieval.

These critical areas in the left cerebral hemisphere are those that are vulnerable to damage or lack of oxygen and glucose carried tirelessly by the network of plumbing known as the cerebral vascular system. These vessels of nourishment are ever-important to the health of neurons. If neurons are deprived of their life-giving nutrients for more than 4 minutes, serious damage can result. First, they weaken and do not fire or transmit neural impulses efficiently, and then after 4 minutes they die. Neurons are extremely fragile. The constant bath of blood that contains glucose, oxygen, and other nutrients perfuses the brain and, if

this perfusion is compromised, the damage begins. This is one of the principal reasons that cardiopulmonary resuscitation (CPR) must be initiated as soon as the heart stops. The heart and cardiac system is responsible for pumping the blood supply into the brain's vascular system and keeping the neurons healthy. By the process of regular chest compressions, the blood can be physically forced into the cerebral blood vessels and thus prevent the neurons from losing their vital perfusion of nutrients. In an emergency, when breathing and the pumping of the heart resumes, the CPR that was initiated may have prevented brain damage during the critical interim. Strokes come in two major types: ischemic and hemorrhagic. Ischemic is a term derived from the word ischemia, meaning a reduction or loss of blood supply. Hemorrhagic is derived from the word hemorrhage, or breaking and leaking of blood.

Hemorrhagic stroke accounts for approximately one out of five strokes and is caused by a blood vessel breaking and leaking blood into or around the brain. This type of stroke is generally more serious than an ischemic stroke, which is caused by a blocked blood vessel. The brain cells normally nourished by the hemorrhaging blood vessel, deprived of oxygen and other nutrients, can perish very quickly. The death of these cells leads to varying states of disability. In the United States, and most likely worldwide, stroke affects women slightly more than it affects men, but the distribution is relatively equal.

Ischemic stroke accounts for the vast majority of cerebrovascular accidents. Ischemic stroke occurs when an artery that carries vital nutrients in blood to the brain is blocked. The brain depends on its arteries to bring refreshing blood from the heart and lungs. The blood carries oxygen, glucose, and other nutrients to keep the brain alive and functioning, and through the system of veins takes away carbon dioxide and cellular waste. If an artery becomes blocked, the brain cells cannot generate enough energy to function properly and may eventually die. Ischemic stroke can be caused by many different kinds of diseases. The most common problem is narrowing of the arteries in the neck or head. This is most often caused by atherosclerosis, or gradual cholesterol or plaque deposits that stick to the insides of the artery. If the arteries become too narrow, blood cells may collect and begin to coagulate or form clots. These blood clots can block the artery where they are formed (thrombosis), or can break loose and become trapped to form little dams that restrict blood flow upstream in the brain (embolism). Blood clots can also form in other parts of the body (legs, heart, lungs) and travel through the maroon stream to the brain. In the heart, for example, clots can occur as a result of irregular heartbeat (atrial fibrillation), heart attack, or abnormalities of the heart valves. Although these are the most common causes of ischemic stroke, there are many other possible causes. Examples include use of recreational street drugs, knife wounds or other traumatic injuries to the blood vessels of the neck, or abnormal blood clotting. Thromboembolic strokes are responsible for more than 50 percent of all strokes.

7.24.1 Mad Cow and other Prion Diseases

Within the last few years, unconventional slow CNS infections, the prion disorders, have been described and defined. In 1997, the second Noble Prize was awarded in this field to Dr. Stanley Prusiner, who has championed the concept of the prion. Our understanding of this group of diseases began with veterinarian virologists and neuropathologists who earlier in this century described spongiform pathology in the disease scrapie, proved it to be transmissible, and developed rodent models that have vastly contributed to our understanding. Other scientists described spongiform pathology in Creutzfeldt-Jacob Disease (C-J disease), which also encouraged the successful transmission experiments. The list of transmissible diseases from animals to humans is large and growing. It includes sporadic, transmissible diseases like kuru and C-J in humans and Scrapie, Mad Cow disease, and mink encephalopathy in animals. All of these diseases can affect the ability to use language and cognition.

7.24.2 Causes and Scope of Brain-Based Disorders

Table 7.6 estimates the incidence and prevalence of the major causes of brain impairment in adulthood in the United States. The estimates are conservative, excluding rare disorders for which reliable data are not available. These statistics are extracted from a very useful website designed for caregivers of persons with brain-based disorders, located at http://www.caregive.org.[8] Worldwide figures on brain-based disorders in general, or neurogenic communication disorders more specifically, are not available, but educated extrapolation can be conducted to get an idea of the scope of the problem. It is not insignificant. If the data presented for the approximate 294,000,000 population of the United States hold, then one can find the population of any given country and determine the incidence or prevalence of a condition. In the United States, for example, one case of aphasia is expected for every 272 residents. Based on the current population, this yields a prevalence of 1,079,600 persons with aphasia. Based on population, we would expect 16,000 Croatians to have aphasia, 10,000 Mongolians, nearly 4 million Indians, 84,000 Taiwanese, 253,000 Turks, and 178,000 South Koreans. Certainly, there are risks to accuracy in extrapolated estimates, but if these data are based on acceptable premises, they can be more useful than having no information, especially for realizing the scope of the problem and planning for the future.[9]

For clarification, incidence refers to the ratio or expected percentage of a condition or disorder relative to a predetermined number of people (e.g., the incidence of pediatric brain tumors in the United States is 2.1 per 1 00,000 children). Prevalence, on the other hand is the actual number of people with a disease or condition in a defined community (e.g., 14,683 people in New Zealand have aphasia). **Table 7.6** shows an estimated 1.2 million people aged 18 years and older who are diagnosed annually with adult-onset brain disease/disorders in the United States. This table also presents an overview of the major etiologies or causes of brain-based disorders. More than 200 diseases or conditions have associated neurogenic diseases. These tables present some of the more frequently observed conditions, syndromes, or causes. Many more rare or relatively obscure brain-based disorders have been documented in the medical literature, but these are the most likely to be encountered. More than one million adults in the United States are

Table 7.6 Incidence of adult-onset brain disorders in the United States

Diagnosis and cause	People diagnosed annually
Alzheimer's disease	250,000
Amyotrophic lateral sclerosis	5,000
Brain tumor	33,039
Epilepsy	135,500
HIV (AIDS) dementia	1,196
Huntington's disease	N/A
Multiple sclerosis	10,400
Parkinson's disease	54,927
Stroke	600,000
Traumatic brain injury	80,000
Total estimated incidence	**1,170,062**

diagnosed annually with a chronic brain disease or disorder.[10] The need for both long-term care and support for family caregivers is dramatic. Many of these conditions—for example, Alzheimer's disease, stroke, and Parkinson's disease—are associated with increasing age. Given the aging of the U.S. population, and extrapolated to similar industrialized countries, global figures will increase drastically in the coming decades. **Table 7.6** illustrates the long-term nature of caregiving for many of these conditions. Although it is estimated that one-quarter of a million people are diagnosed with Alzheimer's disease annually in the United States, there are an estimated four million people living with the disease, many of whom require 24-hour care. Further, the number of households affected by brain impairment only begins to elucidate the impact of brain-based disorders upon family caregivers and the long-term care system. With many individuals requiring 24-hour care, there are often several family members from different households involved in the caregiving process, including spouses, adult children, siblings, and friends. Often these caregivers are juggling the responsibilities of caregiving, child rearing, and employment simultaneously.[9]

The brain can be damaged in many ways. Strokes (CVAs) are the most frequent causes of aphasia, but the zones of language can be compromised by traumatic brain injury, infections, diseases, toxicity or poisons, or any of the other evil influences that can result in malfunction of brain cells.

7.24.3 Pediatric Conditions

Most of the nasty brain diseases that can affect adults can also affect children, though in different proportions and with altered consequence because they occur against the backdrop of physical, mental, communicative, cognitive, and social development.

7.24.4 Cerebral Palsy

Cerebral palsy (CP) is an umbrella term encompassing a group of nonprogressive, noncontagious conditions that cause physical disability in human development. Cerebral refers to the affected area of the brain; the cerebrum (however, the areas of damage have not been localized precisely and the condition most likely involves connections between the cortex and many other parts of the brain such as the cerebellum and basal ganglia). Palsy is the rather antiquated term that refers to a disorder of movement. CP is caused by damage to the motor control centers of the developing brain and can occur during pregnancy (about 75%), during childbirth (about 5%), or after birth (about 15%) up to about age 3. It is a nonprogressive disorder, meaning the brain damage does not worsen, but secondary orthopaedic difficulties are common. There is no known cure for CP. Medical intervention is limited to the treatment and prevention of complications possible from CP's consequences. Along with the other congenital or postnatal neuromuscular conditions such as all the variants of muscular dystrophy, CP can play havoc with the developing communication, swallowing, and sometimes cognitive–linguistic systems, and create barriers to everyday existence.

7.24.5 Autism Spectrum Disorders

Presumably the disorder has always existed, but not until the middle of the twentieth century was there a label for a disorder that now appears to affect an estimated 3.4 of every 1,000 children ages 3 to 10—a disorder that causes disruption in families and discontented lives for many children. In 1943, Dr. Leo Kanner of the Johns Hopkins Hospital studied a group of 11 children and introduced the label "early infantile autism" into the English language. At the same time, a German scientist, Dr. Hans Asperger, described a milder form of the disorder that became known as Asperger's syndrome. These two disorders were described and are today listed in the Diagnostic and Statistical Manual of Mental Disorders DSM-IV as two of the five pervasive developmental disorders (PDD), which are more often referred to today as autism spectrum disorders (ASD).[11] All of these disorders are characterized by varying degrees of impairment in communication skills; social interactions; and restricted, repetitive, and stereotyped patterns of behavior.[12]

The ASDs can often be reliably detected by the age of 3 years and, in some cases, as early as 18 months. Florida State University has an active Center for Autism and Related Disorders, which has pioneered the recognition and development of "red flags" for even earlier identification and intervention. Studies suggest that many children eventually may be accurately identified by the age of 1 year or even younger. The appearance of any of the warning signs of ASD is reason to have a child evaluated by a professional specializing in these disorders. Parents are usually the first to notice unusual behaviors in their child. In some cases, the baby seemed "different" from birth, unresponsive to people or focusing intently on one item for long periods of time. The first signs of an ASD also can be noticed in children who appear to have been developing within normal expectations. Early warning signs are triggered when an engaging, babbling toddler becomes mute, withdrawn, self-abusive, or indifferent to social overtures. Parents notice these changes, but sometimes it is a health care professional who first tunes in to them. The pervasive developmental disorders, or ASDs, range from a severe form called autistic disorder, to a milder form called Asperger's syndrome. If a child has signs or symptoms of either of these disorders but does not meet the specific criteria for either, the diagnosis waffles a bit and is called pervasive developmental disorder not otherwise specified (PDD-NOS). Other rare, very severe disorders that are included in the ASDs are Rett's syndrome and childhood disintegrative disorder.[12] As is apparent in nearly all subdisciplines or areas of neuroscience, brain imaging strategies have advanced our knowledge. These new magical tools—computerized tomography (CT), positron emission tomography (PET), single-photon emission computed tomography (SPECT), and magnetic resonance imaging (MRI), and functional magnetic resonance imaging (fMRI)—have kick-started study of the structure and function of the brain. This new technology and increasing availability of both normal and autism tissue samples for postmortem brain analysis studies has heartened researchers and facilitated the road to clearer understanding of these brain-based disorders. Postmortem and MRI studies have shown that many major brain structures are implicated in autism. These include the cerebellum, cerebral cortex, limbic system, corpus callosum, basal ganglia, and brainstem. Other research is focusing on the role of neurotransmitters such as serotonin, dopamine, and epinephrine, particularly in their possible role in the repetitive behaviors so characteristic of autism. Research into the myriad network of causes of ASDs is being assisted by other recent developments. Evidence points to genetic factors playing a prominent role in the causes for ASD. Twin and family studies point to an underlying genetic vulnerability for the development of ASD. ASD is a web within an enigma, and recent research on this brain-based disorder is beginning to illuminate grains of optimism at the far end of the tunnel.

7.24.6 Risk Factors

Risk factors for brain-based disorders of communication and swallowing are strongly related to the risk factors for the many types of brain damage. Stroke is the leading cause of aphasia and other disorders of communication. The risk factors for this condition are the most salient and sometimes the least understood. Some stroke risk factors are hereditary. Others are a function of natural aging processes. Still others result from a person's lifestyle. You can't choose your gene pool or alter factors related to heredity or natural processes, but those resulting from lifestyle or environment can be changed. Because nutrition and the nature of a person's activities are within the wonderful world of options, people can reduce the lifestyle aspects of risk for stroke and aphasia. Moderate ingestion of gravy and chili-laden French fries and laying off the triple bacon-cheese burgers can go a long way to altering the nutrition time bombs that lurk in our arteries waiting to turn into aphasia-causing strokes.

A better balance of fruits, vegetables, grains, and healthy food choices rather than double rich Chunky Monkey ice cream slathered on death by chocolate cake can help. Similarly, a lifestyle that incorporates heavy smoking, pouring down double Jaggie shots chased with "tastes great, less filling" brew, and an exercise program that consists mostly of chasing little demons around a video game screen is a stroke waiting to happen—in some people, later; in many, sooner. Lifestyle counts. We can't do much about choosing our relatives, but we can influence how we live our life. These decisions can affect our likelihood for stroke and disordered communication.

Similarly, because brain trauma is a frequent cause of aphasia as well, our lifestyle choices can alter our probability of ending up with scrambled sentences. Motor vehicular risk takers who practice the Tokyo drift in high-powered cars or drive in a drunken stupor or while texting or chattering away on a cell phone significantly increase their risk for ending up with a bunch of dead brain cells—not to mention the damage that they can cause to people whom they run into or run over. Brain damage and aphasia arise from many unfortunate sources. We should attempt to control the factors that in fact are under our control. High blood pressure (hypertension), diabetes, smoking, over exuberant alcohol consumption, and buckets of deep fried chicken for breakfast are serious risk factors associated with stroke.

The plates and text in this book have been adapted and created to help students and professionals in the health care disciplines gain an appreciation of the intricacies and complexity of the human nervous system, particularly as it relates to the diseases and disorders described in this book. To appreciate the diseases and help the people who have suffered their ravages, one must have a firm grasp of the normal aspects of this astonishing system of neurons and their connections and organization.

7.25 Neuroanatomy and Neurophysiology of Cognition

Cognition is the alchemy that glues us to being human. It is an amalgamation of mental actions or processes that assimilate knowledge and interpretation through thought, experience, and the senses. Although some writers and researchers fold the concept of language into the rubric of cognition, they can be considered separate and related procedures that are very close cousins. They are no longer thought of as separate or two sides of the same coin. They are utterly intertwined like the DNA double helix or the intricacies of a complex Persian rug. Cognition stands alone, supports, and holds hands with language. One can probably have some aspects of cognition that are devoid of language, but surely one cannot have coherent language that is divorced from cognition.

Attributes and elements of cognition can overlap, fuse, and support each other. Some of these cognitive domains or elements include **arousal**, **attention**, **orientation**, **memory** (in all its flavors), **novel learning**, **organization and categorization of thought**, **reasoning** (interpreting, drawing conclusions, or making rational or purely emotional arguments), **problem solving**, and the choirmaster of cognition, **executive function**. Executive function is perhaps the least understood and in much of the literature an abstruse concept. The executive function(s) are a set of processes that are concerned with managing oneself and one's resources to achieve a goal. It is a parasol term for the neurologically based skills involving mental control and self-regulation. Executive functions allow people to *plan, organize, and complete tasks*. They allow people to access the elements of self-control, emotional control, flexible thinking, working memory (one of the flavors of memory that is far more complex than simple "short-term memory"), self-monitoring, planning and prioritizing, task initiation, and organization. See **Figs. 7.78–7.81**.

7.25.1 Attention

Attention is the queen of cognition. It is the foundation of many other cognitive processes. It can be appreciated as a general concept or as components of the aggregate. It can be generated as *top down*, generated from within the individual, or *bottom up*, generated from stimuli outside the organism or person. Many attempts to precisely define attention have been promoted but a perfect definition is elusive and a bit slimy. A general and serviceable definition infers that attention means unfastening from a current stimulus, reallocating to a new stimulus, and retaining that new or novel stimulus for an interlude of time.

Types or varieties of attention also have attracted creative and sometimes quite different categories. Most expert writers on attention, however, have arrived at a consensus and settled on several subcategories of attention that include the following:

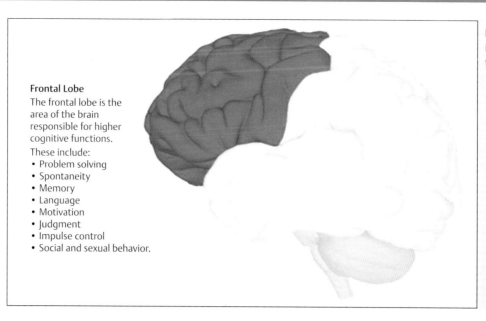

Frontal Lobe
The frontal lobe is the area of the brain responsible for higher cognitive functions.
These include:
• Problem solving
• Spontaneity
• Memory
• Language
• Motivation
• Judgment
• Impulse control
• Social and sexual behavior.

Fig. 7.78 Overview of frontal lobe function, an integral neural component of higher cortical functions such as cognition.

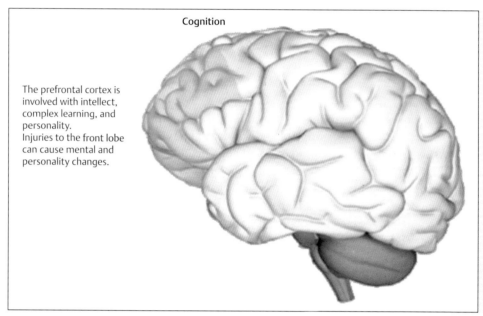

Cognition

The prefrontal cortex is involved with intellect, complex learning, and personality.
Injuries to the front lobe can cause mental and personality changes.

Fig. 7.79 Prefrontal section of the frontal lobes. Involved with specific cognitive functions such as learning, intellect, and personality. Damage to these prefrontal areas can result in drastic personality change.

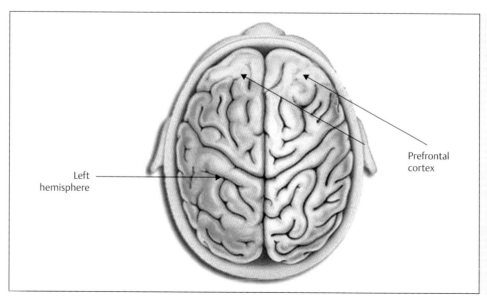

Left hemisphere

Prefrontal cortex

Fig. 7.80 Top view of prefrontal lobes.

Focused attention: The ability to stay engaged on a specific stimulus and maintain it. This focus is on a particular stimulus or stimuli via any of the sensory modalities, be they auditory, visual, tactile, taste, or smell. Focused attention would be necessary, for example, in a wine taster, trying to differentiate the taste of a glass of Two Buck Chuck from Trader Joe's and Penfolds Grange

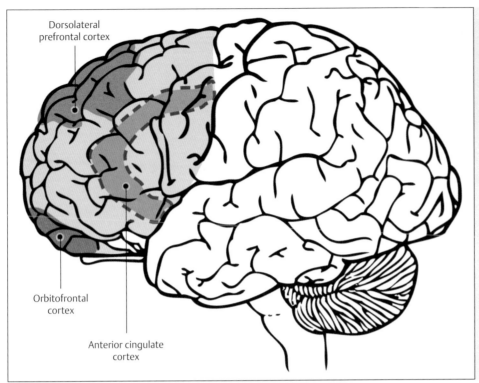

Fig. 7.81 Components and areas of frontal lobes related to higher cortical functions, intellect, personality, and cognition.

Figure labels: Dorsolateral prefrontal cortex; Orbitofrontal cortex; Anterior cingulate cortex

from Australia (for which a collector of specific vintages and varietals recently shelled out nearly $50,000).

Sustained attention: This type of attention allows us to stay engaged for a significant period of time. The amount of time is not demarcated, but it is certainly not fleeting. For example, sustained attention is necessary for tasks such as those required of an air traffic control agent, or more universally for the comprehension necessary in reading long or complicated passages in a book.

Selective attention: Selective attention is the ability to focus on a certain stimulus and at the same time ignore or minimize competing or potentially interfering stimuli. This is a flavor of attention that we use daily. We are constantly surrounded by competing and potentially distracting stimuli, but we must learn to ignore those that are not relevant to the task at hand. Children or adults with attention deficit hyperactivity disorder (ADHD) have difficulty with this type of attention and the spotting of a squirrel might interfere with the primary selected attentional task. Increasingly, the hum, vibration, or buzz of our digital devices is not only compromising our selective attention, but leading us down the subtle path of addiction to the screens we carry so lovingly in our pockets.

Alternating attention: Alternating attention occurs when a person shifts focus between or among two or more stimuli. Shifting tasks is sometimes required for certain chores or responsibilities. Many student tasks such as writing an essay may require reading a bit of research, shifting to writing a few sentences, back to reading or Googling potential sources, and then again to composing nonplagiarized sentences.

Divided attention: The ability to focus on two stimuli or sets of stimuli at the same time is the essence of divided attention. Walking and talking is easy. Walking and texting is not, and can be dangerous. Driving and talking to a passenger is easy. Driving and talking on the cellphone is not and research has shown it is also perilous. The pervasiveness of multitasking has been shown by many research studies to invade the primary task and degrade

cognition. We may think we can multitask well, but depending on the nature of the tasks we simultaneously engage, one is likely to be compromised and degraded. We have studied this phenomenon for years in our laboratory at Florida State and have clarified types of cognitive load that imperil even relatively simple tasks such as ambulation and walking steadily. Some are easy. Walking and counting by ones (14, 15, 16, 17....) is easy. Walking and subtracting from 95 by 3s compromises parameters of gait especially in those with preexisting movement disorders such as Parkinson's disease or multiple sclerosis. This increase in divided attention cognitive load has been shown to result in increased risk of injurious falls. See **Fig. 7.82**.

7.25.2 Memory

Memory is the other stalwart of cognition. If attention is the queen, then memory is the king. Or perhaps the other way around. Royal politics and power are difficult to discern these days and may be as complex as figuring out relative sovereignty in *Game of Thrones*. Memory, like attention, is a cognitive function that is complex and comes in many varieties. The expressions used to describe memory is a terminological maze. One can find frequent and contradictory terms used for different types of memory. How to sort this out? Well, research is progressive, falsifiable, and evolutionary and surely the terms that are used today will change with further knowledge. For today, neuroscientists, neurologists, and those of us in communication science and disorders use three primary categories: working memory, short-term memory, and long-term memory. You may run across another memory term *sensory memory*, a split-second holding tank for all sensory information holding for just an instant. Depending on whether the sensory stimuli are visual, auditory, or through touch, you may see the terms iconic, echoic, or haptic sensory memory. See how the terminological maze of memory begins to muddle and obfuscate.

Working memory: Although short-term and working memory are still used synonymously in some research and writing, the work of current neuroscientists creates a distinction. They take the stance that *short-term memory* is about transitory storage (remembering a phone number that someone told you and then entering it in your contacts section of your iPhone), while *working memory* must have an element of temporary storage to allow *manipulation* in solving a problem. For example, doing a subtraction problem in your head that requires cancellation ("100 minus 9 equals 91"). The classic *n-back test* is frequently used to measure working memory. (Tap the desk when you hear a color that occurred two-back from the current stimulus. "Green, red, orange, blue, red [tap], blue, orange, green, blue [tap]…"). Working memory requires manipulation to solve a forthcoming problem in cognition but is involves the other cognitive functions of executive function, attention,

and short-term memory storage. Working memory brings into play the neural structures of the prefrontal cortex, the cingulate gyrus, and portions of the parietal lobe. See **Fig. 7.83** and **Fig. 7.84**.

Short-term memory: This sometimes catch-all category of memory is now used to indicate how we store small amounts of information (7 units plus or minus two according to some classic research). This type of memory decays rapidly (some say approximately 30 seconds). This decay or loss will happen quickly unless the information is deemed important and the process of rehearsal or practice takes place, setting it up for consolidation and transfer to long-term memory (a process called *encoding*). Examples of short-term memory include going to the refrigerator to get some Korean ginger honey, open the door, and then forget what you were after. This phenomenon of short-term memory is illustrated in the following popular anecdote: Paul: "What do

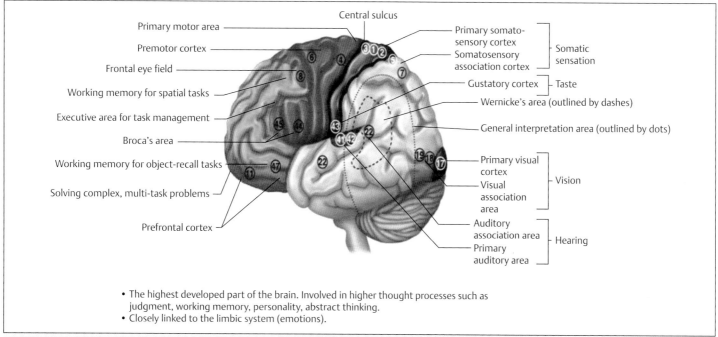

Fig. 7.82 Functional relationships among cortical areas and behaviors. Note the frontal and prefrontal areas related to working memory, solving complex tasks, and elements of cognition.

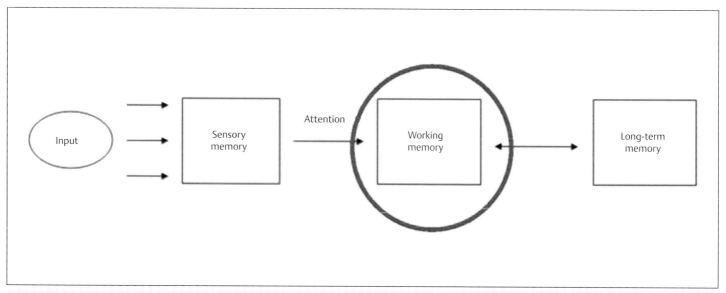

Fig. 7.83 Schematic of elements of cognition including attention and subcomponents of human memory.

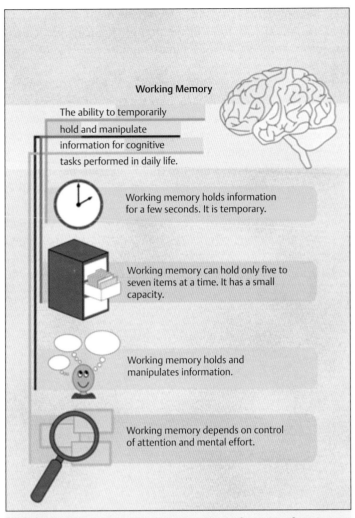

Working Memory

The ability to temporarily hold and manipulate information for cognitive tasks performed in daily life.

Working memory holds information for a few seconds. It is temporary.

Working memory can hold only five to seven items at a time. It has a small capacity.

Working memory holds and manipulates information.

Working memory depends on control of attention and mental effort.

Fig. 7.84 Aspects of working memory as part of cognitive function. Note that working memory inter-relates with other aspects of cognition such as attention and differentiates itself from the older models of memory by requiring manipulation of information.

you and your significant other discuss these days?" Emma: "The hereafter." Paul: "How so?" Emma: "Frequently we enter a room, turn around twice, and then say, 'What am I here after?'"

Long-term memory: Frequently short-term memories undergo consolidation and encoding and transform into long-term memories. Long-term memory can be resilient and robust. It can last for days, weeks, months, or even decades. Your trip to Moorea where you stayed in a thatched hut over the water and watched the fish through the Plexiglas floor; your summer in Paris full of red, sweet strawberries and the medical anomalies of the Dupuytren Museum; your afternoons as a life guard at Sawyer Lake are all examples of strong long-term memories.

In long-term memory, the memory terms fall from the stars and can perplex and bewilder. While terms abound, and you will encounter terms such as declarative and nondeclarative memory, a simplified way of understanding long-term memory is to recall the principal types of this form of memory: *episodic* (mostly involving you and your autobiography); *semantic* (recollection of facts); and *procedural* (how to do something). Examples include Where did you attend grammar school? (episodic); What is the largest mountain in Florida? (semantic); How do you make a peanut butter, jelly, and tuna sandwich? (procedural).

Neuroanatomical areas for memory are not precisely localized but consist of some important specific areas and circuits set up among them. Cortical areas, parahippocampal and rhinal areas, and the hippocampus and the networks that connect them are the primary cores of memory.

Perhaps the most universally recognized cognitive domains are attention and memory, but as one can appreciate from the paragraphs above, this cryptic concept is far more complex than just paying attention and remembering. In the preceding section, we illustrated which portions of the richly complex nervous system are associated with cognition.

References

1. Pollard KS. What makes us human? Sci Am 2009;300(5): 44–49
2. LaPointe LL, Murdoch BE, Stierwalt JAC. Brain-Based Communication Disorders. San Diego, CA: Plural Publishing, Inc; 2010
3. LaPointe LL. Aphasia and Related Neurogenic Language Disorders. 4th ed. New York, NY: Thieme Medical Publishers; 2011
4. Ackerman D. An Alchemy of Mind. New York, NY: Simon and Schuster; 2004
5. Schuenke M, Schulte E, Schumacher U. Atlas of Anatomy: Head and Neuroanatomy. New York, NY: Thieme Medical Publishers; 2007
6. LaPointe LL, Case JL, Duane DD. Perceptual-acoustic speech and voice characteristics of subjects with spasmodic torticollis. In: Till J, Yorkston K, Beukelman D, eds. Motor Speech Disorders: Advances in Assessment and Treatmzent. Baltimore, MD: Brookes Publishing Co; 1994:57–64
7. Klawans HL. Toscanini's Fumble: And Other Tales of Clinical Neurology. Chicago, IL: Contemporary Books; 1988
8. Family Caregiver Alliance. 2009. Available at: http://www.caregiver.org. Accessed December 27, 2017
9. World Health Organization. Neurological Disorders: Public Health Challenges. New York, NY: World Health Organization Press; 2007
10. American Speech-Language-Hearing Association. 2009. Available at: http://www.asha.org. Accessed December 27, 2017
11. American Psychiatric Association. Diagnostic and Statistical Manual of Mental Disorders. 4th ed. New York, NY: American Psychiatric Publishing; 2007
12. Jepson B, Wright K, Johnson J. Changing the Course of Autism: A Scientific Approach for Parents and Physicians. Boulder, CO: Sentient Press; 2007

Suggested Reading

Zraick R, LaPointe LL. Hyperkinetic dysarthria. In: McNeil M, ed. Clinical Management of Sensorimotor Speech Disorders. New York, NY: Thieme Medical Publishers; 2008

Index

Page numbers in *italics* refer to illustrations; those in **bold** refer to tables